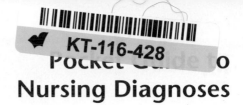

Pocket Guide to Nursing Diagnoses

Mi Ja Kim, RN, PhD, FAAN
Professor and Dean
College of Nursing
University of Illinois at Chicago
Chicago, Illinois

Gertrude Kay McFarland, RN, DNSc, FAAN
Health Scientist Administrator
Nursing Research Study Section
Division of Research Grants
National Institutes of Health
Bethesda, Maryland

Audrey M. McLane, RN, PhD
Professor Emerita
College of Nursing
Marquette University
Milwaukee, Wisconsin

SIXTH EDITION

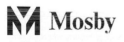

St. Louis Baltimore Boston Carlsbad Chicago Naples New York Philadelphia Portland
London Madrid Mexico City Singapore Sydney Tokyo Toronto Wiesbaden

Mosby
Dedicated to Publishing Excellence

Publisher: Nancy Coon
Editor: Loren Stevenson Wilson
Associate Developmental Editor: Brian Dennison
Project Manager: Gayle Morris
Production Editor: Donna Walls
Designer: Susan Lane
*Manufacturing Supervisor:*Tim Stringham

Sixth Edition
Copyright © 1995 by Mosby–Year Book, Inc.

Previous editions copyrighted 1984, 1987, 1989, 1991, 1993

Printed in the United States of America
Composition by AlphaByte & Co.
Printing/binding by R. R. Donnelley and Sons, Inc.

Mosby–Year Book, Inc.
11830 Westline Industrial Drive
St. Louis, Missouri 63146

Library of Congress Cataloging in Publication Data

Pocket guide to nursing diagnoses / [edited by] Mi Ja Kim, Gertrude
   Kay McFarland, Audrey M. McLane.—6th ed.
     p. cm.
   Includes bibliographical references and index.
   ISBN 0-8016-7886-2 (pbk.)
   1. Nursing diagnosis—Handbooks, manuals, etc. I. Kim, Mi Ja.
II. McFarland, Gertrude K. III. McLane, Audrey M.
IV. Title: Nursing diagnosis
   [DNLM: 1. Nursing Diagnosis—handbooks. 2. Patient Care
   Planning—handbooks. WY 39 P739 1995]
RT48.6.P63 1995
616.07′5—dc20
DNLM/DLC   94-38958
for Library of Congress   CIP

95   96   97   98   99 / 9   8   7   6   5   4   3   2   1

Contributors

Kim Astroth, RN, MS
Clinical Instructor
Mennonite College of Nursing
Bloomington, Illinois

Sarah McNabb Badalamenti, RN, MSN
Clinical Nurse Specialist
St. Joseph's Hospital
Milwaukee, Wisconsin

Thelma I. Bates, RN, CS, MSN
Psychiatric Clinical Specialist
Washington Hospital Center
Washington, DC

Joan M. Caley, RN, MS, CS, CNAA*
Associate Chief, Nursing Service
Department of Veterans Affairs Medical Center
Portland, Oregon

Nancy S. Creason, BSN, MSN, PhD
Dean and Professor
School of Nursing
Southern Illinois University at Edwardsville
Edwardsville, Illinois

Kathryn T. Czurylo, RN, MS, CS
Surgical Clinical Nurse Specialist
Alexian Brothers Medical Center
Elk Grove Village, Illinois

*The opinions expressed herein are those of the authors and do not necessarily reflect those of the National Institutes of Health, U.S. Public Health Service, U.S. Department of Health and Human Services, the Veteran Administration, or the Uniformed Services University of the Health Sciences.

Donna M. Dixon, MS, RN
Doctoral Candidate
University of Illinois at Chicago
Chicago, Illinois

Susan Dudas, RN, MSN, FAAN
Associate Professor
College of Nursing
University of Illinois at Chicago
Chicago, Illinois

Teresa Fadden, MSN, RN, CS
Clinical Nurse IV
St. Joseph's Hospital
Milwaukee, Wisconsin

Richard J. Fehring, DNSc, RN
Associate Professor
Marquette University
College of Nursing
Milwaukee, Wisconsin

Diane M. Fesler, RN, MSN
Periperative Clinical Specialist
Clinical Faculty (Medical–Surgical)
University of Illinois at Chicago
Chicago, Illinois

Margaret I. Fitch, RN, PhD
Oncology Nurse Researcher
Comprehensive Cancer Program at
Toronto–Bayview Regional Cancer Centre/
Sunnybrook Health Sciences Centre
Faculty of Nursing, University of Toronto
Toronto, Ontario, Canada

Margie L. French, RN, MS, CS
Clinical Nurse Specialist, Clinical Manager
Comprehensive Rehabilitation Unit
Veterans Health Administration Medical Center
Vancouver Division
Portland, Oregon

Michele C. Gattuso, RN, MS
Clinical Nurse Specialist
Maternal Child Health
Alexian Brothers Medical Center
Elk Grove Village, Illinois

Elizabeth Kelchner Gerety, MS, RN, CS, FAAN*
Clinical Nurse Specialist
Psychiatry Consultation
Portland Veterans Affairs Medical Center
Portland, Oregon

Wendy Goetter, RN, MS, CNRN
Clinical Specialist Neuroscience
University of Illinois at Chicago Medical Center
Chicago, Illinois

Jane E. Graydon, PhD, RN
Associate Professor and Chair
Graduate Department, Faculty of Nursing
University of Toronto
Toronto, Ontario, Canada

Susan L. Grice, RN, MSN, CS
Psychotherapist—Private Practice
Nurse Consultant
Arlington, Virginia

Terry Griffin, RN, MS
Adjunct Clinical Instructor
University of Illinois at Chicago
Department of Maternal-Child Nursing
Chicago, Illinois

Mary V. Hanley, MA, RN*
Critical Care Nursing Instructor
DVA, VA Medical Center/Outpatient Clinics
Nursing Education
Boston, Massachusetts

Marilyn Harter, RN, MSN, CRRN
Clinical Nurse Specialist
Rehabilitation and Neurology
Columbia Hospital
Milwaukee, Wisconsin

Kathryn A. Hennessy, MS, RN, CNSN
Clinical Network Manager
Caremark, Inc.
Northbrook, Illinois

Pamela D. Hill, RN, BSN, MS, PhD
Associate Professor
Department of Maternal Child Nursing
College of Nursing, Quad–Cities Regional Site
University of Illinois at Chicago
Rock Island, Illinois

Karen E. Inaba, MS, RN, CS
Psychiatric Consultation–Liaison
Clinical Nurse Specialist, University Hospital,
Oregon Health Sciences University
Assistant Professor, Department of Mental Health Nursing
School of Nursing, Oregon Health Sciences University
Portland, Oregon

Joyce H. Johnson, RN, MSN, PhD
Associate Professor
University of Illinois at Chicago
College of Nursing
Chicago, Illinois

Karen Kavanaugh, RN, PhD
Assistant Professor
University of Illinois at Chicago
Chicago, Illinois

Jin H. Kim, RN, MSN
Doctoral Student
College of Nursing
University of Illinois at Chicago
Chicago, Illinois

Mi Ja Kim, RN, PhD, FAAN
Professor and Dean
College of Nursing
University of Illinois at Chicago
Chicago, Illinois

Kristin M. Kleinschmidt, RN, MS
Cardiac Clinical Nurse Specialist
Edward Hines, Jr. Hospital
Department of Veterans Affairs
Hines, Illinois

Pamela Wolfe Kohlbry, RN, MSN
San Marcos, California

Contributors

Patricia A. Koller, RN, MSN
Clinical Care Nurse III, Intensive Care
St. Joseph's Hospital
Milwaukee, Wisconsin

Carol E. Kupperberg, RN, BSN, MSN
Home Care Case Manager
Children's Home Health Care Services
Children's National Medical Center
Washington, DC

Jane Lancour, RN, MSN
Corporate Director
Quality Improvement Accreditation
FHP International, Inc.
Fountain Valley, California

Janet L. Larson, RN, PhD
Associate Professor
University of Illinois at Chicago
College of Nursing
Chicago, Illinois

Lorna A. Larson, DNSc, RN
Formerly Program Analyst
Quality Assurance Division
DC Commission on Mental Health Services
Washington, DC

Marie Maguire, RN, MSN, CNS
Director of Quality Management
Lakeland Nursing Home
Elkhorn, Wisconsin

Mary E. Markert, RN, MN
Acting Branch Chief, Geropsychiatry
DC Commission on Mental Health Services
St. Elizabeths Hospital
Washington, DC

Gertrude K. McFarland, RN, DNSc, FAAN*
Health Scientist Administrator
Nursing Research Study Section
Division of Research Grants
National Institutes of Health
Bethesda, Maryland

Contributors

Audrey M. McLane, RN, PhD
Professor Emerita
College of Nursing
Marquette University
Milwaukee, Wisconsin

Ruth E. McShane, RN, PhD
Assistant Professor
University of Wisconsin at Milwaukee
School of Nursing
Milwaukee, Wisconsin

Karen McWhorter, RN, MN, CS
Clinical Nurse Specialist, Aduld Day Health Care Program
Veterans Health Administration Medical Center
Vancouver Division
Portland, Oregon

Judy Minton, RN, MS, FNP
Nurse Practitioner
Decatur, Illinois

Victoria L. Mock, RN, DNSc, OCN
Director of Oncology Nursing Research
The Johns Hopkins Hospital
Baltimore, Maryland

Martha M. Morris, RN, EdD
Adjunct Associate Professor
St. Louis University School of Nursing
St. Louis, Missouri

Charlotte Naschinski, RN, MS*
Deputy Director, Continuing Health Professional Education
Uniformed Services University of the Health Sciences
Bethesda, Maryland

Emma B. Nemivant, RN, MSN, MEd
Clinical Instructor, Department of Maternal–Child Nursing
University of Illinois at Chicago
College of Nursing
Chicago, Illinois

Colleen M. O'Brien, RN, MSN
Human Resources Development
Bellin Hospital
Green Bay, Wisconsin

Contributors

Linda O'Brien–Pallas, RN, PhD
Associate Professor and Career Scientist
Faculty of Nursing
University of Toronto
Toronto, Ontario, Canada

Annette O'Connor, RN, MScN, PhD
Associate Professor
University of Ottawa
School of Nursing
Ottawa, Canada

Catherine J. Ryan, RN, MS, CCRN
Clinical Nurse Specialist, Critical Care
Alexian Brothers Medical Center
Elk Grove Village, Illinois

Karen V. Scipio–Skinner, MSN, RN, C
Legislative/Practice Specialist
District of Columbia Nurses Association
Washington, DC

Maureen Shekleton, DNSc, RN
Satellite Site Coordinator
DuPage Community Clinic
Wheaton, Illinois
Adjunct Assistant Professor
University of Illinois at Chicago
College of Nursing
Chicago, Illinois

Kathleen C. Sheppard, PhD, RN
Director of Nursing
University of Texas
M.D. Anderson Cancer Center
Houston, Texas

Margaret J. Stafford, MSN, RN, FAAN
Consultant/Lecturer in Cardiac Nursing/Professional Issues
Adjunct Assistant Professor, College of Nursing
University of Illinois at Chicago
Chicago, Illinois

Janet F. Stansberry, RN, MSN
Clinical Nurse Specialist, Infertility
University of Pennsylvania
Philadelphia, Pennsylvania

Rosemarie Suhayda, PhD, RN

Assistant Professor
Rush University
College of Nursing
Chicago, Illinois

Marie L. Talashek, RN, EdD

Associate Professor
University of Illinois at Chicago
College of Nursing
Chicago, Illinois

Alice M. Tse, PhD, RN

Assistant Professor of Nursing and Medicine
University of Hawaii at Manoa
School of Nursing
Honolulu, Hawaii

Evelyn L. Wasli, RN, DNSc

Chief Nurse
Emergency Psychiatric Response Division
DC Commission on Mental Health Services
Washington, DC

Rosemary White–Traut, DnSc, RN

Associate Professor and Coordinator
Graduate Pediatric and Perinatal Programs
University of Illinois at Chicago
Chicago, Illinois

Linda K. Young, RN, MSN

Nursing Faculty, Alverno College
Milwaukee County Medical Center, School of Nursing
Milwaukee, Wisconsin

Contributors

Preface

Since the first edition of the Pocket Guide to Nursing Diagnoses, nursing diagnoses have become integrated into nursing education, research, and practice in the United States. In addition, nursing diagnosis has gained acceptance in countries such as Canada, France, The Netherlands, Australia, Italy, Taiwan, Spain, Slovenia, Denmark, Korea, Japan, Brazil, and other countries. Nursing students find nursing diagnoses to be a useful tool of learning. Both nursing students and practicing nurses find nursing diagnoses a useful way of conceptualizing nursing science and focusing for clinical decision making. Educators have adopted nursing diagnoses as an organizing framework for teaching and practice. Nurse researchers are using nursing diagnoses as a focus for research while the NANDA Taxonomy taken as a whole presents a challenge for systematic validation through research. The nursing profession and its specialty organizations recognize the contribution of a nursing nosology to their ability to demonstrate the effectiveness of nursing practice and to influence health care policy. Given developments in the National Health Care Agenda, nurses will have an expanded role as key health care providers, a trend in which nursing diagnosis can and will play a key role.

Finally, nursing diagnoses do and will continue to influence deliberations at the International level through such organizations as the International Council of Nurses (ICN). Currently, an International Classification for Nursing Practice is being developed by nurse experts under the leadership of the ICN. Nursing diagnoses developed by NANDA played a significant role in the development of this work. The outcome of this work will most likely be submitted to WHO for the next edition of the International Classification of Diseases–Clinical Modification (ICD–CM). This is significant progress at the International level and inclusion of a nursing taxonomy in such a standard classification used worldwide will definitely improve nursing's ability to communicate more effectively, thereby stimulating the growth and dissemination of nursing's knowledge.

The major purposes of the Pocket Guide continue to be:

1. to present the most up–to–date information on NANDA nursing diagnoses terminology, definitions, related/risk factors, and defining characteristics
2. to present a prototype state–of–the–art care plan for each nursing diagnosis
3. to provide an easy–to–use guide for clinicians, faculty, and students in their daily practice
4. to stimulate critical thinking of practice nurses, and
5. to facilitate the use of theory and research–based nursing interventions in the practice setting.

We are deeply indebted to the users of this book who generously provided their suggestions and who continue to endorse this book.

In keeping with the philosophy of the previous editions, every effort has been made to make this Pocket Guide easy to use while providing a theoretical and research base for each prototype care plan. We have chosen to present nursing diagnoses in alphabetical order because the conceptual framework for the organization of nursing diagnoses is still under development. The current NANDA Taxonomy I Revised 1995-1996 version is presented in Appendix A for those who may want to know the taxonomic structure for these diagnoses. All NANDA approved diagnoses are covered in this Pocket Guide, including the 19 new diagnoses approved in 1994.

Defining characteristics and related/risk factors presented are NANDA approved, and the same is true for the majority of definitions. Definitions of nursing diagnoses approved by NANDA have been used to the extent they were developed. For completeness, we developed definitions for diagnoses that do not have definitions.

A concerted effort has been made to present nursing care plans as prototypes rather than standard care plans. By making the care plans prototypes, we have emphasized that they are for specific individuals or a group of patients with specified related/risk factors. Therefore in applying these plans to patients, practicing nurses will need to give specific consideration to individual patient requirements.

Each care plan was developed on the basis of a nursing diagnosis that comprises a diagnostic label and the term related to for related or risk factors. For example, if the nursing diagnosis is Risk for Injury with a risk factor of "emotional lability," the nurse would record this as "Risk for injury related to emotional lability."We used the following guide for the development of the prototype care plans.

- The patient goals/expected outcomes reflect the desired health state of a patient and specify indicators addressing the extent of achievement of the patient goal(s).
- Scientific rationale are specified for interventions or cluster of interventions.
- Clinical conditions or medical diagnosis are specified for each care plan to emphasize the medical diagnosis/ nursing diagnosis link which make the care plans more focused for a specific type of patient.
- Nursing interventions are selected to address related factors or risk factors, to ameliorate/modify defining characteristics, and to assist patients in achieving their goals and optimal health state.
- Prevention is an important component of the care plans where possible.
- Nursing diagnosis and the selected nursing interventions reflect contributions the nurse can make within today's interdisciplinary environment and the importance of interdisciplinary team work.

The care plans were developed from a perspective of persons interacting with their environment in the pursuit of health. The use of nursing diagnoses and relevant nursing interventions that are designed to meet patient goals has sharpened the focus of current practice and has demonstrated the potential of nursing diagnoses for contributing to quality health care.

Contributing authors of the Pocket Guide are clinical experts who reflect the state-of-the-art and science of nursing practice. We acknowledge substantive contributions made by practicing nurses to the development and refinement of nursing diagnoses. Practicing nurses are encouraged to engage in critical thinking while using the prototype care plans. Their participation in research on all nursing diagnoses is essential for the national and international development of nursing diagnoses taxonomy and a scientific base for nursing practice. There is also a critical need to comprehensively evaluate the nursing diagnostic terminology and taxonomy through on going nursing research. There is a critical need to identify and validate nursing diagnoses for use in the various specialty nursing practice areas.

Mi Ja Kim
Gertrude K. McFarland
Audrey M. McLane

Clinical Judgment and Nursing Diagnosis

Nursing diagnoses are made through a series of clinical judgments. Clinical judgment includes: pattern recognition in response to cues within a particular context; validation of the pattern; recognition of factors contributing to its onset; and selection/design of an intervention to achieve desired outcomes.

Pattern recognition in response to cues (defining characteristics) may occur at any point in the assessment process. Assessment data may be gathered to facilitate pattern recognition and/or validate the existence of a previously recognized pattern.

Subjective and objective assessment data are gathered with respect to a presenting situation or longer–term health status, activities and demands of daily living, and internal and external resources (current and potential) of a patient/family. Nursing diagnoses, which are the agreed–upon labels for diagnostic concepts, are assigned to recognized patterns. A nursing diagnosis for a patient/family health care situation includes a diagnostic label and related factors contributing to the onset/maintenance of an actual diagnosis or a diagnostic label and risk factors of a high risk diagnosis. Validation and interpretation of a diagnosis and related/risk factors are on–going processes of cue recognition and pattern recognition. A nursing diagnosis, then, becomes the focal point for developing goals, expected outcomes, interventions, and evaluation.

Practical tips for using The Pocket Guide

- If a nursing diagnosis is suggested by the assessment format you are using, look up the nursing diagnosis in Section One, "Nursing diagnoses: definitions, related/risk factors, and defining characteristics," and review the definition, defining characteristics, and the related/risk factors. Determine if the suggested nursing diagnosis is appropriate. If the nursing diagnosis is not appropriate, you may consult Section three for further possible nursing diagnoses.
- Review the corresponding care plan for the chosen nursing diagnoses in Part Two, "Nursing diagnoses: prototype care plans." Determine which patient goals, expected outcomes, and nursing interventions are applicable to your patient.
- In Section three, medical diagnoses and psychiatric diagnoses with associated nursing diagnoses are listed. This list can help you to determine which nursing diagnoses are most likely to apply to your patient.

North American Nursing Diagnosis Association's (NANDA) Working Definition of Nursing Diagnosis

Nursing diagnosis is a clinical judgment about individual, family, or community responses to actual or potential health problems/life processes. Nursing diagnoses provide the basis for selection of nursing interventions to achieve outcomes for which the nurse is accountable.

Approved at the Ninth Conference on Classification of Nursing Diagnoses.

International Classification of Nursing Practice's (ICNP) Proposed Definition of Nursing Diagnosis

The description or label given by a nurse to the particular condition or human response which the nurse has identified as being the reason for a nursing intervention.

From Nursing's Next Advance: An International Classification for Nursing Practice. ICN Working Paper, April 1993, p. 11.

Contents

NURSING DIAGNOSES

Definitions, Related/Risk Factors, and Defining Characteristics

Activity intolerance

The state in which an individual has insufficient physiological or psychological energy to endure or complete required or desired daily activities.

Related factors
Generalized weakness
Sedentary life-style
Imbalance between oxygen supply and demand
Bed rest or immobility
Defining characteristics
Verbal report of fatigue or weakness
Abnormal heart rate or blood pressure response to activity
Exertional discomfort or dyspnea
Electrocardiographic changes reflecting arrhythmias or ischemia

Activity intolerance, risk for

The state in which an individual is at risk of experiencing insufficient physiological or psychological energy to endure or complete required or desired daily activities.

Risk factors
History of previous intolerance
Deconditioned status
Presence of circulatory/respiratory problems
Inexperience with the activity

Adaptive capacity, decreased: intracranial

A clinical state in which intracranial fluid dynamic mechanisms that normally compensate for increases in intracranial volumes are compromised, resulting in repeated disproportionate increases in intracranial pressure (ICP) in response to a variety of noxious and non-noxious stimuli.

Related factors
Brain injuries
Sustained increase in ICP $\geq$ 10-15 mm Hg
Decreased cerebral perfusion pressure $\leq$ 50-60 mm Hg
Systemic hypotension with intracranial hypertension

Defining characteristics
Major
Repeated increases in ICP of greater than 10 mm Hg for more than 5 minutes following any of a variety of external stimuli.
Minor
Disproportionate increase in ICP following single environmental of nursing maneuver stimulus
Elevated P2 ICP waveform
Volume pressure response test variation (Volume-pressure ratio >2, Pressure-volume index <10
Baseline ICP equal to or greater than 10 mm Hg
Wide amplitude ICP waveform

Adjustment, impaired

The state in which an individual is unable to modify his/her life-style behavior in a manner consistent with a change in health status.

Related factors
Disability requiring change in life-style
Inadequate support systems
Impaired cognition
Sensory overload
Assault to self-esteem
Altered locus of control
Incomplete grieving
Defining characteristics
Verbalization of nonacceptance of health status change
Nonexistent or unsuccessful ability to be involved in problem solving or goal setting
Lack of movement toward independence
Extended period of shock, disbelief, or anger regarding health status change
Lack of future-oriented thinking

Airway clearance, ineffective

The state in which an individual is unable to clear secretions or obstructions from the respiratory tract to maintain airway patency.

Related factors
Decreased energy and fatigue
Tracheobronchial
    Infection
    Obstruction
    Secretion
Perceptual/cognitive impairment
Trauma
Defining characteristics
Abnormal breath sounds—rales (crackles), rhonchi
    (wheezes)
Changes in rate or depth of respiration
Tachypnea
Cough, effective or ineffective, with or without
    sputum
Cyanosis
Dyspnea
Fever

Anxiety

A vague, uneasy feeling, the source of which is often nonspecific or unknown to the individual.

Related factors
Unconscious conflict about essential values and goals
    of life
Threat to self-concept
Threat of death
Threat to or change in health status
Threat to or change in socioeconomic status
Threat to or change in role functioning
Threat to or change in environment
Threat to or change in interaction patterns
Situational and maturational crises
Interpersonal transmission and contagion
Unmet needs
Defining characteristics
Subjective
    Increased tension
    Apprehension
    Increased helplessness

Uncertainty
Fear
Feeling of being scared
Feeling of inadequacy
Shakiness
Fear of unspecific consequences
Regretfulness
Overexcitedness
Feeling of being rattled
Distress
Jitteriness
Objective
Sympathetic stimulation—cardiovascular
excitation, superficial vasoconstriction, pupil
dilation
Restlessness
Insomnia
Glancing about
Poor eye contact
Trembling; hand tremors
Extraneous movements—foot shuffling; hand, arm
movements
Expressed concern regarding changes in life events
Worry
Anxiety
Facial tension
Voice quivering
Focus on self
Increased wariness
Increased perspiration

Aspiration, risk for

The state in which an individual is at risk for entry of gastric
secretions, oropharyngeal secretions, or exogenous food or
fluids into tracheobronchial passages due to dysfunction or
absence of normal protective mechanisms.

Risk factors
Reduced level of consciousness
Depressed cough and gag reflexes
Presence of tracheotomy or endotracheal tube

Overinflated tracheotomy/endotracheal tube cuff
Inadequate tracheotomy/endotracheal tube cuff
    inflation
Gastrointestinal tubes
Bolus tube feedings/medication administration
Situations hindering elevation of upper body
Increased intragastric pressure
Increased gastric residual
Decreased gastrointestinal motility
Delayed gastric emptying
Impaired swallowing
Facial/oral/neck surgery or trauma
Wired jaws

Body image disturbance

Disruption in the way one perceives one's body image

Related factors
Biophysical
Cognitive perceptual
Psychosocial
Cultural or spiritual
Defining characteristics
Either the following A or B must be present to justify
    the diagnosis of body image disturbance:
    A. Verbal response to actual or perceived change in
        structure and/or function
    B. Nonverbal response to actual or perceived
        change in structure and/or function
The following clinical manifestations may be used to
    validate the presence of A or B:
    Objective
        Missing body part
        Actual change in structure and/or function
        Not looking at body part
        Not touching body part
        Hiding or overexposing body part (intentional
            or unintentional)
        Trauma to nonfunctioning part

Change in social involvement
Negative feelings about body
Feelings of helplessness, hopelessness, or
powerlessness
Preoccupation with change or loss
Emphasis on remaining strengths, heightened
achievement
Extension of body boundary to incorporate
environmental objects
Personalization of part or loss by name
Depersonalization of part or loss by impersonal
pronouns
Refusal to verify actual change
It may be possible to identify high-risk populations,
such as those with the following conditions:
Missing body part
Dependence on a machine
Significance of body part or functioning with
regard to age, gender, developmental level, or
basic human needs
Physical change caused by biochemical agents
(drugs)
Physical trauma or mutilation
Pregnancy and/or maturational changes

Body temperature, altered, risk for

The state in which an individual is at risk for failure to maintain
body temperature within normal range.

Risk factors
Extremes of age
Extremes of weight
Exposure to cold/cool or warm/hot environments
Dehydration
Inactivity or vigorous activity
Medications causing vasoconstriction/vasodilation,
altered metabolic rate, sedation
Inappropriate clothing for environmental temperature
Illness or trauma affecting temperature regulation

Bowel incontinence

The state in which an individual experiences a change in normal bowel habits characterized by involuntary passage of stool.

Related factors
Neuromuscular involvement
Musculoskeletal involvement
Depression, severe anxiety
Perception or cognitive impairment
Defining characteristics
Involuntary passage of stool

Breastfeeding, effective

The state in which a mother-infant dyad/family exhibits adequate proficiency and satisfaction with breastfeeding process.

Related factors
Basic breastfeeding knowledge
Normal breast structure
Normal infant oral structure
Infant gestational age greater than 34 weeks
Support sources
Maternal confidence
Defining characteristics
Mother able to position infant at breast to promote a successful latch-on response
Infant is content after feeding
Regular and sustained suckling/swallowing at the breast
Appropriate infant weight patterns for age
Effective mother-infant communication patterns (infant cues, maternal interpretation and response)
Signs and/or symptoms of oxytocin release (let-down or milk ejection reflex)
Adequate infant elimination patterns for age
Eagerness of infant to nurse
Maternal verbalization of satisfaction with the breastfeeding process

Breastfeeding, ineffective

The state in which a mother, infant, and/or family experiences dissatisfaction or difficulty with the breastfeeding process.

Related factors
Prematurity
Infant anomaly
Maternal breast anomaly
Previous breast surgery
Previous history of breastfeeding failure
Infant receiving supplemental feedings with artificial nipple
Poor infant sucking reflex
Nonsupportive partner/family
Knowledge deficit
Interruption in breastfeeding
Defining characteristics
Unsatisfactory breastfeeding process
Actual or perceived inadequate milk supply
Infant's inability to attach on to maternal nipple correctly
No observable signs of oxytocin release
Observable signs of inadequate infant intake
Nonsustained suckling at breast
Nursing less than 7 times in 24 hours
Persistence of sore nipples beyond first week of infant's life
Maternal reluctance to put infant to breast as necessary
Infant exhibiting fussiness and crying within first hour after breastfeeding; unresponsive to other comfort measures
Infant arching and crying at breast; resisting latching on

Breastfeeding, interrupted

A break in the continuity of the breastfeeding process as a result of inability or inadvisability to put baby to breast for feeding.

Related factors
Maternal or infant illness

Prematurity
Maternal employment
Contraindications to breastfeeding (e.g., drugs, true
     breastmilk jaundice)
Need to abruptly wean infant
Defining characteristics
   Major
   Infant does not receive nourishment at the breast
        for some or all of feedings
   Minor
   Maternal desire to maintain lactation and provide
        (or eventually provide) her breastmilk for her
        infant's nutritional needs
   Separation of mother and infant
   Lack of knowledge about expression and storage of
        breastmilk

Breathing pattern, ineffective

The state in which an individual's inhalation and/or exhalation
pattern does not enable adequate ventilation.

Related factors
Neuromuscular impairment
Pain
Musculoskeletal impairment
Perception or cognitive impairment
Anxiety
Decreased energy and fatigue
Inflammatory process
Decreased lung expansion
Tracheobronchial obstruction
Defining characteristics
Dyspnea
Shortness of breath
Tachypnea
Fremitus
Abnormal arterial blood gas levels
Cyanosis
Cough
Nasal flaring
Respiratory depth changes

Assumption of three-point position
Pursed-lip breathing and prolonged expiratory phase
Increased anteroposterior diameter
Use of accessory muscles
Altered chest excursion

Cardiac output, decreased

The state in which the blood pumped by an individual's heart is
sufficiently reduced to the extent that it is inadequate to meet
the needs of the body's tissues.

Related factors
Mechanical
    Alteration in preload
    Alteration in afterload
    Alteration in inotropic changes in heart
Electrical
    Alteration in rate
    Alteration in rhythm
    Alteration in conduction
Structural
Defining characteristics
Variations in hemodynamic readings
Arrhythmias; ECG changes
Fatigue
Jugular vein distention
Cyanosis; pallor of skin and mucous membranes
Oliguria, anuria
Decreased peripheral pulses
Cold, clammy skin
Rales
Dyspnea

Caregiver role strain

A caregiver's felt difficulty in performing the family caregiver
role.

Related factors
    Pathophysiological/physiological
    Severity of illness of the care receiver
    Addiction or codependency

11

Premature birth/congenital defect

Discharge of family member with significant home healthcare needs

Caregiver health impairment

Unpredictable illness course or instability in the care receiver's health

Gender of caregiver (female)

Developmental

Developmental inability to fulfill caregiver role (e.g., a young adult needing to provide care for a middle-aged parent)

Developmental delay or retardation of the care receiver or caregiver

Psychosocial

Psychological or cognitive problems in care receiver

Marginal family adaptation or dysfunction before caregiving became necessary

Marginal coping patterns of caregiver

History of poor relationship with care receiver

Spousal relationship to care receiver

Care receiver exhibits deviant, bizarre behavior

Situational

Presence of abuse or violence

Presence of situational stressors that normally affect families, such as significant loss, disaster or crisis, poverty or economic vulnerability, major life events (e.g., birth, hospitalization, leaving home, returning home, marriage, divorce, employment, retirement, and death)

Duration of caregiving required

Inadequate physical environment for providing care (e.g., housing, transportation, community services, equipment)

Isolation

Lack of respite and recreation

Inexperience with caregiving

Competing role commitments

Complexity/number of caregiving tasks

Defining characteristics

Not having enough resources to provide the care needed

Finding it hard to do specific caregiving activities

Worry about such things as the care receiver's health
and emotional state, having to put the care receiver
in an institution, and who will care for the care receiver if something should happen to the caregiver

Feeling that caregiving interferes with other
important roles in caregiver's life

Feeling loss because the care receiver is like a different
person as compared with before caregiving began
or, in the case of a child, that the care receiver was
never the child the caregiver expected

Family conflict around issues of providing care

Stress or nervousness in the relationship with the care
receiver

Depression

Caregiver role strain, risk for

Vulnerability for feeling difficulty in performing the family
caregiver role.

Risk factors
  Pathophysiological
  Severity of illness of the care receiver
  Addiction or codependency
  Premature birth/congenital defect
  Discharge of family member with significant home
    healthcare needs
  Caregiver health impairment
  Unpredictable illness course or instability in the
    care receiver's health
  Gender of caregiver (female)
  Psychological or cognitive problems in care
    receiver
  Developmental
  Developmental inability to fulfill caregiver role
    (e.g., a young adult needing to provide care for
    middle-aged parent)
  Developmental delay or retardation of the care
    receiver or caregiver
  Psychological
  Marginal family adaptation or dysfunction before
    caregiving became necessary
  Marginal coping patterns of caregiver

History of poor relationship with care receiver
Spousal relationship to care receiver
Care receiver exhibits deviant, bizarre behavior
Situational
Presence of abuse or violence
Presence of situational stressors that normally affect families, such as significant loss, disaster or crisis, poverty or economic vulnerability, major life events (e.g., birth, hospitalization, leaving home, returning home, marriage, divorce, employment, retirement, and death)
Duration of caregiving required
Inadequate physical environment for providing care (e.g., housing, transportation, community services, equipment)
Isolation
Lack of respite and recreation
Inexperience with caregiving
Competing role commitments
Complexity/number of caregiving tasks

Communication, impaired verbal

The state in which an individual experiences a decreased or absent ability to use or understand language in human interaction.

Related factors
Decrease in circulation to brain
Physical barrier, brain tumor, tracheostomy, intubation
Anatomic deficit, cleft palate
Psychological barriers, psychosis, lack of stimuli
Cultural difference
Developmental or age-related
Defining characteristics
Inability to speak dominant language
Refusal or inability to speak
Stuttering; slurring
Impaired articulation
Dyspnea

Disorientation
Inability to modulate speech
Inability to find words
Inability to name words
Inability to identify objects
Loose association of ideas
Flight of ideas
Incessant verbalization
Difficulty with phonation
Inability to speak in sentences

Community coping, potential for enhanced

A pattern of community activities for adaptation and problem solving that is satisfactory for meeting the demands or needs of the community but can be improved for management of current and future problems/stressors.

Related factors
Social supports available
Resources available for problem solving
Community has a sense of power to manage stressors
Defining characteristics
  Major
  Deficits in one or more characteristics that indicate effective coping
  Minor
  Active planning by community for predicted stressors
  Active problem solving by community when faced with issues
  Agreement that community is responsible for stress management
  Positive communication among community members
  Positive communication between community/ aggregates and larger community
  Programs available for recreation and relaxation
  Resources sufficient for managing stressors

Community coping, ineffective

A pattern of community activities for adaptation and problem solving that is unsatisfactory for meeting the demands or needs of the community.

Related factors
Deficits in social support
Inadequate resources for problem solving
Powerlessness
Defining characteristics
   Major
   None
   Minor
   Community does not meet its own expectations
   Deficits of community participation
   Deficits in communication methods
   Excessive community conflicts
   Expressed difficulty in meeting demands for change
   Expressed vulnerability
   High illness rates
   Stressors perceived as excessive

Confusion, acute

The abrupt onset of a cluster of global, transient changes and disturbances in attention, cognition, psychomotor activity level of consciousness, and/or sleep/wake cycle.

Related factors
Over 60 years of age
Dementia
Alcohol abuse
Drug abuse
Delirium
Defining characteristics
   Major
   Fluctuation in cognition
   Fluctuation in sleep-wake cycle
   Fluctuation in level of consciousness
   Fluctuation in psychomotor activity
   Increased agitation or restlessness
   Misperceptions

Lack of motivation to initiate or follow through
with goal-directed or purposeful behavior
Minor
Hallucinations

Confusion, chronic

An irreversible, long-standing and/or progressive deterioration
of intellect and personality characterized by decreased ability to
interpret environmental stimuli, decreased capacity for
intellectual thought processes and manifested by disturbances
of memory, orientation, and behavior

Related factors
Alzheimer's disease
Korsakoff's psychosis
Multi-infarct dementia
Cerebrovascular accident
Head injury
Defining characteristics
  Major
  Clinical evidence of organic impairment
  Altered interpretation of or response to stimuli
  Progressive or long-standing cognitive impairment
  Minor
  No change in level of consciousness
  Impaired socialization
  Impaired memory (short term, long term)
  Altered personality

Constipation

The state in which an individual experiences a change in normal
bowel habits characterized by a decrease in frequency and/or
passage of hard, dry stools.

Related factors
Less than adequate intake
Less than adequate dietary intake and bulk
Less than adequate physical activity or immobility
Personal habits
Medications
Chronic use of medication and enemas
Gastrointestinal obstructive lesions

Neuromuscular impairment
Musculoskeletal impairment
Pain on defecation
Diagnostic procedures
Lack of privacy
Weak abdominal musculature
Pregnancy
Emotional status

Defining characteristics
Frequency less than usual pattern
Hard-formed stool
Palpable mass
Reported feeling of rectal fullness
Straining at stool
Decreased bowel sound
Reported feeling of abdominal or rectal fullness or
    pressure
Less than usual amount of stool
Nausea

Other possible defining characteristics
Abdominal pain
Back pain
Headache
Interference with daily living
Use of laxatives
Decreased appetite
Appetite impairment

Constipation, colonic

The state in which an individual's pattern of elimination is characterized by hard, dry stool that results from a delay in passage of food residue.

Related factors
Less than adequate fluid intake
Less than adequate dietary intake
Less than adequate fiber intake
Less than adequate physical activity
Immobility
Lack of privacy
Emotional disturbances
Chronic use of medication and enemas

...ess
...hange in daily routine
Metabolic problems (e.g., hypothyroidism,
    hypocalcemia, hypokalemia)
Defining characteristics
Decreased frequency
Hard, dry stool
Straining at stool
Painful defecation
Abdominal distention
Palpable mass
Rectal pressure
Headache, appetite impairment
Abdominal pain

Constipation, perceived

The state in which an individual makes a self-diagnosis of
constipation and ensures a daily bowel movement through use
of laxatives, enemas, and suppositories.

Related factors
Cultural/family health beliefs
Faulty appraisal
Impaired thought processes
Defining characteristics
Expectation of a daily bowel movement with resulting
    overuse of laxatives, enemas, and suppositories
Expected passage of stool at same time every day

Coping, defensive

The state in which in individual experiences falsely positive self-
evaluation based on a self-protective pattern that defends
against underlying perceived threats to positive self-regard.

Related factors
To be developed
Defining characteristics
Denial (of obvious problems, weaknesses)
Projection (of blame/responsibility)
Rationalization of failures
Defensiveness (hypersensitivity to criticism)
Grandiosity

Superior attitude toward others
Difficulty establishing/maintaining relationships
Hostile laughter or ridicule of others
Difficulty in reality testing of perceptions
Lack of follow-through or participation in treatment
or therapy

Coping, family: potential for growth

Effective managing of adaptive tasks by family member involved with the patient's health challenge, who now is exhibiting desire and readiness for enhanced health and growth in regard to self and in relation to the patient.

Related factors
Family members attempt to describe growth impact of
crisis on their own values, priorities, goals, or
relationships
Family member is moving in direction of health-
promoting and enriching life-style that supports
and monitors maturational processes, audits and
negotiates treatment programs, and generally
chooses experiences that optimize wellness
Individual expresses interest in making contact on a
one-to-one basis or on a mutual-aid group basis
with another person who has experienced a similar
situation

Coping, ineffective family: compromised

Insufficient, ineffective, or compromised support, comfort, assistance, or encouragement—usually by a supportive primary person (family member or close friend); patient may need it to manage or master adaptive tasks related to his/her health challenge.

Related factors
Inadequate or incorrect information or understanding
by a primary person
Temporary preoccupation by a significant person who
is trying to manage emotional conflicts and
personal suffering and is unable to perceive or act
effectively in regard to patient's needs
Temporary family disorganization and role changes

Other situational or developmental crises or situations
the significant person may be facing
Patient's providing little support for the primary
person
Prolonged disease or disability progression that
exhausts supportive capacity of significant people

Defining characteristics

Subjective

Patient expresses or confirms concern/complaint
about significant other's response to patient's
health problem

Significant person describes preoccupation with
personal reactions (e.g., fear, anticipatory grief,
guilt, anxiety) regarding patient's illness or
disability or to other situational or
developmental crises

Significant person describes or confirms an
inadequate understanding or knowledge base
that interferes with effective assistive or
supportive behaviors

Objective

Significant person attempts assistive or supportive
behaviors with less than satisfactory results

Significant person withdraws or enters into limited
or temporary personal communication with
patient at time of need

Significant person displays protective behavior
disproportionate (too little or too much) to
patient's abilities or need for autonomy

Coping, ineffective family: disabling

Behavior of significant person (family member or other primary
person) that disables his/her own capacities and the patient's
capacities to effectively address tasks essential to either person's
adaptation to the health challenge

Related factors

Significant person with chronically unexpressed
feelings of guilt, anxiety, hostility, despair, etc.

Dissonant discrepancy of coping styles being used to
deal with adaptive tasks by the significant person
and patient or among significant people

Highly ambivalent family relationships

Arbitrary handling of family's resistance to treatment that tends to solidify defensiveness because it fails to deal adequately with underlying anxiety

Defining characteristics

Neglectful care of patient in regard to basic human needs and/or illness treatment

Distortion of reality about patient's health problem, including extreme denial about its existence or severity

Intolerance

Rejection

Abandonment

Desertion

Carrying on usual routines; disregarding patient's needs

Psychosomatic tendency

Taking on illness signs of patient

Decisions and actions by family that are detrimental to economic or social well-being

Agitation, depression, aggression, hostility

Impaired restructuring of a meaningful life for self; impaired individualization; prolonged overconcern for patient

Neglectful relationships with other family members

Patient's development of helpless, inactive dependence

Coping, ineffective individual

Impairment of adaptive behaviors and problem-solving abilities of a person in meeting life's demands and roles.

Related factors

Situational crises

Maturational crises

Personal vulnerability

Multiple life changes

No vacations

Inadequate relaxation

Inadequate support systems

ttle or no exercise
oor nutrition
Unmet expectations
Work overload
Too many deadlines
Unrealistic perceptions
Inadequate coping method

Defining characteristics

Verbalization of inability to cope or inability to ask for
  help
Inability to meet role expectations
Inability to meet basic needs
Inability to problem solve
Alteration in societal participation
Destructive behavior toward self or others
Inappropriate use of defense mechanisms
Change in usual communication patterns
Verbal manipulation
High illness rate
High rate of accidents
Overeating
Lack of appetite
Excessive smoking
Excessive drinking
Overuse of prescribed tranquilizers
Alcohol proneness
High blood pressure
Chronic fatigue
Insomnia
Muscular tension
Ulcers
Frequent headaches
Frequent neckaches
Irritable bowel
Chronic worry
General irritability
Poor self-esteem
Chronic anxiety
Emotional tension
Chronic depression

Decisional conflict (specify)

A state of uncertainty about the course of action to be taken when choice among competing actions involves risk, loss, or challenge to personal life values. (Specify focus of conflict; e.g., choices regarding health, family relationships, career, finances, or other life events).

Related factors
Unclear personal values/beliefs
Perceived threat to value system
Lack of experience or interference with decision making
Lack of relevant information
Support system deficit
Defining characteristics
Verbalized feeling of distress related to uncertainty about choices
Verbalization of undesired consequences of alternative actions being considered
Vacillation between alternative choices
Delayed decision making
Self-focusing
Physical signs of distress or tension (increased heart rate, increased muscle tension, restlessness, etc.)
Questioning personal values and beliefs while attempting to make a decision

Denial, ineffective

A conscious or unconscious attempt to disavow the knowledge or meaning of an event to reduce anxiety/fear to the detriment of health.

Related factors
To be developed
Defining characteristics
Delay in seeking or refusal of medical attention to the detriment of health
Does not perceive personal relevance of symptoms or danger
Use of home remedies (self-treatment) to relieve symptoms

Does not admit fear of death or invalidism
Minimization of symptoms
Displacing source of symptoms to other organs
Inability to admit impact of disease on life pattern
Presence of dismissive gestures or comments when
    speaking of distressing events
Displacing fear of impact of condition
Inappropriate affect

Diarrhea

The state in which an individual experiences a change in normal bowel habits characterized by the frequent passage of loose, fluid, unformed stools.

Related factors
Stress and anxiety
Dietary intake
Medications
Inflammation, irritation, or malabsorption of bowel
Toxins
Contaminants
Radiation
Defining characteristics
Abdominal pain
Cramping
Increased frequency of bowel movements
Increased frequency of bowel sounds
Loose, liquid stools
Urgency
Changes in color

Disuse syndrome, risk for

The state in which an individual is at risk for deterioration of body systems as the result of prescribed or unavoidable inactivity.

Risk factors
Paralysis
Mechanical immobilization
Prescribed immobilization
Severe pain
Altered level of consciousness

Diversional activity deficit

The state in which an individual experiences a decreased stimulation from or interest or engagement in recreational or leisure activities.

Related factors
Environmental lack of diversional activity
Long-term hospitalization
Frequent, lengthy treatments
Defining characteristics
Boredom
Desire for something to do, to read, etc.
Usual hobbies cannot be undertaken in hospital

Dysreflexia

The state in which an individual with a spinal cord injury at T7 or above experiences or is at risk of experiencing a life-threatening uninhibited sympathetic response of the nervous system attributable to a noxious stimulus.

Related factors
To be developed
Defining characteristics
Individual with spinal cord injury (T7 or above) with the following:
Paroxysmal hypertension (sudden periodic elevated blood pressure where systolic pressure is over 140 mm Hg and diastolic pressure is above 90 mm Hg)
Bradycardia or tachycardia (pulse rate of less than 60 or over 100 beats per minute)
Diaphoresis (above injury)
Red splotches on skin (above injury)
Pallor (below injury)
Headache (diffuse pain in different portions of head and not confined to any nerve distribution area)
Chilling (shivering accompanied by sensation of coldness or pallor of skin)
Conjunctival congestion (excessive amount of blood/tissue fluid in conjunctivae)
Horner's syndrome (contraction of pupil, partial

ptosis of eyelid, enophthalmos, and sometimes
loss of sweating over affected side of face due to
paralysis of cervical sympathetic nerve trunk)
Paresthesia (abnormal sensation, such as
numbness, prickling, or tingling; increased
sensitivity)
Pilomotor reflex (gooseflesh formation when skin
is cooled)
Blurred vision
Chest pain
Metallic taste in mouth
Nasal congestion

Energy field disturbance

A disruption of the flow of energy surrounding a person's being,
which results in a disharmony of the body, mind, or spirit.

Defining characteristics
Temperature change (warmth or coolness)
Visual changes (image or color)
Disruption of the field (vacant/hold/spike/bulge)
Movement (wave/spike/tingling/dense/flowing)
Sounds (tone or words)

Environmental interpretation syndrome, impaired

Consistent lack of orientation to person, place, time, or
circumstances over more than from 3 to 6 months, necessitating
a protective environment.

Related factors
Dementia (Alzheimer's disease, multi-infarct
dementia, Pick's disease, AIDS dementia)
Parkinson's disease
Huntington's disease
Depression
Alcoholism
Defining characteristics
  Major
  Consistent disorientation in known and unknown
  environments
  Chronic confusional states

Minor
Loss of occupation or social functioning from memory decline
Inability to follow simple directions or instructions
Inability to reason
Inability to concentrate
Slowness in responding to questions

Family processes, altered: alcoholism

The state in which the psychosocial, spiritual, and physiological functions of the family unit are chronically disorganized, leading to conflict, denial of problems, resistance to change, ineffective problem-solving, and a series of self-perpetuating crises.

Related factors
Abuse of alcohol
Family history of alcoholism, resistance to treatment
Inadequate coping skills
Genetic predisposition
Addictive personality
Lack of problem-solving skills
Biochemical influences

Defining characteristics
  Major
  Feelings
    Decreased self-esteem or sense of worthlessness
    Anger or suppressed rage
    Frustration
    Powerlessness
    Anxiety
    Tension
    Distress
    Insecurity
    Repressed emotions
    Responsibility for alcoholic's behavior
    Lingering resentment
    Shame or embarrassment
    Hurt
    Unhappiness
    Guilt
    Emotional isolation and loneliness
    Vulnerability

Mistrust
Hopelessness
Rejection
Roles and relationships
Deterioration in family relationships or disturbed family dynamics

Ineffective spouse communication or marital problems

Altered role function or disruption of family roles

Inconsistent parenting or low perception of parental support

Family denial

Intimacy dysfunction

Chronic family problems

Closed communication systems

Behaviors
Expression of anger inappropriately

Difficulty with intimate relationships

Loss of control of drinking

Impaired communication

Ineffective problem-solving skills

Enabling alcoholic to maintain drinking

Inability to meet emotional needs of its members

Manipulation

Dependency

Criticizing

Alcohol abuse

Broken promises

Rationalization or denial of problems

Refusal to get help or inability to accept and receive help appropriately

Blaming

Inadequate understanding or knowledge or alcoholism

Minor
Feelings
Being different from other people

Depression

Hostility

Fear

Emotional control by others
Confusion
Dissatisfaction
Loss
Misunderstood
Abandonment
Confused love and pity
Moodiness
Failure
Being unloved
Lack of identity

Roles and relationships

Triangulating family relationships
Reduced ability of family members to relate to each other for mutual growth and maturation
Lack of skills necessary for relationships
Lack of cohesiveness
Disrupted family rituals
Family unable to meet security needs of its members
Family does not demonstrate respect for individuality and autonomy of its members
Pattern of rejection
Economic problems
Neglected obligations

Behaviors

Inability to meet spiritual needs of its members
Inability to express or accept wide range of feelings
Orientation toward tension relief rather than achievement of goals
Family special occasions are alcohol centered
Escalating conflict
Lying
Contradictory, paradoxical communication
Lack of dealing with conflict
Harsh self-judgment
Isolation
Nicotine addiction
Difficulty having fun
Self-blaming
Unresolved grief

Controlling communication and power
struggles
Inability to adapt to change
Immaturity
Stress-related physical illnesses
Inability to deal with traumatic experiences
constructively
Seeking approval and affirmation
Lack of reliability
Disturbances in academic performance in
children
Disturbances in concentration
Chaos
Substance abuse other than alcohol
Failure to accomplish current or past
developmental tasks or difficulty with life
cycle transitions
Verbal abuse of spouse or parent
Agitation
Diminished physical contact

Family processes, altered

The state in which a family that normally functions effectively
experiences a dysfunction.

Related factors
Situational transition and/or crises
Developmental transition and/or crises
Defining characteristics*
Family system unable to meet physical needs of its
members
Family system unable to meet emotional needs of its
members
Family system unable to meet spiritual needs of its
members
Parents do not demonstrate respect for each other's
views on child-rearing practices
Inability to express or accept wide range of feelings

*The first 13 defining characteristics are specifically from Otto H:
Criteria for assessing family strengths, *Fam Process* 2:329-330, Sept
1963

Inability to express or accept feelings of members
Family unable to meet security needs of its members
Inability of family members to relate to each other for
  mutual growth and maturation
Family uninvolved in community activities
Inability to accept or receive help appropriately
Rigidity in function and roles
Family does not demonstrate respect for individuality
  and autonomy of its members
Family unable to adapt to change or to deal with
  traumatic experiences constructively
Family fails to accomplish current or past-
  developmental task
Ineffective family decision-making process
Failure to send and receive clear messages
Inappropriate boundary maintenance
Inappropriate or poorly communicated family rules,
  rituals, symbols
Unexamined family myths
Inappropriate level and direction of energy

Fatigue

An overwhelming sense of exhaustion and decreased capacity
for physical and mental work regardless of adequate sleep.

Related factors
Overwhelming psychological or emotional demands
Increased energy requirements to perform activities of
  daily living
Excessive social/role demands
States of discomfort
Decreased metabolic energy production
Altered body chemistry (e.g., medications, drug
  withdrawal)
Defining characteristics
Verbalization of fatigue/lack of energy
Inability to maintain usual routines
Perceived need for additional energy to accomplish
  routine tasks
Increase in physical complaints
Emotional lability or irritability
Impaired ability to concentrate

Decreased performance
Lethargy or listlessness
Disinterest in surroundings/introspection
Decreased libido
Accident proneness

Fear

Feeling of dread related to an identifiable source that the person validates.

Related factors
Natural or innate origins—sudden noise, loss of
    physical support, height, pain
Learned response—conditioning, modeling from or
    identification with others
Separation from support system in a potentially
    threatening situation (hospitalization, treatments,
    etc.)
Knowledge deficit or unfamiliarity
Language barrier
Sensory impairment
Phobic stimulus or phobia
Environmental stimuli
Defining characteristics
Subjective
    Increased tension
    Apprehension
    Impulsiveness
    Decreased self-assurance
    Afraid
    Scared
    Terrified
    Panicked
    Frightened
    Jittery
Objective
    Increased alertness
    Concentration on source
    Wide-eyed
    Attack behavior
    Focus on "it, out there"
    Fight behavior—aggressive

Flight behavior—withdrawal
Sympathetic stimulation—cardiovascular
excitation, superficial vasoconstriction, pupil
dilation

Fluid volume deficit (1)

The state in which an individual experiences vascular, cellular, or intracellular dehydration related to failure of regulatory mechanisms.

Related factor
Failure of regulatory mechanisms
Defining characteristics
Dilute urine
Increased urine output
Sudden weight loss
Other possible defining characteristics
Possible weight gain
Hypotension
Decreased venous filling
Increased pulse rate
Decreased skin turgor
Decreased pulse volume and pressure
Increased body temperature
Dry skin
Dry mucous membranes
Hemoconcentration
Weakness
Edema
Thirst

Fluid volume deficit (2)

The state in which an individual experiences vascular, cellular, or intracellular dehydration related to active loss.

Related factor
Active loss
Defining characteristics
Decreased urine output
Concentrated urine
Output greater than intake
Sudden weight loss

Decreased venous filling
Hemoconcentration
Increased serum sodium levels
Other possible defining characteristics
Hypotension
Thirst
Increased pulse rate
Decreased skin turgor
Decreased pulse volume and pressure
Change in mental state
Increased body temperature
Dry skin
Dry mucous membranes
Weakness

Fluid volume deficit, risk for

The state in which an individual is at risk for experiencing vascular, cellular, or intracellular dehydration.

Risk factors
Extremes of age
Extremes of weight
Excessive losses through normal routes (e.g., diarrhea)
Loss of fluid through abnormal routes (e.g.,
    indwelling tubes)
Deviations affecting access to, intake of, or absorption
    of fluids (e.g., physical immobility)
Factors influencing fluid needs (e.g., hypermetabolic
    states)
Knowledge deficiency related to fluid volume
Medications (e.g., diuretics)
Increased fluid output
Urinary frequency
Thirst
Altered intake

Fluid volume excess

The state in which an individual experiences increased fluid retention and edema.

Related factors
Compromised regulatory mechanism

Excessive fluid intake
Excessive sodium intake
Defining characteristics
Edema
Effusion
Anasarca
Weight gain
Shortness of breath, orthopnea
Intake greater than output
Third heart sound
Pulmonary congestion on x-ray film
Abnormal breath sounds: crackles (rales)
Change in respiratory pattern
Change in mental status
Decreased hemoglobin, hematocrit levels
Blood pressure changes
Central venous pressure changes
Pulmonary artery pressure changes
Jugular venous distention
Positive hepatojugular reflex
Oliguria
Specific gravity changes
Azoturia
Altered electrolytes
Restlessness and anxiety

Gas exchange, impaired

The state in which an individual experiences an imbalance between oxygen uptake and carbon dioxide elimination at the alveolar-capillary membrane gas exchange area.

Related factors
Altered oxygen supply
Alveolar-capillary membrane changes
Altered blood flow
Altered oxygen-carrying capacity of blood
Defining characteristics
Confusion
Somnolence
Restlessness
Irritability
Inability to move secretions

Hypercapnia
Hypoxia

Grieving, anticipatory

Intellectual and emotional responses and behaviors by which individuals work through the process of modifying self-concept based on the perception of potential loss.

Related factors
Perceived potential loss of significant other
Perceived potential loss of physiopsychosocial well-being
Perceived potential loss of personal possessions
Defining characteristics
Potential loss of significant object
Expression of distress at potential loss
Denial of potential loss
Guilt
Anger
Sorrow
Choked feelings
Changes in eating habits
Alterations in sleep patterns
Alterations in activity level
Altered libido
Altered communication patterns

Grieving, dysfunctional

Extended, unsuccessful use of intellectual and emotional responses by which individuals attempt to work through the process of modifying self-concept based on the perception of loss.

Related factors
Actual or perceived object loss
Thwarted grieving response to a loss
Absence of anticipatory grieving
Chronic fatal illness
Lack of resolution of previous grieving response
Loss of significant others
Loss of physiopsychosocial well-being
Loss of personal possessions

Defining characteristics
Verbal expression of distress at loss
Denial of loss
Expression of guilt
Expression of unresolved issues
Anger
Sadness
Crying
Difficulty in expressing loss
Alterations in
    Eating habits
    Sleep patterns
    Dream patterns
    Activity level
    Libido
Idealization of lost object
Reliving of past experiences
Interference with life functioning
Developmental regression
Labile effect
Alterations in concentration and/or pursuits of tasks

Growth and development, altered

The state in which an individual demonstrates deviations in norms from his/her age-group.

Related factors
Inadequate caretaking: indifference, inconsistent
    responsiveness, multiple caretakers
Separation from significant others
Environmental and stimulation deficiencies
Effects of physical disability
Prescribed dependence
Defining characteristics
Delay or difficulty in performing skills (motor, social,
    or expressive) typical of age-group
Altered physical growth
Inability to perform self-care or self-control activities
    appropriate for age
Flat affect
Listlessness, decreased responses

Health maintenance, altered

Inability to identify, manage, and/or seek help to maintain health.

Related factors

Lack of or significant alteration in communication skills (written, verbal, and/or gestural)

Lack of ability to make deliberate and thoughtful judgments

Perceptual or cognitive impairment

Complete or partial lack of gross and/or fine motor skills

Ineffective individual coping; dysfunctional grieving

Lack of material resources

Unachieved developmental tasks

Ineffective family coping; disabling spiritual distress

Defining characteristics

Demonstrated lack of knowledge regarding basic health practices

Demonstrated lack of adaptive behaviors to internal or external environmental changes

Reported or observed inability to take responsibility for meeting basic health practices in any or all functional pattern areas

History of lack of health-seeking behavior

Expressed interest in improving health behaviors

Reported or observed lack of equipment, financial, and/or other resources

Reported or observed impairment of personal support system

Health-seeking behaviors (specify)

The state in which a patient in stable health is actively seeking ways to alter personal health habits and/or the environment in order to move toward optimal health. (*Stable health status* is defined as age-appropriate illness prevention measures achieved; the patient reports good or excellent health, and signs and symptoms of disease, if present, are controlled.)

Related factors

To be developed

Defining characteristics

Expressed or observed desire to seek higher level of wellness

39

Stated or observed unfamiliarity with wellness
community resources
Demonstrated or observed lack of knowledge in
health promotion behaviors
Expressed or observed desire for increased control of
health practice
Expression of concern about effects of current
environmental conditions on health status

Home maintenance management, impaired

Inability to independently maintain a safe growth-promoting
immediate environment.

Related factors
Disease or injury of individual or family member
Insufficient family organization or planning
Insufficient finances
Unfamiliarity with neighborhood resources
Impaired cognitive or emotional functioning
Lack of knowledge
Lack of role modeling
Inadequate support systems
Defining characteristics
Subjective
Household members express difficulty in
maintaining their home in a comfortable
fashion
Household requests assistance with home
maintenance
Household members describe outstanding debts or
financial crises
Objective
Disorderly surroundings
Unwashed or unavailable cooking equipment,
clothes, or linen
Accumulation of dirt, food wastes, or hygienic
wastes
Offensive odors
Inappropriate household temperature
Overtaxed family members (e.g., exhausted,
anxious family members)

Lack of necessary equipment or aids
Presence of vermin or rodents
Repeated hygienic disorders, infestations, or
    infections

Hopelessness

The subjective state in which an individual sees limited or no
alternatives or personal choices available and is unable to
mobilize energy on own behalf.

Related factors
Prolonged activity restriction creating isolation
Failure or deteriorating physiological condition
Long-term stress
Abandonment
Loss of belief in transcendent values/God
Defining characteristics
Passivity, decreased verbalization
Decreased affect
Verbal cues (indicating despondency, "I can't,"
    sighing)
Lack of initiative
Decreased response to stimuli
Turning away from speaker
Closing eyes
Shrugging in response to speaker
Decreased appetite; increased/decreased sleep
Lack of involvement in care; passively allowing care

Hyperthermia

The state in which an individual's body temperature is elevated
above his/her normal range.

Related factors
Exposure to hot environment
Vigorous activity
Medications/anesthesia
Inappropriate clothing
Increased metabolic rate
Illness or trauma
Dehydration
Inability or decreased ability to perspire

Defining characteristics
Increase in body temperature above normal range
Flushed skin
Warm to touch
Increased respiratory rate
Tachycardia
Seizures/convulsions

Hypothermia

The state in which an individual's body temperature is reduced below his/her normal range but not below 35.6° C (rectal)/36.4° C (rectal, newborn).

Related factors
Exposure to cool or cold environment
Illness or trauma
Inability or decreased ability to shiver
Malnutrition
Inadequate clothing
Consumption of alcohol
Medications causing vasodilation
Evaporation from skin in cool environment
Decreased metabolic rate
Inactivity
Aging
Defining characteristics
Shivering (mild)
Cool skin
Pallor (moderate)
Slow capillary refill
Tachycardia
Cyanotic nail beds
Hypertension
Piloerection

Incontinence, bowel

See Bowel incontinence.

Incontinence, functional

The state in which an individual experiences an involuntary, unpredictable passage of urine.

Related factors
Altered environment
Sensory, cognitive, or mobility deficits
Defining characteristics
Urge to void or bladder contractions sufficiently
  strong to result in loss of urine before reaching an
  appropriate receptacle

Incontinence, reflex

The state in which an individual experiences an involuntary loss
of urine occurring at somewhat predictable intervals when a
specific bladder volume is reached.

Related factor
Neurological impairment (e.g., spinal cord lesion that
  interferes with conduction of cerebral messages
  above level of reflex arc)
Defining characteristics
No awareness of bladder filling
No urge to void or feelings of bladder fullness
Uninhibited bladder contraction/spasm at regular
  intervals

Incontinence, stress

The state in which an individual experiences a loss of urine of
less than 50 ml occurring with increased abdominal pressure.

Related factors
Degenerative changes in pelvic muscles and structural
  supports associated with increased age
High intraabdominal pressure (e.g., obesity, gravid
  uterus)
Incompetent bladder outlet
Overdistention between voidings
Weak pelvic muscles and structural supports
Defining characteristics
Reported or observed dribbling with increased
  abdominal pressure
Urinary urgency
Urinary frequency (more often than every 2 hours)

Incontinence, total

The state in which an individual experiences a continuous and unpredictable loss of urine.

Related factors

Neuropathy preventing transmission of reflex indicating bladder fullness

Neurological dysfunction causing triggering of micturition at unpredictable times

Independent contraction of detrusor reflex due to surgery

Trauma or disease affecting spinal cord nerves

Anatomic (fistula)

Defining characteristics

Constant flow of urine occurring at unpredictable times without distention or uninhibited bladder contractions/spasms

Unsuccessful incontinence refractory to treatments

Nocturia

Lack of perineal or bladder-filling awareness

Unawareness of incontinence

Incontinence, urge

The state in which an individual experiences involuntary passage of urine occurring soon after a strong sense of urgency to void.

Related factors

Decreased bladder capacity (e.g., history of PID, abdominal surgeries, indwelling urinary catheter)

Irritation of bladder stretch receptors, causing spasm (e.g., bladder infection)

Alcohol

Caffeine

Increased fluids

Increased urine concentration

Overdistention of bladder

Defining characteristics

Urinary urgency

Frequency (voiding mcre often than every 2 hours)

Bladder contracture/spasm

Nocturia (more than 2 times per night)

Voiding in small (less than 100 ml) or in large
amounts (more than 550 ml)
Inability to reach toilet in time

Infant behavior, disorganized

Alteration in integration and modulation of the physiological
and behavioral systems of functioning (i.e., autonomic, motor,
state, organizational, self regulatory, and attentional-
interactional systems).

Related factors
Pain
Oral motor problems
Feeding intolerance
Environmental overstimulation
Lack of containment or boundaries
Prematurity
Invasive or painful procedures
Defining characteristics
  Major
  Change from baseline physiologic measures
  Tremors, startles, twitches
  Hyperextension of arms and legs
  Diffuse/unclear sleep
  Deficient self-regulatory behaviors
  Deficient response to visual/auditory stimuli
  Minor
  Yawning
  Apnea

Infant behavior, disorganized: risk for

Risk for alteration in integration and modulation of the
physiological and behavioral systems of functioning (i.e.,
autonomic, motor, state, organizational, self-regulatory, and
attentional-interactional systems)

Risk factors
Pain
Oral motor problems
Environmental overstimulation
Lack of containment or boundaries

Prematurity
Invasive or painful procedures

Infant behavior, organized: potential for enhanced

A pattern of modulation of the physiologic and behavioral systems of functioning of an infant (i.e., autonomic, motor, state, organizational, self-regulatory, and attentional-interactional systems) that is satisfactory but that can be improved, resulting in higher levels of integration in response to environmental stimuli.

Related factors
Prematurity
Pain
Defining characteristics
Stable physiologic measures
Definite sleep-wake states
Use of some self-regulatory behaviors
Response to visual or auditory stimuli

Infant feeding pattern, ineffective

A state in which an infant demonstrates an impaired ability to suck or coordinate the suck-swallow response.

Related factors
Prematurity
Neurological impairment/delay
Oral hypersensitivity
Prolonged NPO status
Anatomic abnormality
Defining characteristics
Inability to initiate or sustain an effective suck
Inability to coordinate sucking, swallowing, and
    breathing

Infection, risk for

The state in which an individual is at increased risk for being invaded by pathogenic organisms.

Risk factors

Inadequate primary defenses (broken skin, traumatized tissue, decrease in ciliary action, stasis of body fluids, change in pH secretions, altered peristalsis)

Inadequate secondary defenses (e.g., decreased hemoglobin level, leukopenia, suppressed inflammatory response, immunosuppression)

Inadequate acquired immunity

Tissue destruction and increased environmental exposure

Chronic disease

Invasive procedures

Malnutrition

Pharmaceutical agents and trauma

Rupture of amniotic membranes

Insufficient knowledge to avoid exposure to pathogens

Injury, perioperative positioning: risk for

A state in which the client is at risk for injury as a result of the environmental conditions found in the perioperative setting.

Risk factors

Disorientation

Immobilization, muscle weakness

Sensory or perceptual disturbances resulting from anesthesia

Obesity

Emaciation

Edema

Injury, risk for

The state in which an individual is at risk of injury as a result of environmental conditions interacting with the individual's adaptive and defensive resources. See also Poisoning, risk for; Suffocation, risk for; Trauma, risk for.

Risk factors

Interactive conditions between individual and environment that impose a risk to defensive and adaptive resources of individual

Internal
Biochemical
   Regulatory function
      Sensory dysfunction
      Integrative dysfunction
      Effector dysfunction
   Tissue hypoxia
   Malnutrition
   Immune-autoimmune
   Abnormal blood profile
      Leukocytosis or leukopenia
      Altered clotting factors
      Thrombocytopenia
      Sickle cell
      Thalassemia
      Decreased hemoglobin level
Physical
   Broken skin
   Altered mobility
Developmental
   Age
      Physiological
      Psychosocial
Psychological
   Affective
   Orientation
External
Biological
   Immunization level of community
   Microorganism
Chemical
   Pollutants
   Poisons
   Drugs
      Pharmaceutical agents
      Alcohol
      Caffeine
      Nicotine
   Preservatives
   Cosmetics and dyes
   Nutrients (vitamins, food types)

Injury, risk for —cont'd

Physical
  Design, structure, and arrangement of
    community, building, and/or equipment
  Mode of transport/transportation
  Nosocomial agents
People-provider
  Nosocomial agents
  Staffing patterns
  Cognitive, affective, and psychomotor factors

Knowledge deficit (specify)

Absence or deficiency of cognitive information related to specific
topic.

Related factors
Lack of exposure
Lack of recall
Information misinterpretation
Cognitive limitation
Lack of interest in learning
Unfamiliarity with information resources
Patient's request for no information
Defining characteristics
Verbalization of the problem
Inaccurate follow-through of instruction
Inadequate performance of test
Inappropriate or exaggerated behaviors (e.g.,
    hysterical, hostile, agitated, apathetic)
Statement of misconception
Request for information

Loneliness, risk for

A subjective state in which an individual is at risk of experiencing
vague dysphoria.

Risk factors
Affectional deprivation
Physical isolation
Cathectic deprivation
Social isolation

Management of therapeutic regimen, community: ineffective

A pattern of regulating and integrating into community processes programs for treatment of illness and the sequelae of illness that are unsatisfactory for meeting health-related goals.

Defining characteristics

Deficits in persons and programs to be accountable for illness care of aggregates

Deficits in advocates for aggregates

Deficits in community activities for secondary and tertiary prevention

Illness symptoms above the norm expected for the number and type of population

Number of health care resources insufficient for the incidence or prevalence of illness(es)

Unavailable health care resources for illness care

Unexpected acceleration of illness

Management of therapeutic regimen, families: ineffective

A pattern of regulating and integrating into family processes a program for treatment of illness and the sequelae of illness that is unsatisfactory for meeting specific health goals.

Related factors

Complexity of health care system

Complexity of therapeutic regimen

Decisional conflicts

Economic difficulties

Excessive demands made on individual or family

Family conflict

Defining characteristics

Major

Inappropriate family activities for meeting the goals of a treatment or prevention program

Minor

Acceleration (expected or unexpected) of illness symptoms of a family member

Lack of attention to illness and its sequelae

Verbalized desire to manage the treatment of illness and prevention of the sequelae

Verbalized difficulty with regulation/integration of
one or more effects or prevention of
complications
Verbalizes that family did not take action to reduce
risk factors for progression of illness and
sequelae

Management of therapeutic regimen, individual: effective

A pattern of regulating and integrating into daily living a
program for treatment of illness and its sequelae that is
satisfactory for meeting specific health goals.

Defining characteristics
Appropriate choices of daily activities for meeting the
goals of a treatment or prevention program
Illness symptoms within a normal range of
expectation
Verbalized desire to manage the treatment of illness
and prevention of sequelae
Verbalized intent to reduce risk factors for progression
of illness and sequelae

Management of therapeutic regimen, individuals: ineffective

A pattern of regulating and integrating into daily living a
program for treatment of illness and the sequelae of illness that
is unsatisfactory for meeting specific health goals.

Related factors
Complexity of health care system
Complexity of therapeutic regimen
Decisional conflicts
Economic difficulties
Excessive demands made on individual or family
Family conflict
Family patterns of health care
Inadequate number and types of cues to action
Knowledge deficits
Mistrust of regimen and/or health care personnel
Perceived seriousness
Perceived susceptibility

Perceived barriers
Perceived benefits
Powerlessness
Social support deficits
Defining characteristics
  Major
  Choices of daily living ineffective for meeting the
    goals of a treatment or prevention program
  Minor
  Acceleration (expected or unexpected) of illness
    symptoms
  Verbalized desire to manage the treatment of illness
    and prevention of sequelae
  Verbalized difficulty with regulation/integration of
    one or more prescribed regimens for treatment
    of illness and its effects or prevention of
    complications
  Verbalization that intimated that patient would not
    attempt to include treatment regimens in daily
    routines
  Verbalization that intimated that patient would not
    attempt to reduce risk factors for progression of
    illness and sequelae

Memory, impaired

The state in which an individual experiences the inability to
remember or recall bits of information or behavioral skills.
Impaired memory may be attributed to pathophysiological or
situational causes that are either temporary or permanent.

Related factors
Acute or chronic hypoxia
Anemia
Decreased cardiac output
Fluid and electrolyte imbalance
Neurologic disturbances
Excessive environmental disturbances
Defining characteristics
  Major
  Observed or reported experiences of forgetting
  Inability to determine whether a behavior was
    performed

Inability to learn or retain new skills or
    information
Inability to perform a previously learned skill
Inability to recall factual information
Inability to recall recent or past events
Minor
Forgets to perform a behavior at a scheduled time

Mobility, impaired physical

The state in which an individual experiences a limitation of
ability for independent physical movement.

Related factors
Intolerance to activity; decreased strength and
    endurance
Pain and discomfort
Perceptual or cognitive impairment
Neuromuscular impairment
Musculoskeletal impairment
Depression; severe anxiety
Defining characteristics
Inability to purposefully move within physical
    environment, including bed mobility, transfer, and
    ambulation
Reluctance to attempt movement
Limited range of motion
Decreased muscle strength, control, and/or mass
Imposed restrictions of movement, including
    mechanical; medical protocol
Impaired coordination

Noncompliance (specify)

A person's informed decision not to adhere to a therapeutic
recommendation.

Related factors
Patient's value system
    Health beliefs
    Cultural influences
    Spiritual values
Client and provider relationships

Defining characteristics
Behavior indicative of failure to adhere by direct
   observation or statements by patient or significant
   others
Objective tests (physiological measures, detection of
   markers)
Evidence of development of complications
Evidence of exacerbation of symptoms
Failure to keep appointments
Failure to progress
Inability to set or attain mutual goals

Nutrition, altered: less than body requirements

The state in which an individual experiences an intake of
nutrients insufficient to meet metabolic needs.

Related factor
Inability to ingest or digest food or absorb nutrients
   because of biological, psychological, or economic
   factors
Defining characteristics
Loss of body weight with adequate food intake
Body weight 20% or more under ideal for height and
   frame
Reported inadequate food intake less than
   Recommended Daily Allowance
Weakness of muscles required for swallowing or
   mastication
Reported or evidence of lack of food
Lack of interest in food
Perceived inability to ingest food
Aversion to eating
Reported altered taste sensation
Satiety immediately after ingesting food
Abdominal pain with or without pathological
   conditions
Sore, inflamed buccal cavity

Noncompliance (specify) —cont'd

Nutrition, altered: more than body requirements

The state in which an individual is experiencing an intake of nutrients that exceeds metabolic needs.

Related factor
Excessive intake in relationship to metabolic need

Defining characteristics
Weight 10%-20% over ideal for height and frame
Triceps skinfold greater than 15 mm in men and 25 mm in women
Sedentary activity level
Reported or observed dysfunctional eating patterns
  Pairing food with other activities
  Concentrating food intake at end of day
  Eating in response to external cues (e.g., time of day, social situation)
  Eating in response to internal cues other than hunger (e.g., anxiety)

Nutrition, altered: risk for more than body requirements

The state in which an individual is at risk of experiencing an intake of nutrients that exceeds metabolic needs.

Risk factors
Hereditary predisposition
Excessive energy intake during late gestational life, early infancy, and adolescence
Frequent, closely spaced pregnancies
Dysfunctional psychological conditioning in relationship to food
Membership in lower socioeconomic group
Reported or observed obesity in one or both parents
Rapid transition across growth percentiles in infants or children
Reported use of solid food as major food source before 5 months of age
Observed use of food as reward or comfort measure
Reported or observed higher baseline weight at beginning of each pregnancy

Dysfunctional eating patterns
Pairing food with other activities
Concentrating food intake at end of day
Eating in response to external cues (e.g., time of day or social situation)
Eating in response to internal cues other than hunger (e.g., anxiety)

Oral mucous membrane, altered

The state in which an individual experiences disruptions in the tissue layers of the oral cavity.

Related factors
Pathological conditions—oral cavity (radiation to head and/or neck)
Dehydration
Trauma
Chemical (e.g., acidic foods, drugs, noxious agents, alcohol)
Mechanical (e.g., ill-fitting dentures; braces; tubes—endotracheal, nasogastric; surgery in oral cavity)
NPO instructions for more than 24 hours
Ineffective oral hygiene
Mouth breathing
Malnutrition
Infection
Lack of or decreased salivation
Medication
Defining characteristics
Coated tongue
Xerostomia (dry mouth)
Stomatitis
Oral lesions or ulcers
Lack of or decreased salivation
Leukoplakia
Edema
Hyperemia
Oral plaque
Oral pain or discomfort
Desquamation
Vesicles

Hemorrhagic gingivitis
Carious teeth
Halitosis

Pain

The state in which an individual experiences and reports the presence of severe discomfort or an uncomfortable sensation.

Related factors
Injuring agents
    Biological
    Chemical
    Physical
    Psychological
Defining characteristics
    Subjective
    Communication (verbal or coded) of pain descriptors
    Objective
    Guarding behavior; protective
    Self-focusing
    Narrowed focus (altered time perception, withdrawal from social contact, impaired thought process)
    Distraction behavior (moaning, crying, pacing, seeking other people and/or activities, restlessness)
    Facial mask of pain (eyes lack luster, "beaten look," fixed or scattered movement, grimace)
    Alteration in muscle tone (may span from listless to rigid)
    Autonomic responses not seen in chronic, stable pain (diaphoresis, blood pressure and pulse rate change, pupillary dilation, increased or decreased respiratory rate)

Pain, chronic

The state in which an individual experiences pain that continues for more than 6 months.

Related factor
Chronic physical/psychosocial disability

Defining characteristics
Verbal report or observed evidence of pain
    experienced for more than 6 months
Fear of reinjury
Physical and social withdrawal
Altered ability to continue previous activities
Anorexia
Weight changes
Changes in sleep patterns
Facial masks
Guarded movement

Parent/infant/child attachment, altered: risk for

Disruption of the interactive process between parent or significant other and infant that fosters the development of a protective and nurturing reciprocal relationship.

Risk factors
Inability of parents to meet the personal needs
Anxiety associated with the parent role
Substance abuse
Premature infant
Ill infant or child who is unable to effectively initiate
    parental contact because of altered behavioral
    organization
Separation
Physical barriers
Lack of privacy

Parental role conflict

The state in which a parent experiences role confusion and conflict in response to a crisis.

Related factors
Separation from child due to chronic illness
Intimidation with invasive or restrictive modalities
    (e.g., isolation, intubation)
Specialized care centers, policies
Home care of a child with special needs (e.g., apnea
    monitoring, postural drainage, hyperalimentation)
Change in marital status

Interruptions of family life due to home health-care
regimen (treatments, caregivers, lack of respite)
Defining characteristics
Parent(s) expresses concerns/feelings of inadequacy to
provide for child's physical and emotional needs
during hospitalization or in home
Demonstrated disruption in caretaking routines
Parent(s) expresses concerns about changes in
parental role, family functioning, family
communication, and/or family health
Expresses concern about perceived loss of control over
decisions relating to child
Reluctant to participate in normal caretaking activities
even with encouragement and support
Verbalizes/demonstrates feelings of guilt, anger, fear,
anxiety, and/or frustrations about effect of child's
illness on family process

Parenting, altered

Parenting, altered, risk for

The state in which the ability of nurturing figure(s) to create an
environment that promotes the optimal growth and
development of another human being is altered or at risk.

Related/risk factors
Lack of available role model
Ineffective role model
Physical and psychosocial abuse of nurturing figure
Lack of support between or from significant other(s)
Unmet social and emotional maturation needs of
parenting figures
Interruption in bonding process (e.g., maternal,
paternal, other)
Perceived threat to own survival: physical and
emotional
Mental and/or physical illness
Presence of stress: financial or legal problems, recent
crisis, cultural move
Lack of knowledge
Limited cognitive functioning
Lack of role identity

Lack of appropriate response of child to relationship
Multiple pregnancies
Unrealistic expectation of self, infant, partner
Defining characteristics
Actual and potential
Lack of parental attachment behaviors
Inappropriate visual, tactile, auditory stimulation
Negative identification of characteristics of infant/child
Negative attachment of meanings to characteristics of infant/child
Constant verbalization of disappointment in gender or physical characteristics of infant/child
Verbalization of resentment toward infant/child
Verbalization of role inadequacy
Inattention to needs of infant/child
Verbal disgust at body functions of infant/child
Noncompliance with health appointments for self and/or infant/child
Inappropriate caretaking behaviors (toilet training, sleep and rest, feeding)
Inappropriate or inconsistent discipline practices
Frequent accidents
Frequent illness
Growth and development lag in child
History of child abuse or abandonment by primary caretaker
Verbalizes desire to have child call parent by first name despite traditional cultural tendencies
Child receives care from multiple caretakers without consideration for needs of child
Compulsive seeking of role approval from others
Actual
Abandonment
Runaway
Verbalization of inability to control child
Evidence of physical and psychological trauma

Peripheral neurovascular dysfunction, risk for

A state in which an individual is at risk of experiencing a disruption in circulation, sensation, or motion of an extremity.

Risk factors
Fractures
Mechanical compression (e.g., tourniquet, cast, brace, dressing, or restraint)
Orthopedic surgery
Trauma
Immobilization
Burns
Vascular obstruction

Personal identity disturbance

Inability to distinguish between self and nonself.

Related factors
To be developed
Defining characteristics
To be developed

Poisoning, risk for

Accentuated risk of accidental exposure to or ingestion of drugs or dangerous products in doses sufficient to cause poisoning.

Risk factors
  Internal (individual) factors
  Reduced vision
  Verbalization of occupational setting without adequate safeguards
  Lack of safety or drug education
  Lack of proper precaution
  Cognitive or emotional difficulties
  Insufficient finances
  External (environmental) factors
  Large supplies of drugs in house
  Medicines stored in unlocked cabinets accessible to children or confused persons
  Dangerous products placed or stored within reach of children or confused persons

Availability of illicit drugs potentially
    contaminated by poisonous additives
Flaking, peeling paint or plaster in presence of
    young children
Chemical contamination of food and water
Unprotected contact with heavy metals or
    chemicals
Paint, lacquer, etc., in poorly ventilated areas or
    without effective protection
Presence of poisonous vegetation
Presence of atmospheric pollutants

Post-trauma response

The state in which an individual experiences a sustained painful
response to (an) overwhelming traumatic event(s)

Related factors
Disaster
War
Epidemic
Rape
Assault
Torture
Catastrophic illness
Accident
Defining characteristics
Reexperience of traumatic event, which may be
    identified in cognitive, affective, and/or sensory
    motor activities (flashbacks, intrusive thoughts,
    repetitive dreams or nightmares, excessive
    verbalization of traumatic event, verbalization of
    survival guilt or guilt about behavior required for
    survival)
Psychic/emotional numbness (impaired interpretation
    of reality, confusion, dissociation or amnesia, vague-
    ness about traumatic event, constricted affect)
Altered life-style (self-destructiveness, such as
    substance abuse, suicide attempt, or other acting-
    out behavior; difficulty with interpersonal
    relationships; development of phobia regarding
    trauma; poor impulse control/irritability;
    explosiveness)

Powerlessness

Perception that one's own action will not significantly affect an outcome; a perceived lack of control over a current situation or immediate happening.

Related factors
Health-care environment
Interpersonal interaction
Illness-related regimen
Life-style of helplessness
Defining characteristics
Severe
Verbal expressions of having no control or influence over situation
Verbal expressions of having no control or influence over outcome
Verbal expressions of having no control over self-care
Depression over physical deterioration that occurs despite patient compliance with regimens
Apathy
Moderate
Nonparticipation in care or decision making when opportunities are provided
Expressions of dissatisfaction and frustration over inability to perform previous tasks and/or activities
Does not monitor progress
Expression of doubt regarding role performance
Reluctance to express true feelings, fearing alienation from caregivers
Inability to seek information regarding care
Dependence on others that may result in irritability, resentment, anger, and guilt
Does not defend self-care practices when challenged
Low
Passivity
Expressions of uncertainty about fluctuating energy levels

Protection, altered

The state in which an individual experiences a decrease in the ability to guard the self from internal or external threats, such as illness or injury.

Related factors
Extremes of age
Inadequate nutrition
Alcohol abuse
Abnormal blood profiles (leukopenia, thrombocytopenia, anemia, coagulation)
Drug therapies (antineoplastic, corticosteroid, immune, anticoagulant, thrombolytic)
Treatments (surgery, radiation)
Diseases such as cancer and immune disorders
Defining characteristics
Deficient immunity
Impaired healing
Altered clotting
Maladaptive stress response
Neurosensory alterations
Chilling
Perspiring
Dyspnea
Cough
Itching
Restlessness
Insomnia
Fatigue
Anorexia
Weakness
Immobility
Disorientation
Pressure sores

Rape-trauma syndrome

Forced, violent sexual penetration against the victim's will and consent. The trauma syndrome that develops from this attack or attempted attack includes an acute phase or disorganization of the victim's life-style and a long-term process of reorganization of life-style.

Related factors
Inadequate support systems
Spouse-family blaming
Fear of reprisal, pregnancy, going out alone
Anxiety about potential health problems (e.g., AIDS,
 venereal disease, herpes)
Defining characteristics
 Acute phase
 Emotional reactions
  Anger
  Embarrassment
  Fear of physical violence and death
  Humiliation
  Revenge
  Self-blame
 Multiple physical symptoms
 Gastrointestinal irritability
 Genitourinary discomfort
 Muscle tension
 Sleep pattern disturbance
 Long-term phase
 Changes in life-style (changes in residence; dealing
 with repetitive nightmares and phobias; seeking
 family support; seeking social network support)

Rape-trauma syndrome: compound reaction

An acute stress reaction to a rape or attempted rape,
experienced along with other major stressors, that can include
reactivation of symptoms of a previous condition.*

Related factors
Drug or alcohol abuse
History of and/or current psychiatric illness
History of and/or current physical illness
Defining characteristics
All defining characteristics listed under Rape-trauma
 syndrome
Reactivated symptoms of such previous conditions
 (i.e., physical illness, psychiatric illness)
Reliance on alcohol and/or drugs

*Definition developed by Kim, McFarland, and McLane.

Rape-trauma syndrome: silent reaction

A complex stress reaction to a rape in which an individual is unable to describe or discuss the rape.*

Related factors
Fear of retaliation
Intense shame
Excessive denial
Lack of support
Defining characteristics
Abrupt changes in relationships with members of the
    opposite sex
Increase in nightmares
Increasing anxiety during interview (e.g., blocking of
    associations, long periods of silence, minor
    stuttering, physical distress)
Marked changes in sexual behavior
No verbalization of occurrence of the rape
Sudden onset of phobic reactions

Relocation stress syndrome

Physiological and/or psychosocial disturbances as a result of transfer from one environment to another.

Related factors
Past, concurrent, and recent losses
Losses involved with decision to move
Feeling of powerlessness
Lack of adequate support system
Little or no preparation for the impending move
Moderate to high degree of environmental change
History and types of previous transfers
Impaired psychosocial health status
Decreased physical health status
Defining characteristics
    Major
    Change in environment/location
    Anxiety
    Apprehension
    Increased confusion (elderly population)

*Definition developed by Kim, McFarland, and McLane.

Depression
Loneliness
Minor
Verbalization of unwillingness to relocate
Sleep disturbance
Change in eating habits
Dependency
Gastrointestinal disturbances
Increased verbalization of needs
Insecurity
Lack of trust
Restlessness
Sad affect
Unfavorable comparison of post/pre-transfer staff
Verbalization of being concerned/upset about
    transfer
Vigilance
Weight change
Withdrawal

Role performance, altered

Disruption in the way one perceives one's role performance.

Related factors
To be developed
Defining characteristics
Change in self-perception of role
Denial of role
Change in others' perception of role
Conflict in roles
Change in physical capacity to resume role
Lack of knowledge of role
Change in usual patterns or responsibility

Self-care deficit, bathing/hygiene

The state in which one experiences an impaired ability to
perform or complete bathing/hygiene activities for oneself.

Related factors
To be developed
Defining characteristics
Inability to wash body or body parts

Inability to obtain or get to water source
Inability to regulate temperature or flow

Self-care deficit, dressing/grooming

The state in which one experiences an impaired ability to perform or complete dressing and grooming activities for oneself.

Related factors
To be developed
Defining characteristics
Impaired ability to put on or take off necessary items of clothing
Impaired ability to obtain or replace articles of clothing
Impaired ability to fasten clothing
Inability to maintain appearance at satisfactory level

Self-care deficit, feeding

The state in which one experiences an impaired ability to perform or complete feeding activities for oneself.

Related factors
To be developed
Defining characteristics
Inability to bring food from receptacle to mouth

Self-care deficit, toileting

The state in which one experiences an impaired ability to perform or complete toileting activities for oneself.

Related factors
Impaired transfer ability
Impaired mobility status
Intolerance to activity; decreased strength and endurance
Pain, discomfort
Perceptual or cognitive impairment
Neuromuscular impairment
Musculoskeletal impairment
Depression, severe anxiety

Defining characteristics
Inability to get to toilet or commode
Inability to sit on or rise from toilet or commode
Inability to manipulate clothing for toileting
Inability to carry out proper toilet hygiene
Inability to flush toilet or empty commode

Self-concept, disturbance in

See Body image disturbance; Personal identity disturbance; Self-esteem disturbance.

Self-esteem disturbance

Negative self-evaluation/feelings about self or self-capabilities, which may be directly or indirectly expressed.

Related factors
To be developed
Defining characteristics
Self-negating verbalization
Expressions of shame/guilt
Evaluation of self as unable to deal with events
Rationalization/rejection of positive feedback and
    exaggeration of negative feedback about self
Hesitancy to try new things/situations
Denial of problems obvious to others
Projection of blame/responsibility for problems
Rationalization of personal failures
Hypersensitivity to criticism
Grandiosity

Self esteem, chronic low

Long-standing negative self-evaluation/feelings about self or self-capabilities.

Related factors
To be developed
Defining characteristics
Self-negating verbalization
Expressions of shame/guilt
Evaluation of self as unable to deal with events
Rationalization/rejection of positive feedback and
    exaggeration of negative feedback about self

Hesitancy to try new things/situations
Frequent lack of success in work or other life events
Overly conforming; dependence on others' opinions
Lack of eye contact
Nonassertive/passive
Indecisive
Excessively seeks reassurance

Self-esteem, situational low

Negative self-evaluation/feelings about self that develop in response to a loss or change in an individual who previously had a positive self-evaluation.

Related factors
To be developed
Defining characteristics
Episodic occurrence of negative self-appraisal in response to life events in a person with a previous positive self-evaluation
Verbalization of negative feelings about self (helplessness, uselessness)
Self-negating verbalizations
Expressions of shame/guilt
Evaluation of self as unable to handle situations/events
Difficulty making decisions

Self-mutilation, risk for

A state in which an individual is at high risk to perform an act on the self to injure, not kill, that produces tissue damage and tension relief.

Risk factors
Groups at risk:
Clients with borderline personality disorder, especially females 16 to 25 years of age
Clients in psychotic state—frequently males in young adulthood
Emotionally disturbed and/or battered children
Mentally retarded and autistic children

Clients with a history of self-injury
History of physical, emotional, or sexual abuse
  Inability to cope with increased psychological/
    physiological tension in a healthy manner
Feelings of depression, rejection, self-hatred,
  separation anxiety, guilt, and depersonalization
Fluctuating emotions
Command hallucinations
Need for sensory stimuli
Parental emotional deprivation
Dysfunctional family

Sensory/perceptual alterations (specify) (visual, auditory, kinesthetic, gustatory, tactile, olfactory)

The state in which an individual experiences a change in the amount or patterning of incoming stimuli accompanied by a diminished, exaggerated, distorted, or impaired response to such stimuli.

Related factors
Environmental factors
Therapeutically restricted environments (isolation,
  intensive care, bed rest, traction, confining
  illnesses, incubator)
Socially restricted environment
  (institutionalization, homebound, aging,
  chronic illness, dying, infant deprivation);
  stigmatized (mentally ill, mentally retarded,
  mentally handicapped); bereaved
Altered sensory reception, transmission, and/or
  integration
  Neurological disease, trauma, or deficit
  Altered status of sense organs
  Inability to communicate, understand, speak, or
    respond
  Sleep deprivation
  Pain
Chemical alteration
Endogenous (electrolyte imbalance, elevated BUN
  level, elevated ammonia, hypoxia)

71

Exogenous (central nervous system stimulants or depressants, mind-altering drugs)
Psychological stress (narrowed perceptual fields caused by anxiety)

Defining characteristics
Disoriented in time, in place, or with persons
Altered abstraction
Altered conceptualization
Change in problem-solving abilities
Reported or measured change in sensory acuity
Change in behavior pattern
Anxiety
Apathy
Change in usual response to stimuli
Indication of body image alteration
Restlessness
Irritability
Altered communication patterns
Disorientation
Lack of concentration
Daydreaming
Hallucinations
Noncompliance
Fear
Depression
Rapid mood swings
Anger
Exaggerated emotional responses
Poor concentration
Disordered thought sequencing
Bizarre thinking
Visual and auditory distortions
Motor incoordination

Other possible defining characteristics
Complaints of fatigue
Alteration in posture
Change in muscular tension
Inappropriate responses
Hallucinations

Sensory/perceptual alterations (specify)—cont'd

Sexual dysfunction

The state in which an individual experiences a change in sexual function that is viewed as unsatisfying, unrewarding, or inadequate

Related factors
Biopsychosocial alteration of sexuality
  Ineffectual or absent role models
  Physical abuse
  Psychosocial abuse (e.g., harmful relationships)
  Vulnerability
  Misinformation or lack of knowledge
  Values conflict
  Lack of privacy
  Lack of significant other
  Altered body structure or function: pregnancy, recent childbirth, drugs, surgery, anomalies, disease process, trauma, radiation

Defining characteristics
Verbalization of problem
Alterations in achieving perceived sex role
Actual or perceived limitation imposed by disease and/or therapy
Conflicts involving values
Alterations in achieving sexual satisfaction
Inability to achieve desired satisfaction
Seeking of confirmation of desirability
Alteration in relationship with significant other
Change in interest in self and others

Sexuality patterns, altered

The state in which an individual expresses concern regarding his/her sexuality.

Related factors
Knowledge/skill deficit about alternative responses to health-related transitions, altered body function or structure, illness, or medical treatment
Lack of privacy
Lack of significant other
Ineffective or absent role models

Conflicts with sexual orientation or variant
  preferences
Fear of pregnancy or of acquiring sexually transmitted
  disease
Impaired relationship with significant other
Defining characteristics
Reported difficulties, limitations, or changes in sexual
  behaviors or activities

Skin integrity, impaired

The state in which an individual's skin is adversely altered.

Related factors
  External (environmental)
  Hyperthermia or hypothermia
  Chemical substance
  Mechanical factors
    Shearing forces
    Pressure
    Restraint
    Radiation
    Physical immobilization
    Humidity
  Internal (somatic)
  Medication
  Altered nutritional state: obesity, emaciation
  Altered metabolic state
  Altered circulation
  Altered sensation
  Altered pigmentation
  Skeletal prominence
  Developmental factors
  Immunological deficit
  Alterations in turgor (change in elasticity)
  Excretions/secretions
  Psychogenic
  Edema
Defining characteristics
Disruption of skin surface
Destruction of skin layers
Invasion of body structures

Skin integrity, impaired, risk for

The state in which an individual's skin is at risk of being adversely altered.

Risk factors
   External (environmental)
   Hypothermia or hyperthermia
   Chemical substance
   Mechanical factors
      Shearing forces
      Pressure
      Restraint
   Radiation
   Physical immobilization
   Excretions and secretions
   Humidity
   Internal (somatic)
   Medication
   Alterations in nutritional state (obesity, emaciation)
   Altered metabolic state
   Altered circulation
   Altered sensation
   Altered pigmentation
   Skeletal prominence
   Developmental factors
   Alterations in skin turgor (change in elasticity)
   Psychogenic
   Immunological

Sleep pattern disturbance

Disruption of sleep time causes discomfort or interferes with desired life-style.

Related factors
Sensory alterations
   Internal factors
      Illness
      Psychological stress
   External factors
      Environmental changes
      Social cues

Defining characteristics
Verbal complaints of difficulty in falling asleep
Awakening earlier or later than desired
Interrupted sleep
Verbal complaints of not feeling well rested
Changes in behavior and performance
    Increasing irritability
    Restlessness
    Disorientation
    Lethargy
    Listlessness
Physical signs
    Mild, fleeting nystagmus
    Slight hand tremor
    Ptosis of eyelid
    Expressionless face
Thick speech with mispronunciation and incorrect
    words
Dark circles under eyes
Frequent yawning
Changes in posture
Not feeling well rested

Social interaction, impaired

The state in which an individual participates in an insufficient or excessive quantity or ineffective quality of social exchange.

Related factors
Knowledge/skill deficit about ways to enhance
    mutuality
Communication barriers
Self-concept disturbance
Absence of available significant others or peers
Limited physical mobility
Therapeutic isolation
Sociocultural dissonance
Environmental barriers
Altered thought processes
Defining characteristics
Verbalized or observed discomfort in social situations

Verbalized or observed inability to receive or
   communicate a satisfying sense of belonging,
   caring, interest, or shared history
Observed use of unsuccessful social interaction
   behaviors
Dysfunctional interaction with peers, family, and/or
   others
Family report of change in style or pattern of
   interaction

Social isolation

Aloneness experienced by an individual and perceived as
imposed by others and as a negative or threatened state.

Related factors
Factors contributing to the absence of satisfying
   personal relationships, such as the following:
   Delay in accomplishing developmental tasks
   Immature interests
   Alterations in physical appearance
   Alterations in mental status
   Unaccepted social behavior
   Unaccepted social values
   Altered state of wellness
   Inadequate personal resources
   Inability to engage in satisfying personal
      relationships
Defining characteristics
   Objective
   Absence of supportive significant other(s)—family,
      friends, group
   Sad, dull affect
   Inappropriate or immature interests and activities
      for developmental age or stage
   Uncommunicative, withdrawn; no eye contact
   Preoccupation with own thoughts, repetitive,
      meaningless actions
   Projects hostility in voice, behavior
   Seeks to be alone or exists in subculture
   Evidence of physical and/or mental handicap or
      altered state of wellness

Shows behavior unaccepted by dominant cultural group

Subjective

Expresses feeling of aloneness imposed by others

Expresses feelings of rejection

Experiences feelings of indifference of others

Expresses values acceptable to subculture but is unable to accept values of dominant culture

Inadequacy in or absence of significant purpose in life

Inability to meet expectations of others

Insecurity in public

Expresses interests inappropriate to developmental age or stage

Spiritual distress (distress of the human spirit)

Disruption in the life principle that pervades a person's entire being and that integrates and transcends one's biological and psychosocial nature.

Related factors

Separation from religious and cultural ties

Challenged belief and value system (e.g., result of moral or ethical implications of therapy or result of intense suffering)

Defining characteristics

Expresses concern with meaning of life and death and/or belief systems

Anger toward God (as defined by the person)

Questions meaning of suffering

Verbalizes inner conflict about beliefs

Verbalizes concern about relationship with deity

Questions meaning of own existence

Inability to choose or chooses not to participate in usual religious practices

Seeks spiritual assistance

Questions moral and ethical implications of therapeutic regimen

Displacement of anger toward religious representatives

Description of nightmares or sleep disturbances

Alteration in behavior or mood evidenced by anger,
     crying, withdrawal, preoccupation, anxiety,
     hostility, apathy, etc.
Regards illness as punishment
Does not experience that God is forgiving
Inability to accept self
Engages in self-blame
Denies responsibilities for problems
Description of somatic complaints

Spiritual well-being, potential for enhanced

Spiritual well-being is the process of an individual's developing
or unfolding of mystery through harmonious
interconnectedness that springs from inner strengths.

Defining characteristics
Inner strengths
A sense of awareness, self consciousness, sacred source,
     unifying force, inner core, and transcendence
Unfolding mystery
One's experience about life's purpose and meaning,
     mystery, uncertainty, and struggles
Harmonious interconnectedness
Relatedness, connectedness, harmony with self,
     others, higher power or God, and the environment

Suffocation, risk for

Accentuated risk of accidental suffocation (inadequate air
available for inhalation).

Risk factors
   Internal (individual) factors
   Reduced olfactory sensation
   Reduced motor abilities
   Lack of safety education
   Lack of safety precautions
   Cognitive or emotional difficulties
   Disease or injury process
   External (environmental) factors
   Pillow placed in infant's crib
   Vehicle warming in closed garage

Children playing with plastic bags or inserting
    small objects into their mouths or noses
Discarded or unused refrigerators or freezers
    without doors removed
Children left unattended in bathtubs or pools
Household gas leaks
Smoking in bed
Use of fuel-burning heaters not vented to outside
Low-strung clothesline
Pacifier hung around infant's head
Eating of large mouthfuls of food
Propped bottle placed in infant's crib

Swallowing, impaired

The state in which an individual has decreased ability to
voluntarily pass fluids and/or solids from the mouth to the
stomach.

Related factors
Neuromuscular impairment (e.g., decreased or absent
    gag reflex, decreased strength or excursion of
    muscles involved in mastication, perceptual
    impairment, facial paralysis)
Mechanical obstruction (e.g., edema, tracheotomy
    tube, tumor)
Fatigue
Limited awareness
Reddened, irritated oropharyngeal cavity
Defining characteristics
Observed evidence of difficulty in swallowing (e.g.,
    stasis of food in oral cavity, cough/choking)
Evidence of aspiration

Thermoregulation, ineffective

The state in which an individual's temperature fluctuates
between hypothermia and hyperthermia

Related factors
Trauma or illness
Immaturity
Aging
Fluctuating environmental temperature

Defining characteristics

Fluctuations in body temperature above or below
   normal range

See also defining characteristics of hypothermia and
   hyperthermia

Thought processes, altered

The state in which an individual experiences a disruption in
cognitive operations and activities.

Related factors
Physiological changes
Psychological conflicts
Loss of memory
Impaired judgment
Sleep deprivation
Defining characteristics
Inaccurate interpretation of environment
   Cognitive dissonance
   Distractibility
   Memory deficit or problems
   Egocentricity
   Hypervigilance/hypovigilance
   Decreased ability to grasp ideas
   Impaired ability to make decisions
   Impaired ability to problem solve
   Impaired ability to reason
   Impaired ability to abstract or conceptualize
   Impaired ability to calculate
   Altered attention span—distractibility
   Obsessions
   Inability to follow commands
   Disorientation to time, place, person,
      circumstances, and events
   Changes in remote, recent, or immediate memory
   Delusions
   Ideas of reference
   Hallucinations
   Confabulation
   Inappropriate social behavior
   Altered sleep patterns
   Inappropriate affect

Other possible defining characteristic
Inappropriate/nonreality-based thinking

Tissue integrity, impaired

The state in which an individual experiences damage to mucous membrane or corneal, integumentary, or subcutaneous tissue. See also Oral Mucous Membrane, Altered.

Related factors
Altered circulation
Nutritional deficit/excess
Fluid deficit/excess
Knowledge deficit
Impaired physical mobility
Irritants
    Chemical (including body excretions, secretions, medications)
    Thermal (temperature extremes)
    Mechanical (pressure, shear, friction)
    Radiation (including therapeutic radiation)
Defining characteristics
Damaged or destroyed tissue (cornea, mucous membrane, integumentary, or subcutaneous)

Tissue perfusion, altered (specify type) (renal, cerebral, cardiopulmonary, gastrointestinal, peripheral)

The state in which an individual experiences a decrease in nutrition and oxygenation at the cellular level due to a deficit in capillary blood supply.

Related factors
Interruption of flow, arterial
Interruption of flow, venous
Exchange problems
Hypervolemia
Hypovolemia
Defining characteristics
Skin temperature: cold extremities
Skin color
    Dependent, blue or purple

Pale on elevation, and color does not return on
lowering leg
Diminished arterial pulsations
Skin quality: shining
Lack of lanugo
Round scars covered with atrophied skin
Gangrene
Slow-growing, dry, thick, brittle nails
Claudication
Blood pressure changes in extremities
Bruits
Slow healing of lesions

Trauma, risk for

Accentuated risk of accidental tissue injury (e.g., wound, burn,
fracture)

Risk factors
Internal (individual) factors
Weakness
Poor vision
Balancing difficulties
Reduced temperature and/or tactile sensation
Reduced large—or small—muscle coordination
Reduced hand-eye coordination
Lack of safety education
Lack of safety precautions
Insufficient finances to purchase safety equipment
or effect repairs
Cognitive or emotional difficulties
History of previous trauma
External (environmental) factors
Slippery floors (e.g., wet or highly waxed)
Snow or ice on stairs, walkways
Unanchored rugs
Bathtub without hand grip or antislip equipment
Use of unsteady ladder or chairs
Entering unlighted rooms
Unsturdy or absent stair rails
Unanchored electric wires
Litter or liquid spills on floors or stairways
High beds

Children playing without gates at tops of stairs
Obstructed passageways
Unsafe window protection in homes with young children
Inappropriate call-for-aid mechanisms for bed-resting client
Pot handles facing toward front of stove
Bathing in very hot water (e.g., unsupervised bathing of young children)
Potential igniting of gas leaks
Delayed lighting of gas burner or oven
Experimenting with chemicals or gasoline
Unscreened fires or heaters
Wearing of plastic aprons or flowing clothing around open flame
Children playing with matches, candles, cigarettes
Inadequately stored combustibles or corrosives (e.g., matches, oily rags, lye)
Highly flammable children's toys or clothing
Overloaded fuse boxes
Contact with rapidly moving machinery, industrial belts, or pulleys
Sliding on coarse bed linen or struggling within bed restraints
Faulty electrical plugs, frayed wires, or defective appliances
Contact with acids or alkalis
Playing with fireworks or gunpowder
Contact with intense cold
Overexposure to sun, sun lamps, radiotherapy
Use of cracked dishware or glasses
Knives stored uncovered
Guns or ammunition stored unlocked
Large icicles hanging from roof
Exposure to dangerous machinery
Children playing with sharp-edged toys
High-crime neighborhood and vulnerable patient
Driving a mechanically unsafe vehicle
Driving after partaking of alcoholic beverages or drugs
Driving at excessive speeds

Driving without necessary visual aids
Children riding in front seat of car
Smoking in bed or near oxygen
Overloaded electrical outlets
Grease waste collected on stoves
Use of thin or worn pot holders or mitts
Unrestrained babies riding in car
Nonuse or misuse of seat restraints
Nonuse or misuse of necessary headgear for
    motorized cyclists or young children carried on
    adult bicycles
Unsafe road or road-crossing conditions
Play or work near vehicle pathways (e.g.,
    driveways, lanes, railroad tracks)

Unilateral neglect

The state in which an individual is perceptually unaware of and inattentive to one side of the body.

Related factors
Effects of disturbed perceptual abilities (e.g.,
    hemianopsia)
One-sided blindness
Neurological illness or trauma
Defining characteristics
Consistent inattention to stimuli on affected side
Inadequate self-care
Positioning and/or safety precautions in regard to
    affected side
Does not look toward affected side
Leaves food on plate on affected side

Urinary elimination, altered

The state in which an individual experiences a disturbance in urine elimination. See also Incontinence (functional, reflex, stress, total, urge).

Related factors
Sensory motor impairment
Neuromuscular impairment
Mechanical trauma

Defining characteristics
Dysuria
Frequency
Hesitancy
Incontinence
Nocturia
Retention
Urgency

Urinary retention

The state in which an individual experiences incomplete emptying of the bladder.

Related factors
High urethral pressure caused by weak detrusor
Inhibition of reflex arc
Strong sphincter
Blockage
Defining characteristics
Bladder distention
Small, frequent voiding or absence of urine output
Sensation of bladder fullness
Dribbling
Residual urine
Dysuria
Overflow incontinence

Ventilation, inability to sustain spontaneous

A state in which the response pattern of decreased energy reserves results in an individual's inability to maintain breathing adequate to support life.

Related factors
Metabolic factors
Respiratory muscle fatigue
Defining characteristics
  Major
  Dyspnea
  Increased metabolic rate
  Minor
  Increased restlessness

Apprehension
Increased use of accessory muscles
Decreased tidal volume
Increased heart rate
Decreased pO_2 level
Increased pCO_2 level
Decreased cooperation
Decreased SaO_2 level

Ventilatory weaning response, dysfunction (DVWR)

A state in which an individual cannot adjust to lowered levels of mechanical ventilator support, which interrupts and prolongs the weaning process.

Related factors
Physical
Ineffective airway clearance
Sleep pattern disturbance
Inadequate nutrition
Uncontrolled pain or discomfort
Psychological
Knowledge deficit of the weaning process/patient
    role
Patient-perceived inefficacy about the ability to
    wean
Decreased motivation
Decreased self-esteem
Anxiety: moderate, severe
Fear
Hopelessness
Powerlessness
Insufficient trust in the nurse
Situational
Uncontrolled episodic energy demands or
    problems
Inappropriate pacing of diminished ventilator
    support
Inadequate social support
Adverse environment (noisy, active environment;
    negative events in the room; low nurse-patient

ratio; extended nurse absence from bedside;
unfamiliar nursing staff)
History of ventilator dependence >1 week
History of multiple unsuccessful weaning attempts
Defining characteristics
Mild DVWR
Major
Responds to lowered levels of mechanical
ventilator support with the following:
Restlessness
Slight increased respiratory rate from baseline
Minor
Responds to lowered levels of mechanical
ventilator support with the following:
Expressed feelings of increased need for oxygen;
breathing discomfort; fatigue; warmth
Queries about possible machine malfunction
Increased concentration on breathing
Moderate DVWR
Major
Responds to lowered levels of mechanical
ventilator support with the following:
Slight increase from baseline blood pressure
<20mm Hg
Slight increase from baseline heart rate <20
beats/minute
Baseline increase in respiratory rate <5
breaths/minute
Minor
Hypervigilance to activities
Inability to respond to coaching
Inability to cooperate
Apprehension
Diaphoresis
Eye widening
Decreased air entry on auscultation
Color changes; pale; slight cyanosis
Slight respiratory accessory muscle use
Severe DVWR
Major
Responds to lowered levels of mechanical
ventilator support with the following:

Agitation

Deterioration in arterial blood gas levels from current baseline

Increase from baseline blood pressure >20mm Hg

Increase from baseline heart rate >20 beats/minute

Respiratory rate increases significantly from baseline

Minor

Profuse diaphoresis

Full respiratory accessory muscle use

Shallow, gasping breaths

Paradoxical abdominal breathing

Discoordinated breathing with the ventilator

Decreased level of consciousness

Adventitious breath sounds, audible airway secretions

Cyanosis

Violence, risk for: self-directed or directed at others

The state in which an individual experiences behaviors that can be physically harmful either to the self or others.

Risk factors

Antisocial character

Battered women

Catatonic excitement

Child abuse

Manic excitement

Organic brain syndrome

Panic states

Rage reactions

Suicidal behavior

Temporal lobe epilepsy

Toxic reactions to medication

NURSING DIAGNOSES

Prototype Care Plans

Key to the Care Plan Format

Patient goals
Expected outcomes
    Associated nursing/collaborative interventions *and*
      scientific rationale

LINDA K. YOUNG, MARIE MAGUIRE, MARILYN HARTER,
AND AUDREY M. MCLANE.

Activity intolerance

CLINICAL CONDITIONS/ MEDICAL DIAGNOSES	RELATED FACTORS
Myocardial infarction; nearing discharge from acute care hospital	Imbalance between oxygen supply and demand; ineffective pain management

Patient goals
Expected outcomes
> Associated nursing/collaborative interventions *and scientific rationale*

Develop activity/rest pattern consistent with physiological limitations as evidenced by the following:

Monitors physiological response to activity
Manages pain effectively
Engages in regular exercise of 4 METs or less
Tolerates job-related activities without pain or fatigue

> Teach patient to monitor physiological responses to activity, e.g., pulse rate, shortness of breath *Self-monitoring facilitates determination/evaluation of activity level consistent with physical status.*

> Develop individualized activity/exercise program including home exercises. *Patients are more likely to follow individualized programs of activity/exercise to obtain the beneficial effects on cardiac performance.*

> Collaborate with patient to tailor medication taking to demands of activities. *Taking medications as prescribed can enhance activity tolerance and reduce pain.*

> Assist patient to identify factors that decrease/increase activity tolerance. *Accurate determination of factors that decrease/increase activity tolerance provides a foundation for effective problem solving.*

Activity intolerance

Teach patient to eliminate/reduce activities that cause pain or fatigue.

Discuss necessity to pace activities. *Pacing activity levels lessens cardiac workload.*

Teach patient use of exercise log to record exercise activities and responses (pulse, shortness of breath, anxiety). *Keeping a log may increase compliance.*

Teach patient warning signs of cardiac decompensation; e.g., difficulty breathing, dependent edema.

Recognize influences of emotional responses on exercise tolerance as evidenced by the following:

Discusses emotional responses with significant other
Learns/practices relaxation techniques
Significant other understands reasons for use of cognitive coping strategies

Teach patient/significant other influence of fears/anxiety on exercise tolerance. *Fear and anxiety may decrease activity tolerance.*

Teach/monitor use of cognitive coping strategies, e.g., imagery relaxation, controlled breathing. *Emotional responses to activity may be managed through the use of cognitive coping strategies.*

Encourage significant other to learn coping strategies and/or assist patient in use of the strategies.

Use social support network to maintain desired life-style as evidenced by the following:

Significant other assists with activities of daily living to prevent activity level from exceeding 4 METs
Friends/family/neighbors help with home maintenance activities

Collaborate with patient/significant other to establish a plan of daily activities consistent with desired life-style and exercise prescription of <4 METs.

Teach significant other to help patient pace activities.

Encourage patient/significant other to seek assistance with home maintenance activities from friends, family, neighbors. *Social support enhances compliance and recovery.*

Determine interest of patient/significant other in sexual counseling. *Sexual activity is often a great concern to patients and their sexual partners.*

REFERENCES

Buchannan L and others: Measurement of recovery from myocardial infarction using heart rate variability and psychological outcomes, *Nurs Res* 42(2):74, 1993.

Cowan MJ: Cardiovascular nursing research, *Ann Rev Nurs Res* 8:3-33.

Davis M, Eshel E: *The relaxation and stress reduction workbook*, Oakland, Cal, 1988, Hew Herbinger.

Holm K, Penckofer SM: Women's cardiovascular health. In *Annual review of women's health*, New York, 1993, National League for Nursing Press, pp 289-310.

Johnson JC, Mouse JM, Regaining control: the process of adjustment after myocardial infarction, *Heart Lung* 19(2):126, 1990.

McCaffery M, Beebe A: *Pain: clinical manual for nursing*, St. Louis, 1989, Mosby.

Miller P and others: Influence of a nursing intervention on regimen adherence and societal adjustment post myocardial infarction, *Nurs Res* 37(5):297, 1988.

Squires R and others: *Cardiovascular rehabilitation: status, 1990*, Rochester, Minn, 1990, Mayo Clinic Proc 6S:731.

Activity intolerance—cont'd

AUDREY MCLANE, LINDA K. YOUNG, MARIE MAGUIRE,
AND MARILYN HARTER

Activity intolerance, risk for

CLINICAL CONDITION/ MEDICAL DIAGNOSIS	RISK FACTORS
Myocardial infarction	Fatigue, >15%

> **Patient goals**
> **Expected outcomes**
> Associated nursing/collaborative interventions *and scientific rationale*

Participate in cardiac rehabilitation program as evidenced by the following:

Enrolls in cardiac rehabilitation program
Negotiate with patient to participate in cardiac rehabilitation program. *Cardiac rehabilitation programs can facilitate the patient's ability to achieve and maintain a vital and productive life while remaining within the heart's ability to respond to increases in activity and stress.*

Encourage spouse to accompany patient on walks. *Social support may enhance participation in this activity.*

Clarifies values with nurse's assistance
Assist patient and significant other with clarification of values. *Becoming aware of one's own values may enhance compliance with prescribed regime.*

Teach patient long-term value of increased activity. *Highlighting positive long-term effects may increase compliance.*

Verbalizes fears about increasing level of activity
Assist patient in verbalizing anxiety/fear/concerns about engaging in exercise. *Recognizing fears and anxiety is the first step to managing them.*

Integrate exercise prescription into daily living by the following:

Experiences less fatigue after exercise regime over a period of time

Teach patient/significant other benefits of exercise
regimen in decreasing fatigue/weakness.

**Uses written list of activities with MET levels to guide
activities**

Teach patient/significant other the importance of
using MET levels to guide and prioritize
activities.

Provide written specifications for duration,
intensity, frequency, and METs levels of ADLs
and recreational activities. Knowledge of METs
of ADLs and recreational activities promotes safe
functioning.

**Uses exercise log to record distance walked and
symptoms experienced**

Teach patient/significant other use of exercise log
to record activities, time, duration, intensity,
and physiologic responses (e.g., pulse rate,
shortness of breath, lightheadedness). *Use of log
may increase compliance.*

Teach self-monitoring of heart rate during exercise.
Self-monitoring promotes self-care.

Teach self-evaluation of response to activity,
including actions for specific signs and
symptoms.

**Gradually reduce body weight as evidenced by the
following:**

**Consults with dietitian to begin weight reduction
program**

Negotiate with patient to make decision to lose
weight. *Client input and motivation are factors
affecting patient participation in weight reduction.*

Refer to dietitian for diet instruction and for
recommending caloric requirements.

Encourage spouse to participate in weight
reduction instructions

Assist patient/significant other in preparing
shopping list for low-caloric meals. *Predetermined
low-caloric meals and snacks help increase the
likelihood of limited caloric intake.*

Discuss low-caloric food preparation, e.g., broiling,
baking, and poaching.

Achieves desired body weight
Set realistic weekly weight-loss goal.

Monitor weight twice a week *to help patient realize weight loss and gain, which can reinforce changed behavior.*

Encourage spouse to support patient effort in weight loss.

REFERENCES

Buchannan L and others: Measurement of recovery from myocardial infarction using heart rate variability and psychological outcomes, *Nurs Res* 42(2):74, 1993.

Christ J: Weight management. In Bulechek GM, McCloskey JC, eds: *Nursing interventions: essential nursing treatments*, ed 2, Philadelphia, 1992, WB Saunders.

Johnson JC, Mouse JM: Regaining control: the process of adjustment after myocardial infarction, *Heart Lung* 19(2):126, 1990.

Miller P and others: Influence of a nursing intervention on regimen adherence and societal adjustment post myocardial infarction, *Nurs Res* 37(5):297, 1988.

Mol V, Baker C: Activity intolerance in the geriatric stroke patient, *Rehab Nurs* 16(6):337, 1991.

Squires R and others: *Cardiovascular rehabilitation: status, 1990*, Rochester, Minn, 1990, Mayo Clinic Proc 6S:731.

Adaptive capacity, decreased: intracranial

CLINICAL CONDITION/ MEDICAL DIAGNOSIS	RELATED FACTORS
Traumatic, closed head injury	Sustained increase in intracranial pressure (ICP of ≥ 15 mm Hg and decreased cerebral perfusion pressure (CPP) of ≤50-60 mm Hg.

Patient goals
Expected outcomes
Associated nursing/collaborative interventions *and scientific rationale*

Experience reduced ICP as evidenced by the following:

Decreased or no evidence of deleterious effects of increased ICP

Perform neurologic assessment every hour or PRN in order to detect progressive signs of increased ICP.

Observe for decreasing levels of consciousness, including restlessness, irritability, drowsiness, lethargy, confusion, obtundation, stupor, lower Glasgow Coma Score (GCS), and ability to follow commands.

Assess pupillary responses: ovoid pupil, hippus, sluggish reactivity progressing to fixed, unilateral change in pupil size (midposition to gradual dilation).

Assess for visual deficits: decreased visual acuity, blurred vision, papilledema, field cuts, diplopia, nystagmus, and ptosis.

Assess motor function: progressive paresis, hemiplegia, Babinski sign, or decorticate or decerebrate posturing.

Observe for headache, vomiting, and seizures.

Monitor vital signs every hour or PRN: watch for elevation in blood pressure with widening pulse pressure and bradycardia. Signs of

Adaptive capacity, decreased: intracranial

decompensation include a decrease in blood pressure, tachycardia, and irregular respirations (Cheyne-stokes respiration progressing to neurogenic hyperventilation to irregular brainstem patterns). *Cushing reflex is seen when ICP approaches systemic arterial pressure (SAP), producing pressure and ischemia on the vasomotor center. This triggers a sympathetic response, causing a rise in systolic BP, widening pulse pressure, pulse slowing, and irregular respirations.*

Monitor for cardiac arrhythmias. *Cardiac dysrhythmias are frequently associated with intracranial pathologic conditions and result in decreased cerebral blood flow (CBF) and ischemia, contributing further to cerebral edema and increased ICP.*

Observe for loss of brainstem reflexes: corneal, gag and swallow, oculocephalic, and oculovestibular reflexes.

Report to physician any evidence of deterioration in neurologic status and initiate interventions to reverse process immediately. *Changes in neurologic status indicate increasing ICP. Early intervention to increase intracranial adaptive capacity and decrease demands prevents deleterious effects of ICP.*

Experience reduced or no elevations in ICP and maintain CCP as evidenced by the following:

ICP within normal limit of 10-15 mm Hg
Repeated or sustained elevations in ICP are prevented or minimized
CPP within normal limit of 60-100 mm Hg
Patent airway and adequate gas exchange maintained (e.g., PaO_2 80-100 mm Hg, $PaCO_2$ 25-30 mm Hg, and ability to manage secretions)
Normothermia to hypothermia maintained

Accurately measure ICP and monitor trends continuously.

Regulate CSF drainage through ventricular catheter.

Calculate CPP every hour and PRN.

Maintain blood pressure within accepted patient parameters. *Hypotension causes ischemia, whereas hypertension causes edema leading to increased ICP and tissue damage.*

Maintain neutral body alignment at all times with head of bed elevated 30 degrees unless contraindicated. *Neutral head position maintains CSF flow and prevents obstruction of the jugular veins, increasing venous return and lowering ICP.*

Avoid securing endotracheal tube to neck area. *Prevents obstruction of the jugular veins, increasing venous return and lowering ICP.*

Avoid procedures that increase thoracic and abdominal pressure (e.g., turning and positioning, hip flexion, coughing, restraints, isometric exercises, noxious stimuli, and Valsalva maneuver). Log roll and instruct patient to exhale during activity. Use narcotics, sedating or paralyzing agents, hyperventilation, or local anesthetics to blunt response to stimuli. Assess ICP waves during activity and avoid stimulation when elevation of P_2 component occurs. *Increases in thoracic pressure decrease venous return, increase CSF pressure, decrease cardiac output and increase blood pressure, causing additional rise in ICP. Elevation of P_2 occurs with rise in ICP. Analysis of waveforms allows individualization of care.*

Minimize patient activity levels: provide nonstimulating environment, administer anticonvulsants, avoid clustering patient care activities, and prevent shivering. Individualize care on the basis of physiologic responses—ICP, CPP, SAP, and cerebral blood flow. *Continued stimulation may lead to undesirable increases in physiologic parameters and deleterious effects on brain function.*

Administer oxygen to maintain paO_2 above 80-100 mm Hg. Monitor arterial blood gases (ABGs), O_2 saturations, and jugular bulb O_2 extraction. *Hypoxia and hypercapnia produce synergistic effects and increase CBF more than either factor alone.*

Adaptive capacity, decreased: intracranial—cont'd

Monitor ABGs and regulate ventilator to keep PaCO$_2$ 25-30 mm Hg.

Synchronize manual hyperventilation with inspiration. *Hyperventilation lowers paCO$_2$ levels, leading to vasoconstriction and a decreased ICP. Synchronization of manual hyperventilation prevents increases in intrathoracic pressure and ICP.*

Closely monitor physiologic parameters when using positive end-expiratory pressure (PEEP). *PEEP reduces arterial BP, thereby reducing CPP. PEEP decreases cerebral venous outflow, increasing ICP.*

Suction patient to maintain patent airway only PRN, adhering to the following guidelines:

Preoxygenate patient with 100% FiO$_2$ prior to suctioning. *Hyperoxygenation prevents hypoxemia during suctioning.*

Limit suction duration to 10 seconds and suction passes to 1 or 2. *Limiting suction time and number of suction passes avoids or minimizes cerebral hypertension.*

Allow 2 minutes of undisturbed rest between catheter passes. *Two minutes of undisturbed rest is needed to allow mean SAP, mean ICP, CPP and heart rate to reach baseline levels. MICP increases in a step-wise fashion from baseline to first suctioning episode and from first to second suctioning episode.*

Do not rotate head from side to side. *Passive rotation of head to the right and left is known to increase ICP, with return to baseline levels taking more than 10 minutes.*

Keep negative suction pressure < 120 mm Hg. *Negative suction pressure of < 120 mm Hg is sufficient to remove secretion without reducing residual capacity or contributing to excessive tracheal mucosal damage.*

Use suction catheters with outer to inner diameter ratios < 0.50. *Suction catheters with an OD/ID ratio of < 0.50 allows for passive influx of air into the endotracheal tube.*

Adaptive capacity, decreased: intracranial—cont'd

Use hyperventilation combined with hyperoxygenation *with caution* in head-injured patients with low paCO$_2$. *Reduction of paCO$_2$ to below 25 mm Hg significantly decreases CBF further and may actually cause cerebral ischemia.*

Use hyperosmotics, corticosteroids, and diuretics as directed.

Limit fluid intake to a slightly dehydrated level (1500 to 2000 ml). Monitor fluid balance every hour, and electrolytes, CVP or pulmonary artery catheter, urine or serum osmolality, specific gravity, and blood count PRN. Observe for diabetes insipidus or syndrome of inappropriate diuretic hormone. Replace fluids with isotonic fluids, crystalloids, or colloids. *Decrease in intracellular volume decreases cerebral edema and ICP. Hypotonic fluids increase cerebral edema.*

Maintain temperature at normothermic levels or lower by using cooling blanket, antipyretics, antibiotics, aseptic technique. *Each degree centigrade rise in body temperature raises the metabolic demands of the brain by 10%.*

REFERENCES

Barker E: *Neuroscience nursing.* St. Louis, 1994, Mosby.

Crosby CJ, Parsons LC: Cerebrovascular response of closed head-injured patients to a standardized endotracheal tube suctioning and manual hyperventilation procedure, *J Neurosci Nurs* 24(1):40, 1992.

Keller C, Williams A: Cardiac dysrhythmias associated with central nervous system dysfunction, *J Neurosci Nurs* 25(6):349, 1993.

Kerr ME, Rudy EB, Brucia J, Stone KS: Head-injured adults: Recommendations for endotracheal suctioning, *J Neurosci Nurs* 25(2):86, 1993.

March K, Mitchell P, Grady S, Winn R: Effect of backrest position on intracranial and cerebral perfusion pressures. *J Neurosci Nurs* 22(6):375, 1990.

Prendergast V: Current trends in research and treatment of intracranial hypertension, *Crit Care Nurs Q* 17(1):1, 1994.

Rudy EB, Turner BS, Baun M, Stone KS, Brucia J: Endotracheal suctioning in adults with head injury, *Heart Lung* 20(6):667, 1991.

Adjustment, impaired

CLINICAL CONDITION/ MEDICAL DIAGNOSIS	RELATED FACTORS
Myocardial infarction, MI	Disabliity requiring change in lifestyle

---

Patient goals
Expected outcomes
Associated nursing/collaborative interventions *and scientific rationale*

Modify life-style to decrease impact of disability and increase independence within limits imposed by changed health status as evidenced by the following:

Recognizes that choice of self-care practices can influence adjustment to disability

Assist patient in working through emotional responses to MI (e.g., denial, anxiety, or depression) by using communication techniques that help patient to maintain appropriate control over own care and health.

Provide opportunity for expression of fears related to MI and potential physical limitations; *the patient's perception of disability associated with the MI influences the patient's adaptation to the change in health status.*

Teach patient and family to differentiate between denial of the presence of change in health status due to MI and denial of possible limitations *to maximize physiological and psychosocial adaptation.*

Consistently convey value of self-directive behavior on patient's part.

Assist patient in identifying and understanding how choice of health care practices can influence adjustment from MI.

Encourage use of problem-focused coping strategies, (e.g., discussing own health problems with others in a similar situation, pacing

Adjustment, impaired

changes in health care and life-style by setting monthly goals with related daily activities). *Patients who use problem-focused coping strategies experience increased perception of self-control, and appear to have less psychosocial difficulty with post-MI adjustment.*

Demonstrates self-care practices that are within prescribed treatment regimen

Provide information about MI and what to expect during and after hospitalization, based on assessment of learning readiness, *to reduce fear and anxiety associated with hospitalization and to reinforce positive psychological and social outcomes.*

Promote patient's making decisions related to specific aspects of care, sharing observations of physical status and progress with caregivers, and assuming responsibility for selected aspects of care *to maximize patient's achieving and maintaining a sense of control (within physical limitations).*

Assist patient to select self-care practices that enhance adjustment to disability (e.g., maintaining balanced exercise/rest regimen).

Uses strengths and potential to engage in maximally independent and constructive life-style

Convey hope that patient is able to overcome difficulties in current situation.

Use the patient's family as a resource to promote discussion of topics that are not related to disability (e.g., current events, family activities, hobbies, recreational interests).

Encourage identification of personal strengths and intact roles *to maximize sense of ability for regaining control and minimizing perception of disability as a handicap.*

Have patient identify previous coping behaviors and support systems used for past problem solving *to help patient mobilize previous coping strengths and skills that can be used in current situation.*

Makes future plans that are congruent with changed health status

Assess for possible correlation between extent of family's willingness to support patient's changed life-style and patient's ability to adapt to changes in health status.

Actively include family and significant others in entire cardiac rehabilitation process. *The perceived beliefs of significant others are important for patient's adherence to medical regimen.*

Collaborate with patient and other staff *to assist in determining factors that will promote control and management of patient's health status change.*

Facilitate compromise when patient's identified goals differ from goals developed by health-care providers or from family expectations.

Uses available health-care system and community resources

Assess for presence of closed networks (e.g., closed family system or closed cultural system). *Social support plays a significant role in coping with disability and life-style management. Closed family or closed cultural systems may influence appropriate help-seeking by patient and/or family.*

Encourage patient and family to explore such resources as Medicare, Social Security, and disability insurance.

Refer patient and significant other to community resources, such as cardiac support groups or the American Heart Association for assistance with ongoing informational needs, advocacy issues, and current developments in treatment and research.

REFERENCES

Belgrave FZ: Psychosocial predictors of adjustment to disability in African Americans, *J Rehabil* 57(1):37, 1991.

Burckhardt CS: Coping strategies of the chronically ill, *Nurs Clin North Am* 22(3):543, 1987.

Call JG, Davis LL: The effect of hardiness on coping strategies and adjustment to illness in chronically ill individuals, *Appl Nurs Res* 2(4):187, 1989.

Forsyth GL, Delaney KD, Gresham ML: Vying for a winning position: management style of the chronically ill, *Res Nurs Health* 7:181, 1984.

Adjustment, impaired—cont'd

Johnson JL, Morse JM: Regaining control: the process of adjustment after myocardial infarction, *Heart Lung* 19(2):126, 1990.

Keckeisen ME, Nyamathi AM: Coping and adjustment to illness in the acute myocardial infarction patient, *J Cardiovasc Nurs* 5(1):25, 1990.

Lamm B, Dungan JM, Hiromoto B: Long-term lifestyle management, *Clin Nurse Spec* 5(4):182, 1991.

Lowery BJ: Psychological stress, denial and myocardial infarction outcomes, *Image: J Nurs Sch* 23(1):51, 1991.

Milier P and others: Influence of a nursing intervention on regimen adherence and societal adjustments post myocardial infarction, *Nurs Res* 37(5):297, 1988.

White NE and others: Coping, social support, and adaptation to chronic illness, *West J Nurs Res* 14(2):211, 1992.

Airway clearance, ineffective

CLINICAL CONDITION/ MEDICAL DIAGNOSIS	RELATED FACTORS
Tracheostomy with tracheal intubation	Ineffective coughing; excessive secretions with intubated trachea

> **Patient goals**
> Expected outcomes
> > Associated nursing/collaborative interventions *and scientific rationale*

Manage secretions more effectively as evidenced by the following:

Secretions are easily expectorated or suctioned
Breath sounds are clear following treatments

Assist patient to cough after several deep breaths.

Help patient to assume a comfortable cough position (e.g., high Fowler's with knees bent and a light weight pillow over abdomen) *to augment expiratory pressures and minimize discomfort. Effective cough requires a deep breath and contraction of expiratory muscles especially the abdominal muscles to increase the intrathoracic pressure and expel secretions.*

Remove expectorated secretions from opening of tracheostomy tube using aseptic technique. Use clean technique in home. Note volume, viscosity, and color of secretions.

Avoid deep suctioning; if patient can cough secretions to tracheal tube, suction the tube only.

Perform chest physical therapy maneuvers to drain remote areas of lung by gravity (add percussion, if not contraindicated). *Chest physical therapy consists of vibration, percussion, and postural drainage of selected lung units, e.g., segments. Vibration applied to chest wall, together with gravity and slow exhalation after deep breathing, dislodges retained secretions from the underlying airways and facilitates mucous clearance.*

Airway clearance, ineffective

Vibrate affected area during exhalation; be prepared to collect expectorated secretions or suction as described later.

Initiate cough assists (as described previously) or provide a fast manual resuscitative bag breath to stimulate cough receptors. Quickly release hand pressure on bag and again be ready to collect secretions.

Adjust frequency of therapy according to achievement of expected outcomes, target times, and patient comfort.

Tracheal tube is free of plugs

Provide systemic hydration which is calculated from patient's intake, output, and body weight. *The usual water loss from expired gas is 300 ml per day, depending on respiratory rate and route of inspiration. Systemic dehydration or fluid excess adversely affects the mucociliary escalator (i.e., relationship of cilia, sol, and gel layers) and impairs mucociliary clearance.*

Provide humidified gas at 37° C and 100% saturation via ventilator, T-piece connector attached to wide-bore tubing or tracheostomy mask. *Normally inspired gas is filtered, warmed, and humidified by the upper airway, primarily the nose. By the time the inspired gas reaches the trachea it is 37° C and 100% humidified. When the normal host defenses are bypassed, dryer and cooler air dehydrates the respiratory mucous membranes and impairs mucociliary clearance and causes inspissated tracheobronchial secretions.*

Remove condensed vapor from inspiratory line p.r.n. and change humidifier, connectors, and tubing every day.

Protect opening of tracheal tube from unfiltered ambient air and avoid introduction of foreign objects and blind instillation of fluids (e.g., saline).

Perform intratracheal suctioning only when secretions are reachable by catheter and patient cannot cough effectively.

Prepare patient for this uncomfortable and potentially traumatic procedure and explain purpose and sequence of maneuvers.

Use aseptic technique during suctioning; clean technique is appropriate in home.

Preoxygenate with 100% oxygen before suctioning.

If patient is spontaneously breathing and has a dominant hypoxic drive to breathe, adjust FiO_2 accordingly.

After preoxygenation and hyperinflations, use a sterile catheter which is one half the diameter of the tracheal tube and apply intermittent negative pressure for less than 15 seconds per pass; reoxygenate and remain with patient until return to baseline vital signs. *Suctioning removes air as well as secretions from the airways and induces hypoxemia.*

Use minimal cuff inflation. If patient is spontaneously breathing and can swallow oropharyngeal secretions and oral feedings without aspiration, the cuff can be left deflated to minimize tracheal damage.

Consult physician for adjunctive therapies and further assessment, mucolytics, bronchodilators, antibiotics, fiberoptic bronchoscopy, diagnostic tests (e.g., sputum for culture, sensitivity and Gram stain, or chest x-ray).

Patient or significant other is able to perform airway clearance procedures

Provide patient with cues/devices to motivate independent deep breathing exercises (e.g., visual or tactile feedback).

Teach patient to cough after several deep breaths.

Teach patient alternate cough techniques (e.g., huff or quad) if patient is having difficulty.

Teach patient or significant other airway clearance procedure and administration of medical adjunctive therapies as appropriate.

REFERENCES

Ackerman MH: The effect of saline lavage prior to suctioning, *Am J Crit Care* 2(4):326-330, 1993.

Bostwick J, Wendelgass ST: Normal saline instillation as part of the suctioning procedure: effects on PaO$_2$ and amount of secretions, *Heart Lung* 16:532-537, 1987.

Hanley MV, Rudd T, Butler J: What happens to intratracheal saline instillations? *Am Rev Respir Dis* 117(part 2 suppl):124, 1978.

Hanley MV, Tyler ML: Ineffective airway clearance related to airway infection, *Nurs Clin North Am* 22(1):135-150, 1987.

Kirilloff LH and others.: Does chest physical therapy work? *Chest* 88:436-444, 1985.

Preusser BA and others: Effects of two methods of preoxygenation on mean arterial pressure, cardiac output, peak airway pressure, and postsuctioning hypoxemia, *Heart Lung* 17(3):290-299, 1988.

Rogge JA, Bunde L, Baun MM: Effectiveness of oxygen concentrations of less than 100% before and after endotracheal suction in patients with chronic obstructive pulmonary disease, *Heart Lung* 18(1):64-71, 1989.

Shekleton ME, Nield M: Ineffective airway clearance related to artificial airway, *Nurs Clin North Am* 22(1):167-178, 1987.

Stone KS and others: The effect of lung hyperinflation and endotracheal suctioning on cardiopulmonary hemodynamics, *Nurs Res* 40(2):76-80, 1991.

Traver GA: Ineffective airway clearance, physiology and clinical application, *Dimens Crit Care Nurs* 4(4):198-208, 1985.

Airway clearance, ineffective—cont'd

Anxiety

CLINICAL CONDITION/ MEDICAL DIAGNOSIS	RELATED FACTORS
Major depression, single episode	Maturational crisis (mid-life/aging process)

Patient goals
Expected outcomes
 Associated nursing/collaborative interventions *and scientific rationale*

Experience reduced anxiety of at least one level as evidenced by the following:

Experiences a decrease in symptoms, e.g., decreased tension, apprehension, insomnia, tremors, irritability, isolation, fatigue, restlessness, perceptual distortions, physical reactions to anxiety

Assess level of anxiety associated with crisis experience, e.g.,
- Ability to comprehend
- Problem-solving ability
- Narrowing perceptual field
- Level of functioning
- Ability to perform ADLs
- Appropriateness of response to situation

Maintain calm and safe environment

Decrease stimuli

Talk to and reassure patient

Encourage involvement in activities, depending on level of anxiety

Guide participation in self-care

Redirect activities and attention as necessary

Assist patient in identifying possible sources of stress

Provide health teaching about anxiety in the following areas:
- Impact of anxiety on body
- Levels of anxiety
- Impact of chemicals on the body

Anxiety

112

Assess use of alcohol, caffeine, nicotine, and other drugs

Recognize own anxiety and participate in developing plan of care to effect change as evidenced by the following:

Discusses and monitors own behavior every shift
Identifies stressors
Actively participates in unit activities
Initiates interactions with peers
Develops realistic goals
Connects behavior with feelings
> Help patient to connect behavior with feelings
> Encourage patient to discuss feelings about anxiety
> Obtain patient's perception of anxiety experienced
> Focus on the "here and now"
> Develop room plan with patient, e.g., remain out of room for 50 minutes each hour
> Help patient to identify how anxiety is manifested through behavior
> Explore with patient ways of anticipating anxiety
> Provide health teaching in the following areas:
>> • Stress management
>> • Goal setting

Accept physical and emotional changes of the aging process as evidenced by the following:

Acknowledges limitations
Verbalizes fears of aging process
Functions at optimal level
Utilizes strengths to develop ways of coping with the aging process
> Provide health teaching about the aging process
> Encourage patient to function as independently as possible
> Encourage patient to discuss feelings/fears
> Assist patient in identifying effective coping strategies

Demonstrate effective coping strategies in relation to maturation crisis as evidenced by the following:

Develops a personal plan to decrease anxiety utilizing problem-solving process
Identifies community resources/support
Demonstrates relaxation techniques
Meets self-care needs
Forms interpersonal relationships
Participates in discharge planning

Explore coping mechanisms with patient; help patient to identify those coping mechanisms that were successful in decreasing anxiety

Help patient to identify adaptive coping mechanisms within patient's own cultural expectations

Discuss importance of regular exercise program

Provide health teaching in the following areas:

- Teach the problem-solving process, e.g., organize, prioritize, implement, and evaluate
- Teach relaxation techniques including deep breathing
- Instruct patient to take slow, deep breaths (eyes may be opened or closed) repeat and demonstrate as necessary, progressive relaxation
- Tell patient to sit or lie in a comfortable position in a quiet area (patient should close eyes unless that makes him/her uncomfortable)
- At periods throughout exercise ask patient to focus on breathing (slow and deep)
- To begin exercise, instruct patient to get in a comfortable position and imagine being in a quiet, comfortable place (e.g., on a beach, listening to a gentle rain). Then instruct patient to tense gently for 5 seconds and then relax each muscle group for 10 to 15 seconds. Begin with toes and feet and move progressively upward—calf of leg, thigh, buttock, lower back, hands (make fist), lower arm, upper arm, shoulders, neck, and ending with face (grimace). After relaxing face, patient should remain quiet for 15 minutes (or as

patient can tolerate), concentrating on peace, quiet, and breathing.

- Instruct patient to use entire exercise or just for areas of tension.

REFERENCES

Coplan J, Tiffon L, Gorman J: Therapeutic strategies for the patient with treatment resistant anxiety, *J Clin Psychiatry* 54:5 (suppl.):69, 1993.

Davis M, Eshelman ER, McKay M: *The relaxation and stress reduction workbook*, Oakland, Cal, 1982, New Harbinger.

Flannery RB Jr: *Becoming stress resistant: through the project smart program*, New York, 1990, Continuum.

Peplau H: *Interpersonal relationships in nursing*, New York, 1952, GP Putnam's Sons.

Stinemetz J and others: *Rx for stress: a nurses' guide*, Palo Alto, Cal, 1984, Bull Publishing.

Whitley GG: Anxiety: defining the diagnosis, *J Psychosoc Nurs Ment Health Serv* 27(10):7, 1989.

Aspiration, risk for

CLINICAL CONDITION/ MEDICAL DIAGNOSIS	RISK FACTORS
Decreased level of consciousness as a result of severe trauma	Enteral feeding via nasoenteric tubes

---

Patient goals
Expected outcomes
    Associated nursing/collaborative interventions *and scientific rationale*

Tolerate nasoenteric feedings without complication, as evidenced by the following:

No signs or symptoms of aspiration related to nasoenteric feedings

Orient patient and teach significant other about procedure for enteral feeding via nasoenteric tube. Emphasize the use of frequent hand washing and clean techniques when handling enteral feeding and related equipment *to decrease formula contamination.*

Confirm tube placement after insertion and at regular intervals at least every 4 hours with continuous feeding or before each intermittent feeding.

Confirm initial tube placement by chest x-ray examination in collaboration with physician.

Aspirate stomach contents. If needed, check aspirate for acidic pH level to confirm initial tube placement. *An acidic pH indicates that the nasogastric tube is in the stomach. If patient is on H_2 blockers, the gastric pH may be as high as 5.5.* If the tube becomes dislodged after feedings are initiated, check the respiratory secretions for presence of glucose. *Glucose is not usually present in tracheal or pulmonary secretions. Diabetics may exhibit glucose in respiratory secretions due to high serum levels. False positives for glucose can occur if* *blood is visible in the pulmonary secretions and the presence of complex carbohydrates may cause erroneous results.*

Inject 10 cc of air using at least a 20 to 30 cc syringe before aspiration, if aspiration of stomach contents is difficult. *This will prevent tube from collapsing during aspiration.* Position patient on the right side to help pool secretions, *making it easier to obtain gastric contents when aspirating through a small-bore feeding tube.*

Monitor potential risk factors, such as decreased levels of consciousness, sedated state, decreased cough/gag reflex, and incompetent lower esophageal sphincter.

To avoid dislodging tube:
- Monitor coughing, vomiting, and suctioning.
- Tape feeding tube securely and monitor external tube markings for possible tube migration every 4 hours and before each feeding.

Assess for gastric retention every 4 hours through the following procedures: Check gastric residuals. If residuals are 50% greater than prescribed volume, hold tube feeding and recheck residual in 1 hour; notify physician if this occurs for two consecutive measurements of residuals (tube feedings may need to be discontinued or a prokinetic agent may need to be ordered).

Evaluate gastric motility at least every 4 hours through the following procedures:
- Auscultate bowel sounds
- Percuss abdomen for air
- Assess for nausea/vomiting
- Assess for diarrhea/constipation
- Assess for gastric distention by checking abdominal girths serially. Measure from one anterior iliac crest to the other. An increase of 8 to 10 cm above baseline should be considered significant, and tube feeding should be stopped and physician notified.

Hold the tube feedings and notify the physician if bowel sounds are absent, distention is present, or there is nausea/vomiting. *The absence of bowel sounds with abdominal distention and nausea and/or vomiting may indicate a paralytic ileus and thus contraindicate tube feedings. Jejunal feedings can be administered in the absence of bowel sounds.*

Maintain proper patient positioning during tube feeding administration through the following procedures:

- Elevate head of bed 30 to 45 degrees during feeding *to minimize amount of feeding in stomach and reduce the chance of aspirating.*
- Turn patient to right side to facilitate passage of stomach contents through pylorus, if unable to elevate head of bed. *The side lying position also allows emesis to drain from the mouth rather than be aspirated into the lungs. (When side lying is not possible, consider an alternate feeding method.)*
- Stop tube feeding 30 to 60 minutes before physical activity and procedures that require lowering of patient's head.

Monitor patient for signs of aspiration (cyanosis, dyspnea, cough, wheezing, tachycardia, fever, massive atelectasis with pulmonary edema, hypoxemia, temperature greater than 38° C for 24 hours).

Check vital signs, temperature every 4 to 8 hours.

Auscultate breath sounds every 4 to 8 hours.

Observe and record color and character of sputum every 8 hours. Add blue food coloring to tube feedings. *The presence of blue food coloring in the pulmonary secretions indicates that tube feeding has been aspirated. Blue food coloring may cause false positive hemocult readings for stool.*

Check pulmonary-tracheal secretions for glucose with reagent strip every 4 to 8 hours in high risk patients. *Positive glucose indicates presence of formula in pulmonary secretions (false-positive may occur with presence of blood in pulmonary secretions, or an increase in glucose in the blood).*

Consider use of combination gastric-jejunal tubes to decompress the stomach while feeding into the jejunum *to prevent gastric secretion aspiration.*

REFERENCES

Ibanez J and others: Gastroesophageal reflux in intubated patients receiving enteral nutrition: effect of supine and semi-recumbent positions, *JPEN* 16·419-422, 1992.

Kinsey GC and others: Tracheal glucose as a detector of enteral feeding aspiration, *JPEN* 16 (Suppl)35S (From 16th Clinical Congress Program Summary & Abstracts, Abstract No. 105), 1992.

Kohn CL: The relationship between enteral formula contamination and length of enteral delivery set usage, *JPEN* 15(5):567-571, 1991.

McClave S and others: Use of residual volume as a marker for enteral feeding intolerance: prospective blinded comparison with physical examination and radiographic findings, *JPEN* 16(2):99, 1992.

Metheny NA and others: Effectiveness of pH measurements in predicting feeding tube placement, *Nurs Res* 38(5):280-285, 1989.

Metheny NA and others: Aspiration pneumonia in patients fed through nasoenteric tubes. *Heart and Lung* 15(3):256, 1986.

Montecalvo MA and others: Nutritional outcome and pneumonia in critical care patients randomized to gastric versus jejunal tube feedings, *Crit Care Med* 20(10):1377-1387, 1992.

Mullan H and others: Risks of pulmonary aspiration among patients receiving enteral nutrition support, *JPEN* 16(2):160, 1992.

Potts RG and others: Comparison of blue dye visualization and glucose oxidase test strip methods for detecting pulmonary aspiration of enteral feedings in intubated adults, *Chest* 103(1):117-121, 1993.

Strong RM and others: Equal aspiration rates from postpylorus and intragastric-placed small-bore nasoenteric feedings tubes: a randomized prospective study, *JPEN* 16:59-63, 1992.

Body image disturbance

CLINICAL CONDITION/ MEDICAL DIAGNOSIS	RELATED FACTORS
Mastectomy for breast cancer	Difficulty accepting postoperative body image

Patient goals
Expected outcomes
  Associated nursing/collaborative interventions *and*
    scientific rationale

Accept body image change and incorporate into self-concept as evidenced by the following:

Verbalizes feelings related to disfigurement and loss of body part

Acknowledge feelings expressed by patient and communicate acceptance *in order to support normal grieving and adjustment.*

Encourage patient to verbalize feelings about perceived changes and meaning of altered body image.

Assess patient's perception of impact of mastectomy on relationship with present or future partner *to determine patient's fears and possible distortions.*

Respect patient's need for privacy, emotional withdrawal, or denial (e.g., concealing or minimizing change). *These behaviors are consistent with normal grieving, and intrusiveness may increase vulnerability of the patient.*

Personalizes loss of body part and acknowledges changes

Encourage patient to view and touch altered body part and participate in self-care activities.

Provide information about cosmetic aids and use of clothing styles *to improve self-image of patient.*

Acknowledge patient's problem-solving efforts to enhance own appearance *to reinforce adaptive behaviors.*

Body image disturbance

Uses available resources for information and support

Provide information about support services and self-help groups in the community and encourage participation *to connect with peers for information and validation.*

Include partners and family members when providing support and education to patient, and make referrals for additional follow-up, if indicated.

REFERENCES

Cronan L: Management of the patient with altered body image, *Brit J Nurs* 2:257, 1993.

Newell B: Body image disturbance: cognitive behavioral formulation and intervention, *J Adv Nurs* 16:1400, 1991.

Northouse LL, Cracchiolo-Caraway A, Appel CP: Psychological consequences of breast cancer on partner and family, *Semin Onc Nurs* 7(3):216, 1991.

Price B: A model for body-image care, *J Adv Nurs* 15:585, 1990.

Price B: *Body image, nursing concepts and care*, London, 1990, Prentice Hall.

Rice MA, Szopa TJ: Group intervention for reinforcing self-worth following mastectomy, *Oncol Nurs Forum* 15(1):33, 1988.

Royak-Schaler R: Psychological processes in breast cancer: a review of selected research, *J Psychosoc Oncol* 9(4):71, 1991.

Wainstock JM: Breast cancer: psychosocial consequences for the patient, *Semin Onc Nurs* 7(3):207, 1991.

Wong CA, Bramwell L: Uncertainty and anxiety after mastectomy for breast cancer, *Cancer Nurs* 15(5):363, 1992.

Body image disturbance—cont'd

Body temperature, altered, risk for

CLINICAL CONDITION/ MEDICAL DIAGNOSIS	RISK FACTORS
Head injury	Trauma affecting hypothalamus

Patient goals
Expected outcomes
  Associated nursing/collaborative interventions *and scientific rationale*

Maintain normothermia as evidenced by the following:

Temperature remains within normal range

Monitor temperature every 4 hours; if elevated, monitor more frequently, or use continuous rectal or pulmonary artery temperatures.

Administer steroids as ordered *in order to decrease edema around the area of hypothalamus.*

Administer antipyretic agents as ordered; *antipyretics reduce fever by affecting hypothalamic response to pyrogens.*

Apply external cooling measures: cooling blankets should be kept at a temperature of 23.9° C. *This temperature causes less shivering and is effective in reducing febrile temperatures.*

Apply ice packs in axillae and groin. *Axillae and groin are close to large blood vessels that will lose heat readily by conduction.*

Wrap hands and feet in terry-cloth toweling to prevent shivering: *hands and feet have many nerve endings sensitive to heat loss; shivering should be avoided as it causes increases in metabolic rate, CO_2 production, oxygen consumption and myocardial work and decreases in O_2 saturation and glycogen stores.*

Administer IV fluids at room temperature.

Consider other causes of fever, including drug fever (check liver function studies) and infectious process (check CBC/cultures).

REFERENCES

Bruce J, Grove S: Fever: pathology and treatment, *Crit Care Nurs* 12(1):40, 1992.

Caruso C and others: Cooling effects and comfort of four cooling blanket temperatures in humans with fever, *Nurs Res* 41(2):68, 1992.

Cunha B, Tu R: Fever in the neurosurgical patient, *Heart and Lung* 17(6)608, 1988.

Holtzclaw B: Shivering, *Nurs Clin North Am* 25(4):977, 1990.

Holtzclaw B: The febrile response in critical care: state of the science, *Heart and Lung* 21(5):482, 1992.

Sherman DW: Managing an acute head injury, *Nursing* 20(4):47, 1990.

Body temperature, altered, risk for—cont'd

Bowel incontinence

CLINICAL CONDITION/ MEDICAL DIAGNOSIS	RELATED FACTORS
Pelvic floor trauma	Defecation pain; excessive use of laxatives

> **Patient goals**
> **Expected outcomes**
> > Associated nursing/collaborative interventions *and scientific rationale*

Take an active role in pain management as evidenced by the following:

Records pain experienced during defecation, measures used to control pain, and pain relief

Use lubricated gloved finger to examine rectum for presence of stool, areas of pain/tenderness, and impairment of external anal sphincter; use local anesthetic cream if necessary. Place lubricated index finger approximately 7 cm into the rectum and hook posteriorly. Instruct patient to tighten the muscles to avoid defecation. The puborectalis muscle will move anteriorly and narrow the anal canal constricting the finger.

Teach/monitor patient's ability to rate pain on a scale of 1 to 10, and to use pain log and measures to obtain pain relief. *Participation in pain management increases patient's perception of control.*

Elicit from patient measures used to increase comfort prior to seeking assistance, e.g., warm soaks.

Refer to physician to evaluate resolution of pelvic trauma.

Establish a regular pattern of bowel elimination as evidenced by the following:

Gradually decreases reliance on laxatives to control stool consistency

Provide written information about use of bulk forming agents and a high-fiber diet *to achieve desired stool consistency.*

Teach/monitor use of food diary *to gain awareness of pattern of food intake.*

Collaborate with patient to develop/monitor a plan for increasing fluid intake to 6 to 8 glasses of water a day.

Practices pelvic floor exercises 3 times a day

Discuss with physician patient's readiness to begin pelvic floor exercises (PFEs).

Teach PFEs and coach practice sessions. *PFEs strengthen the external anal sphincter and help prevent incontinence.*

Instruct patient to maintain contractions for 3 to 4 seconds and then repeat without tensing muscles of legs, buttocks, or abdomen. *If contractions are maintained for 1 minute, sphincters tend to fatigue and go into a refractory stage.*

Reports easy passage of soft formed stool and decrease in episodes of bowel incontinence

Collaborate with patient to plan and implement a toileting routine.

Teach patient to respond immediately to urge to defecate. *Stool will harden in rectum when evacuation is delayed.*

Alert patient to avoid fatty acids in triggering meal (usually breakfast). *Fatty acids delay stimulation of the gastrocolic and duodenocolic reflexes.*

REFERENCES

Alterescu V: Theoretical foundations for an approach to fecal incontinence, *J Enterost Ther* 13:44, 1986.

Davis A and others: Bowel management: a quality assurance approach to upgrading programs, *J Gerontol Nurs* 12(5):13, 1986.

Lewis NA: Nursing management of altered patterns of elimination, *J Home Health Care Prac* 1:35, 1988.

Maas M, Specht J: Bowel incontinence. In Maas M, Buckwalter KC, Hardy M, eds: *Nursing diagnosis and interventions for the elderly,* ed 2, Redwood City, Cal, 1991, Addison-Wesley, pp 169-180.

McLane AM, McShane RE: Bowel management. In Bulechek GM, McCloskey JC, eds: *Nursing interventions: essential nursing treatments*, Philadelphia, 1992, WB Saunders, pp 73-85.

McLane AM, McShane RE: Bowel incontinence. In Thompson JM and others: *Mosby's Clinical Nursing*, ed 3, St. Louis, 1993, Mosby, pp 1481-1482.

McCormick KA, Burgio KL: Incontinence: update on nursing care measures, *J Gerontol Nurs* 10:16, 1984.

McShane RE, McLane AM: Constipation: impact of etiological factors, *J Gerontol Nurs* 14(4):31, 1988.

Bowel incontinence—cont'd

Breastfeeding, effective

CLINICAL CONDITION/ MEDICAL DIAGNOSIS	RELATED FACTORS
Adequate lactation and transfer	Appropriate knowledge; support sources

Patient goals
Expected outcomes
> Associated nursing/collaborative interventions *and scientific rationale*

Adequate lactation is maintained as evidenced by the following:

Infant demonstrates adequate weight gain appropriate to age.
Mother meets her intended breastfeeding goal

> Review present pattern of breastfeeding. *Knowledge of physiology of milk production is crucial in the management of lactation.*

> Discuss nutritious diet from all four major food groups.

> Instruct to avoid intentional weight loss. *Proper nutrition is necessary to maintain health of mother and infant and maintain adequate lactation.*

> Encourage to maintain adequate fluid intake and drink to satisfy thirst; discourage taking excessive fluids. *Forcing fluids negatively affects milk production.*

> Encourage frequent rest or nap while the baby is asleep. *Fatigue may inhibit the milk ejection reflex and diminish milk supply.*

> Encourage mother to avoid use of cigarettes, caffeine, alcohol, and illegal drugs. *These substances may enter breastmilk and be harmful to the infant. Nicotine may decrease prolactin levels and inhibit milk ejection reflex.*

> Provide anticipatory guidance for infant developmental changes that affect lactation (growth spurts at 2 to 3 weeks, 6 weeks, and 3

Breastfeeding effective

months). *Mother may misperceive an inadequate milk supply due to increased infant feedings.*

Avoid introducing solids until infant is 5 to 6 months of age. *Current recommendations stress delaying the addition of solids; solids may diminish milk supply.*

Demonstrate how to express/pump breastmilk and store properly. *Adequate stimulation of the breasts is necessary to maintain lactation when mother and infant are separated.*

Discuss with mother her feelings about breastfeeding outside the home.

Prevent breast complications as evidenced by the following:

Mother develops no breast or nipple complications

Encourage use of supportive bra 24 hours a day.

Advise how to choose correct bra and bra size. Bra should give support and not bind.

Avoid underwires and elastic around the cups, *which may prevent sufficient drainage by pressing on milk ducts.*

Advise to wash the breasts and nipples with warm water daily. Avoid soaps and other drying agents *that may irritate the nipple and remove natural oils.*

Stress importance of preventing engorgement via unrestricted feeding. *Breast engorgement can be painful, may predispose to the development of nipple fissures and breast abscesses, and is associated with lactation failure.*

Encourage mother to use both breasts at a feeding. *Inadequate drainage of milk sinuses can lead to a diminished milk production.*

Encourage mother to nurse at least 10 minutes per breast before switching. Allow adequate time for the milk ejection reflex to occur *to ensure that the infant receives the hindmilk and not only the low-calorie foremilk.*

Demonstrate how to massage breasts during feeding. *Breast massage causes the hindmilk to move from the alveoli to the lactiferous sinuses, thus facilitating the milk ejection reflex and emptying of the breasts.*

Encourage mother to alternate infant's feeding positions. *Changing positions will help alleviate stress on the nipples and minimize irritation.*

Stress importance of the infant getting as much of the areola as possible in his/her mouth *to compress the lactiferous sinuses, not just the nipple.*

Instruct mother to avoid external pressure on the breasts (e.g., positions that put pressure on one spot for long periods).

Demonstrate how to empty breast manually or with pump if baby does not drain breast adequately. *Ducts may become plugged and mastitis develop if inadequate emptying occurs.*

Maintain family adaptation to breastfeeding process as evidenced by the following:

Family members verbalize support of the breastfeeding mother

Provide age-appropriate literature about breastfeeding to family members. *Support and encouragement from the partner and family significantly influence breastfeeding duration and the maintenance of lactation.*

Encourage mother to answer questions from her other children.

Role play with mother possible situations related to questions of her child(ren).

Family sleep patterns are maintained with minimal disruption

Discuss sleep pattern disruptions that may occur.

Encourage significant others to demonstrate their support by assisting with household duties.

Provide praise and positive reinforcement to family members.

Family activities are not curtailed

Discuss how to plan family activities, including trips, conducive to breastfeeding.

Discuss selection of clothing that allows for discreet breastfeeding such as loose-knit pullovers, button-fronted blouses, and shawl.

REFERENCES

Auerbach K: Assisting the employed breast-feeding mother, *J Nurs Midwifery* 35:1:26, 1990.

Dusdieker L and others: Prolonged maternal fluid supplementation in breastfeeding, *Pediatrics* 86:5:737, 1990.

Hill PD: The enigma of insufficient milk supply, *Am J Matern Child Nurs* 16:6:313, 1991.

Hill PD, Humenick SS: Nipple pain during breastfeeding: the first two weeks and beyond, *J Hum Lact* 2:2:21, 1993.

Matich JR, Sims LS: A comparison of social support variables between women who intend to breast or bottle feed, *Soc Sci Med* 34:8:919, 1992.

Newton N: The quantitative effect of oxytocin (pitocin) on human milk yield, *Ann N Y Acad Sci* 652:597, 1992.

Righard L, Alade MO: Sucking technique and its effect on success of breastfeeding, *Birth* 19:4:185, 1992.

Breastfeeding, effective—cont'd

Breastfeeding, ineffective

CLINICAL CONDITION/ MEDICAL DIAGNOSIS	RELATED FACTORS
Insufficient milk supply syndrome	Previous history of breastfeeding failure; poor infant suck reflex

---

Patient goals
Expected outcomes
   Associated nursing/collaborative interventions *and scientific rationale*

Establish optimal lactation as evidenced by:

Verbalizes accurate information related to breastfeeding

   Interview patient to assess patient's level of knowledge.

   Initiate teaching to reduce patient's inadequate knowledge about breastfeeding. *Patients who are knowledgeable about breastfeeding tend to be more successful at breastfeeding.*

   Include patient's significant other in teaching.

Identifies personal and family support for breastfeeding

   Identify cultural barriers to breastfeeding. *The acceptance/success of breastfeeding may be negatively influenced in certain cultures.*

   Encourage patient/significant others to verbalize emotional attitudes about breastfeeding. *The acceptance/success of breastfeeding can positively influence successful breastfeeding.*

Feeds infant with minimal assistance

   Use nipple shells if nipples are flat or inverted. *The nipple protrudes through a hole in the center and constant gentle pressure around the nipple causes it to evert.*

   Demonstrate colostrum expression to entice infant.

   Promote appropriate positioning for feeding; side lying, football hold, sitting, or across abdomen.

   Provide suggestions for waking a sleepy baby

Breastfeeding, ineffective

Demonstrate techniques to help infant "latch on" correctly. *Incorrect position of the infant's mouth abrades the nipple, causes soreness, and contributes to early weaning.*

Observe infant during feeding for faulty sucking mechanism.

Do not restrict sucking time.

Offer both breasts at each feeding.

Provide for frequent feedings on demand every 2 to 3 hours.

Has fewer breast complications as evidenced by:

No evidence of breast/nipple trauma

Observe breast for engorgement, warmth, redness of nipple, cracks or fissures in nipple, or anomaly of breast.

Monitor for frequency of analgesia use.

Patient demonstrates breast care techniques utilized to decrease breast complications

Encourage frequent feedings with proper positioning.

Encourage patient to apply warm, moist packs 10 to 15 minutes before feeding or encourage patient to take warm showers before feeding.

Assist patient with hand expression or by pumping breast to soften areola and make nipple protrude.

Encourage use of varying positions of baby's mouth on breast by changing holding position with each feeding.

Teach proper technique to break suction of nursing infant.

Encourage air drying nipples after feeding and use of a supportive bra.

Discourage use of soaps or lotions containing alcohol; use ointments as prescribed.

Maintains the breastfeeding process as evidenced by:

Expresses confidence in ability to handle future situations

Encourage appropriate changes in nutrition and rest.

Discuss implications for using medications while breastfeeding. *Passive diffusion causes passage of a drug from plasma to milk.*

Discourage delaying or skipping feedings.

Discuss observing for signs of adequate letdown reflex.

Teach patient how to evaluate if infant is getting enough. *Perceived insufficient milk supply leads to supplementing and early discontinuation of breastfeeding.*

Discourage supplements. *Substitute bottles may confuse infant. Supplementation can negatively affect milk production.*

Identifies resources for problems and/or support

Provide consistent information, support and positive reinforcement. *Patients who have support in their network tend to be more successful in breastfeeding.*

Provide anticipatory guidance for developmental changes that affect breastfeeding (i.e., growth spurts).

Provide written information about resources/support groups for breastfeeding.

Demonstrate use of assistive devices for infants with problems.

Discuss strategies to continue breastfeeding after returning to work. *Knowledge about methods to facilitate breastfeeding can delay discontinuation of breastfeeding after returning to work.*

Discuss role of father/significant other while breastfeeding.

Discuss effects of breastfeeding on sexuality.

REFERENCES

Abramson R: Cultural sensitivity in the promotion of breastfeeding, *NAACOG Clin Issues Perinat Women Health Nurs* 3(4):717-22, 1992.

Bono BJ: Assessment and documentation of the breastfeeding couple, *J Hum Lact* 8(1):17-22, 1992.

Duckett L, Henly SJ, Garvis M: Predicting breastfeeding duration during the postpartum hospitalization, *West J Nurs Res* 15(2):177-198, 1993.

Breastfeeding, ineffective—cont'd

Hill PD, Aldag JC: Insufficient milk supply among black and white breastfeeding mothers, *Res Nurs Health* 16(3):203-11, 1993.

Hill PD, Aldag JC: Potential indicators of insufficient milk supply syndrome, *Res Nurs Health* 14(1):11-19, 1991.

Lawrence RA: *Breastfeeding: a guide for the medical profession*, ed 3, St. Louis, 1989, Mosby.

O'Campo P and others: Prenatal factors associated with breastfeeding duration: recommendations for prenatal interventions, *Birth* 19(4):195-201, 1992.

Rentschler DD: Correlates of successful breastfeeding, *Image: J Nurs Sch* 23(3):151-154, 1991.

Breastfeeding, interrupted

CLINICAL CONDITION/ MEDICAL DIAGNOSIS	RELATED FACTORS
Prematurity	Uncoordinated sucking, swallowing, and breathing mechanisms

Patient goals
Expected outcomes
> Associated nursing/collaborative interventions *and scientific rationale*

Demonstrate a commitment to provide adequate and bacteriologically safe breast milk to the preterm infant for gavage feeding as evidenced by the following:

Participates in initial consultation with nurse with expertise in breastfeeding premature infants

> Encourage mother to consult (NICU) breastfeeding specialist. *NICU breastfeeding specialist has expertise in both lactation and in the clinical care of high risk infants.*

> Provide privacy during consultation.

Recognizes the immunological, nutritional, and emotional benefits of breastfeeding as they relate to the infant's special condition

> Reinforce the mother's knowledge about the immunological and nutritional benefits of breastfeeding. *Milk produced by mothers who deliver preterm infants differs in composition from milk produced by mothers who deliver at term. It has higher concentration of protein, sodium, calcium, lipids, and selected antiinfective properties, which is consistent with the unique nutritional needs of preterm infants. Evidence indicates that breastfeeding affords protection against illness, such as respiratory and gastrointestinal infections, specifically, during infancy.*

> Discuss the emotional benefits of breastfeeding. *Mothers of preterm infants have stated repeatedly that breastfeeding is the one thing they can do for*

their preterm infants when professionals have assumed other caregiving activities.

Recognizes that the expressed milk will be given to the infant by artificial feeding method such as gavage

Provide information to the mother that most small, preterm infants cannot be breastfed directly. Therefore, preterm infants receive expressed mother's milk (EMM) by artificial feeding such as gavage infusion until they have demonstrated the ability to feed orally. *Preterm infant's ability to coordinate sucking, swallowing, and breathing varies from 32 to 36 weeks of gestation depending on feeding method.*

Discuss two major problems that may occur during gavage feeding, such as significant nutrient loss and bacterial growth of already colonized milk, *to understand the risks in gavage feeding.*

Maintains adequate milk supply by pumping breasts correctly 8 to 12 times daily in the early postpartum period

Develop a workable plan that incorporates physiological principles of early and frequent milk expression in the postpartum period. *Stimulating lactation is easier in the early postpartum period than it is several days later. Milk produced in early lactation, especially colostrum, contains antiinfective properties that are more beneficial to the infant. Frequent pumping contributes to adequate milk supply.*

Uses recommended pump and collecting equipment for optimal production of milk

Encourage the patient to rent an electric breast pump with a double pump collecting kit for home use, *to optimize prolactin levels and decrease pumping times.*

Help with breast pump rentals and purchases from referral agencies, *to relieve mother of the burden of phone calls at a stressful time. Nurse's assistance ensures services from the agencies that benefit the mother, such as (1) delivery of appropriate pump and collecting equipment, (2) direct billing of third-party*

Breastfeeding, interrupted—cont'd

payers, if the mother so desires, and (3) picking up pump from the home, when no longer needed.

Teach mother the correct use of pump, proper cleaning, and the assembly and disassembly of the equipment.

Inform mother that with few exceptions, pumping will continue for at least 2 weeks after the infant has been discharged from NICU, *to empty breasts completely and increase prolactin levels.*

Recognizes importance of adequate nutrition and implications of drugs for safe milk supply

Reinforce the importance of adequate nutrition, fluids, and rest, *to ensure adequate milk supply.*

Discuss on individual basis concerns related to medications, smoking, or alcohol ingestion while mother is expressing milk for her preterm infant. *Depending on maternal dosage and clinical condition of the infant, a drug that is considered "safe" if present in EMM for full-term healthy infants may not be equally safe for a 750-g, 26-week infant.*

Produces expressed mother's milk (EMM) with "abnormally" low bacteriological contamination, e.g., an absence of all bacteria except skin flora in minimal concentrations (10^2 to 10^4 colony-forming units per ml)

Develop protocol for maternal breast care and bacteriologic surveillance of EMM. *EMM is never sterile and contains Staphylococcus epidermidis that may be pathogenic to preterm infants.*

Explain the milk expression techniques and the reasons for special precautions. *Assure mother that her hygiene is not being questioned but that precautions are needed to reduce the bacteria to "abnormally" low levels.*

Complies with the established protocol for milk expression

Teach mothers about bacteria-reducing techniques for milk expression as recommended by Meier and Wilks. *The smaller, sicker preterm infant has a compromised immune system and may be more susceptible to bacteria in EMM.*

Send mother's EMM for culture per protocol *to ensure that mother is exercising appropriate expression techniques.*

Uses recommended containers for storage of EMM to minimize the bacteriologic contamination except skin flora concentration at 10^2 to 10^4 colony forming units per ml

Instruct mothers to collect EMM in sterile, graduated plastic feeders with twist-on, air-tight caps. This EMM can be refrigerated or frozen for later use, by the nurses who will prepare the milk for gavage or bottle feeding. *Such feeders are ideal for EMM storage and easier to defrost and handle without contaminating the contents.*

Label each bottle with baby's name, date, time milk was pumped, and any medication the mother is taking.

Uses EMM within 24 hours after refrigeration

Advise mothers to use fresh and/or previously frozen EMM for feeding within 24 hours after refrigeration. *No definitive guidelines are available for the length of time EMM can remain refrigerated until it is fed to the infant, except for conservative policy based on American Academy of Pediatrics Committee on Nutrition.*

Encourage mother to express milk just before each feeding. *This approach is optimal in minimizing bacterial growth and maximizing antiinfective properties of the milk received by the infant.*

Take an active role in the management of in-hospital breastfeeding sessions as evidenced by:

Recognizes that the intended outcomes of early breast-feeding sessions are positioning the infant correctly at breast and physiologic stability during feeding

Determine the readiness to breastfeed by assessing whether the infant can coordinate the suck-swallow-breathe mechanisms *rather than currently used criteria, such as infant weight, ability to bottle-feed, type of thermal support an infant requires, and gestational age.*

Initiate breastfeeding according to the criteria currently being used for initiating bottle-feeding, *until the time a research based tool is available to enable the nurse and the physician to make decisions about readiness to feed. Specific NICU policy, such as bottle-feeding at 34 weeks of gestation when an infant weighs a minimum of 1500 gms, can be used for breastfeeding.*

Delay bottle-feeding for at least 1 week while the infant learns to breastfeed, *to introduce the preterm infant to breastfeeding before bottle-feeding.*

Assess prefeeding vital signs of the preterm infant *to provide baseline data.*

Explain rationale for test-weighing to the mothers. *Mothers should understand that test-weighing is not being used as a determinant of a "successful" breastfeeding session and that adequate infant intake is not the goal of early breastfeeding.*

Perform test-weighing by using electronic scales *to determine the volume of milk the preterm infant consumes during breastfeeding so that other fluids, e.g., supplemental gavage feeding or parenteral fluids, can be adjusted accordingly.*

Prepare the breast for feeding by cleansing it with sterile water and gauze pads.

Assist in positioning the infant (cross-chest position) at breast *to facilitate "latch-on."*

Consider skin-to-skin contact by positioning the infant chest-to-chest with the mother *Preterm infants held skin-to-skin (kangaroo care) are warm enough and have regular heart rate and respiration. Breastfeeding may be enhanced by skin-to-skin contact where lactation becomes more productive and lasts longer. Parents may become attached to their infants and feel confident about caring for them.*

Monitor physiologic variables during breastfeeding *to determine infant's responses.*

Provide gavage supplementation during or after the feeding as needed.

Recognizes that the intended outcome of *later breastfeeding* sessions is the infant's consumption of adequate volumes of milk in order to prepare for discharge

Implement the same nursing interventions as in early breastfeeding.

Conduct and evaluate serial test weighing by using electronic scales. *Ideally, volume of intake during breastfeeding should approximate that consumed by the infant during gavage or bottle feeding and should demonstrate a trend of increasing volume over time. If mothers are concerned that their infants do not consume volumes comparable to those they receive by gavage or bottle, they should be reassured that small volumes of intake are normal, especially until milk ejection and mature infant sucking patterns are synchronized.*

Implement cue-based feeding during the last 1 to 2 weeks of the infant's hospitalization. *Mothers will experience what "demand" feeding is and will have an opportunity to observe their infants awaken in response to hunger.*

Utilize postdischarge consultation services to support breastfeeding at home as evidenced by:

Recognizes that postdischarge consultation can influence successful adjustment in breastfeeding at home

Provide an individualized written plan for breastfeeding management at home.

Allow for liberal complementation/supplementation of breastfeeding in the individualized plan.

Develop a schedule for telephone consultation and an occasional home visit.

REFERENCES

Anderson GC: Current knowledge about skin-to-skin (kangaroo) care for preterm infants, *J Perinatol* 11(3):216, 1991.

Blaymore-Bier J and others: Breast-feeding of very low birthweight infants, *J Pediatr* 123(5):773, 1993.

Kavanaugh KL and others: Getting enough: Mothers' concern about breast feeding a preterm infant post-discharge (In press, *JOGNN*).

Breastfeeding, interrupted—cont'd

Meier P: Bottle and breast-feeding: effects on transcutaneous oxygen pressure and temperature in preterm infants, *Nurs Res* 137:36-44, 1988.

Meier P, Anderson G: Responses of small preterm infants to bottle- and breast-feeding, *MCN Am J Matern Child Nurs* 12:97-105, 1987.

Meier P, Pugh E: Breast-feeding behavior of small preterm infants, *MCN Am J Matern Child Nurs* 10:396-401, 1985.

Meier PP and others: Breastfeeding support services in the neonatal intensive care, *J Obstet Gynecol Neonatal Nurs* 22(4):338, 1993.

Meier PP, Mangurten HH: Breastfeeding the preterm infant. In Riordan J, Auerbach KG, eds: *Breastfeeding and human lactation*, Boston, 1993, Jones and Bartlett.

Meier PP, Wilks SO: The bacteria in expressed mothers milk, *MCN Am J Matern Child Nurs* 12:420-423, 1987.

Breathing pattern, ineffective

CLINICAL CONDITION/ MEDICAL DIAGNOSIS	RELATED FACTORS
Stable chronic obstructive pulmonary disease	Respiratory muscle fatigue, impaired respiratory mechanics

Patient goals
Expected outcomes
    Associated nursing/collaborative interventions *and scientific rationale*

Minimize energy expenditure of respiratory muscles as evidenced by the following:

Respiratory rate and tidal volume within normal limits, minimal dyspnea

Teach pursed-lip breathing, abdominal stabilization, and controlled coughing techniques; provide optimal care for mechanical assistance (e.g., ventilatory) if necessary. *Pursed-lip breathing forces patients to breathe more slowly and deeply and reduces dyspnea during exertion. Coughing can be fatiguing, hence abdominal stabilization and controlled coughing techniques are used to provide support to the expiratory muscles and assist in removing airway secretions while minimizing energy expenditure. These techniques will be beneficial only to patients who are producing excessive mucus.*

Increase inspiratory muscle strength and endurance as evidenced by the following:

Increases maximal inspiratory pressure and reports decreased exertional dyspnea

Evaluate status of inspiratory muscle for training and, if appropriate, initiate inspiratory muscle training. *Inspiratory muscle training improves conscious control of respiratory muscles and decreases anxiety associated with increased inspiratory effort. Increased strength of the inspiratory muscles may allow some patients to tolerate submaximal levels of activity for longer periods with less dyspnea.*

Monitor oxygen saturation with pulse oximeter during training session to verify that patient does not desaturate. Encourage patient to breathe as deeply as possible during inspiratory muscle training. *Use of very small tidal volumes during inspiratory muscle training could decrease alveolar ventilation and cause some patients to experience oxyhemoglobin desaturation.*

Limit work of breathing as evidenced by the following:

Reports taking prn antibiotics when sputum color changes (yellow or green)

Teach patient to monitor color, consistency, and volume of sputum *because respiratory infections increase work of breathing. Early treatment of bacterial infection of the lungs may speed recovery and thereby reduce the work of breathing.*

Reports taking bronchodilator medications as prescribed

Teach patient name, dosage, method of administration, schedule, and appropriate behavior if side effects occur, and teach consequences of improper use of medications. *Anticholinergics (ipratropium bromide), beta agonists, and methylxanthines are commonly prescribed bronchodilators that can be beneficial in decreasing airway resistance and work of breathing.*

Evaluate patient's technique for taking inhaled medications. Recommend a spacer device for patients who have difficulty with timing during the procedure. *Under optimal conditions, no more than 10% of the drug from each puff is deposited into the lungs; with a spacer device, as much as 15% of the drug will be deposited.*

Demonstrates ability to pace ADLs in line with ventilatory function

Teach patient to modify ADLs within ventilatory limits.

Induce periodic hyperinflation of lungs with a series of slow, deep breaths. *Hyperinflation works like a deep sigh, expanding alveoli that are partially closed, mobilizing airway secretions, and increasing lung tissue compliance.*

REFERENCES

Anthonisen M and others: Antibiotic therapy in exacerbations of chronic obstructive pulmonary disease, *Ann Intern Med* 106:196-203, 1987.

Ferguson GT, Cherniack RM: Management of chronic obstructive pulmonary disease, *N Engl J Med* 328:1017-1022, 1993.

Harris RS, Lawson TV: The relative mechanical effectiveness and efficiency of successive voluntary coughs in healthy young adults, *Clin Sci* 34:569-577, 1968.

Kim MJ and others: Inspiratory muscle training in patients with chronic obstructive pulmonary disease, *Nurs Res* 42:356-362, 1993.

Larson JL and others: Maximal inspiratory pressure: Learning effect and test-retest reliability in patients with chronic obstructive pulmonary disease, *Chest* 104:448-453, 1993.

Larson JL and others: Inspiratory muscle training with a pressure threshold breathing device in patients with chronic obstructive pulmonary disease, *Am Rev Respir Dis* 138:689-696, 1988.

Mueller RE, Petty TL, Filley GF: Ventilation and arterial blood gas changes induced by pursed lips breathing, *J Appl Physiol* 29: 784-789, 1970.

Sharp JT and others: Postural relief of dyspnea in severe chronic obstructive pulmonary disease, *Am Rev Respir Dis* 122:201-211, 1980.

Sutton PP and others: Assessment of forced expiration technique, postural drainage and directed coughing in chest physiotherapy, *Eur J Respir Dis* 64:62-68, 1983.

Tiep BL and others: Pursed lips breathing training using ear oximetry, *Chest* 90:218-221, 1986.

Breathing pattern, ineffective—cont'd

KRISTIN M. KLEINSCHMIDT, MARGARET J. STAFFORD,
AND MI JA KIM

Cardiac output, decreased

CLINICAL CONDITION/ MEDICAL DIAGNOSIS	RELATED FACTORS
Myocardial infarction (MI) Congestive heart failure (CHF)	Electrophysiologic rhythm disturbances: bradyarrhythmias (heart rate $\leq$ 60/minute), tachyarrhythmias (heart rate $\geq$ 160/minute), or pulseless electrical activity (PEA)

Patient goals
Expected outcomes
    Associated nursing/collaborative interventions *and*
        scientific rationale

Regain normal range of cardiac output (CO) as evidenced by the following:

Has normal blood pressure (BP)

Review history of patient's BP to determine normal range.

Monitor BP at regular intervals and when there is a significant heart rate/rhythm change.

Assess for change in sensorium in presence of hypotension because a decrease in cardiac output will reduce cerebral blood flow.

Consult with physician in presence of significant heart rate/rhythm changes or BP changes for indicated drug therapy or treatment (e.g., cardiac pacing).

Has cardiac rate/rhythm within normal range, free of bradyarrhythmias and/or tachyarrhythmias without IV medication; with or without maintenance oral medications; with or without pacemaker therapy; with or without support of implantable cardioverter defibrillator (ICD)

Monitor the patient's physiologic responses to the bradyarrhythmias or tachyarrhythmias (e.g., altered mentation, hypotension, pallor, diaphoresis, abnormal breath sounds or heart sounds, hypoxia, change in the quality of pulse, and loss of consciousness).

Cardiac output, decreased

Set alarm limits on ECG monitor (rate, rhythm, S-T trending).

Monitor for ECG changes that increase the risk for development of arrhythmias (e.g., prolonged P-R, QRS, or Q-T interval; frequent premature atrial or ventricular beats; or R on T phenomenon).

Determine the need for continuous monitoring in collaboration with the physician.

If the patient's rate is ≤ 60 beats/minute, evaluate the patient's response to the slow rate and hemodynamic disorders. *Bradycardia (≤ 60 beats/minute) may cause symptoms of decreased perfusion as CO is compromised due to the slow rate (CO=SV × HR).*

If the patient has hypotension or a syncopal episode, lower the patient's head and raise the legs *to facilitate cerebral circulation.* Encourage deep breaths and coughing *to stimulate cardiac activity and improve CO.* Notify the physician immediately.

Initiate an IV and administer drugs (according to hospital policy/protocol), e.g., a bolus of atropine sulfate, 0.5 to 1 mg. If rate does not increase, repeat 0.5-mg doses every 3 to 5 minutes up to a maximum of .04 mg/kg of body weight. *Atropine is a parasympatholytic agent that blocks the action of the vagus nerve, increasing heart rate and enhancing atrioventricular (AV) conduction.*

Monitor side effects of atropine sulfate (e.g., urinary retention, headache, dizziness, dryness of mouth, abdominal distention and pain, photophobia/glaucoma, and ectopic ventricular beats). Give with caution *because excessive increases in rate may worsen myocardial ischemia.*

Initiate transcutaneous pacing (according to protocol), if available. *Transcutaneous pacing is a convenient and effective intervention. It may be used as a temporary measure when hemodynamic problems persist and until a temporary or permanent pacemaker can be inserted.*

Titrate dopamine IV (5 to 20 mcg/kg/min) if ordered. *Dopamine is an endogenous catecholamine that increases cardiac output and blood pressure.*

Titrate epinephrine IV (2 to 10 mcg/min) if ordered.

Cardiac output, decreased—cont'd

Epinephrine is a sympathomimetic drug with potent inotropic and chronotropic properties, increasing the heart rate and force of cardiac contractions.

Titrate isoproterenol HCl (Isuprel) IV (2 to 10 mcg/min) if ordered. *Isoproterenol is a synthetic sympathomimetic drug with potent inotropic and chronotropic properties. Isoproterenol should be used, if at all, with extreme caution because it may increase myocardial oxygen consumption and cause peripheral vasodilatation, and precipitate ventricular arrhythmias.*

Review patient's current medications *to identify drugs that could decrease the heart rate* e.g., morphine sulfate, a vagomimetic agent; verapamil, a calcium channel blocker; propranolol, a beta blocker; amiodarone, an antiarrhythmic with a potential side effect of bradycardia; or digoxin, a cardiac glycoside with potential side effects of bradycardia and AV block). Discuss with the physician the feasibility of modifying the drug therapy.

Monitor serum potassium levels. *Hyperkalemia may cause AV blocks, ventricular arrhythmias, and asystole.*

Provide adequate ventilation and administer oxygen as indicated *because hypoxia may contribute to bradycardia.*

Assist with insertion of a transvenous, temporary pacemaker if indicated and reassuringly explain its purpose and describe the sensory aspects of the procedure to the patient. Temporary pacing *is indicated for the patient with severe bradycardia but with a palpable pulse and for the patient who has high-grade heart block whose conducted beat results in a palpable pulse.* When symptoms persist, a permanent pacemaker is considered.

If pulseless electrical activity (PEA) is present (cardiac rhythm without a pulse), initiate CPR and administer epinephrine IV 1 mg and, if no response, atropine IV 1 mg (according to protocol). The underlying cause of PEA is identified and treated.

If electrophysiology study (EPS) is indicated, explain the treatment to the patient, secure a consent, and assist as indicated. *EPS is an invasive, diagnostic procedure in which two to five catheters are placed inside the heart to determine conduction intervals and to identify sites of origin of heart blocks.*

In the presence of a tachycardia, analyze the rhythm for regularity and the morphology of the complexes. Determine the site of origin of the tachyarrhythmia in the conduction system (sinus, atrial, junctional, or ventricular). *In general, the treatment for sinus tachycardia is to determine and treat the cause. However, in the presence of an MI, a beta blocker may be used. Heart rates > 160 that originate above the ventricles, atrial or junctional, referred to as supraventricular tachycardia (SVT), are not imminently life-threatening but may seriously compromise CO. The diastolic filling time is shortened, diminishing preload, stroke volume, and ultimately decreasing CO (CO = SV × HR).*

In the presence of a supraventricular tachycardia (SVT), assess the following: (1) Assess the rate and quality of peripheral pulses and detect pulse deficits. *In atrial fibrillation (and other atrial rhythms that are extremely fast and/or uncoordinated) the atrial contribution to CO (the "atrial kick") is lost by as much as 30%.* (2) Monitor blood pressure for hypotension and signs of decreased perfusion and auscultate for extra heart sounds, specifically S_3. *When the left ventricle is failing and noncompliant, the sudden deceleration of the filling wave produces an audible third sound.* (3) Monitor and evaluate the 12-lead ECG for precipitous changes and signs of myocardial ischemia (e.g., depressed ST segments and significant T-wave changes). (4) Determine the presence of and evaluate chest pain/discomfort. *With sustained tachycardia, there is the potential for decreased cardiac perfusion (related to the shortened diastolic filling time), decreased oxygen to the myocardium, and increased myocardial workload.* (5) Monitor pulmonary status, respiratory rate and effort, and adverse behavioral changes, *all of which indicate a serious decrease in oxygen delivery to the tissues*. If pulse oximetry is available, monitor oxygen saturation. (6) If the patient is being anticoagulated *(disorganized atrial activity may result in thrombus formation and emboli)*, monitor partial thromboplastin and prothrombin times and, if not, discuss with the physician the feasibility of anticoagulation.

Heart rates $\geq$ 160 that originate above the ventricles (atrial or junctional), referred to as supraventricular tachycardia (SVT), are not imminently life-threatening but may seriously compromise CO. The diastolic filling time is shortened, diminishing preload, stroke volume, and ultimately decreasing CO. (CO=SV $\times$ HR). In general, the treatment for sinus tachycardia is to determine and treat the cause. However, in the presence of an MI, a beta blocker may be used.

Initiate oxygen therapy, an IV, and hemodynamic monitoring as indicated and ordered.

Notify the physician of significant changes and discuss therapeutic options.

Monitor the patient's response to valsalva maneuver or carotid sinus stimulation as indicated. *These actions increase parasympathetic (vagal) responses, producing a block in the AV node and reducing the ventricular rate.*

Administer medication as ordered (e.g., adenosine IV *which interrupts the re-entrant circuit*, verapamil or diltiazem IV *which interrupt the re-entrant circuit and increase the delay in the AV node; digoxin, to slow AV conduction, increasing degrees of heart block and slowing the ventricular rate;* and/or metoprolol, esmolol, or propranolol IV *to decrease automaticity and conduction velocity slowing the heart rate)*. Monitor response to drug therapy and report untoward reactions to the physician.

Prepare the patient for electrical cardioversion if indicated and ordered. *Cardioversion delivers a*

Cardiac output, decreased—cont'd

149

synchronized direct current charge to the myocardium causing all the cells to depolarize simultaneously and allowing the sinus node to gain control. Assist as indicated with synchronizing the charge with the patient's QRS to avoid the vulnerable period of the cardiac cycle and potential ventricular fibrillation. Initial charge is 100 joules (j), followed by 200 j, 300 j, and 360 j.

Explain the procedure in accurate but nonthreatening terms, secure a written consent, and reassure the patient that he/she will receive a medication before the treatment to avoid pain and discomfort.

Monitor blood pressure, heart rate, rhythm, and level of consciousness until stable, after cardioversion.

If overdrive pacing is ordered, explain the treatment to the patient, secure a consent, and assist as indicated. *Overdrive pacing is usually effective in controlling the fast rate and may convert some SVTs to normal sinus rhythm.*

If electrophysiology study (EPS) is indicated, explain the treatment to the patient, secure a consent, and assist as indicated. *EPS is an invasive, diagnostic procedure to determine not only the sites of origin of heart blocks, but also tachyarrhythmias.*

If radiofrequency ablation (RFA) is indicated, explain the treatment to the patient, secure a consent, and assist as indicated. *RFA is an invasive, therapeutic procedure in which radiofrequency energy is delivered to a small portion of the heart, causing necrosis of the tissue that is responsible for the tachyarrhythmia.*

In the presence of ventricular tachycardia (VT), assess level of consciousness and presence of carotid pulse. *Ventricular tachycardia (VT) not only causes a decrease in CO as described with SVTs, but may also rapidly progress to ventricular fibrillation (VF) and death.* In the monitored patient who is unresponsive, not breathing, and pulseless, initiate CPR, administer chest thump, and alert the CPR team. Thump chest only if a defibrillator is not available, *because doing so could precipitate ventricular fibrillation.* If a defibrillator is available, immediately deliver unsynchronized countershock stat at 200 j, followed by 300 j and 360 j, and proceed with CPR/ACLS as outlined in hospital policy.

If the patient is conscious and hemodynamically stable, initiate drug regimen according to hospital policy (e.g., a lidocaine bolus 1.5 mg/kg, followed by an IV infusion with lidocaine). *Lidocaine reduces ventricular automaticity and may terminate VT.*

Administer procainamide 20 to 30 mg/min IV and, if no response, bretylium IV 5 to 10 mg/kg IV, as ordered, if VT persists. *Procainamide reduces automaticity and slows AV conduction and may terminate VT. Bretylium raises the VF threshold.* Monitor response to drug therapy and report untoward reactions to the physician.

Prepare the patient for synchronized cardioversion if indicated. Talk with the patient throughout the procedure, calmly and reassuringly explaining the treatment.

Monitor serum potassium and magnesium levels and replace as indicated. *Hypokalemia may cause AV blocks, ventricular arrhythmias, and asystole. Hypomagnesemia may cause ventricular arrhythmias.*

If EPS or RFA is indicated, explain the treatment to the patient, secure a consent, and assist as indicated.

If an implantable cardioverter defibrillator (ICD) is implanted, a detailed teaching plan with the patient and family should include purpose, restrictions, how it works, what to do when it doesn't, how a shock feels, how to perform CPR, and follow-up care. *An ICD is a programmable device designed to deliver burst or ramp overdrive pacing, synchronized cardioversion shocks, or defibrillation shocks for VT or defibrillation shocks for VF episodes.*

Expresses freedom from chest pain/discomfort, dyspnea, dizziness, lightheadedness, palpitations, and syncope

Assess/document/evaluate the patient's perceptions related to the bradyarrhythmias or tachyarrhythmias (e.g., dizziness or lightheadedness, dyspnea, feelings of anxiety or alarm, fatigue, palpitations, chest pain).

Experience less stress as evidenced by the following:

Verbalizes understanding of and acceptance of therapy, drugs, and treatment

Explain, if indicated, the purpose of ICU or surveillance unit to patient/significant others and reassuringly discuss the advantages of "having your heartbeat watched continuously."

Assess emotional response to bradyarrhythmias, tachyarrhythmias, and the environment.

Individualize patient teaching appropriate to age, reading level, and ethnic background.

Review all medications, i.e., purpose, side effects, diet, and activity restrictions, if indicated, and promote positive "upbeat" attitude/behavior.

Explain the procedural and describe the sensory aspects of therapies (e.g., how the instrument is placed and how it will feel). *Preparation for stressful events, particularly description of the sensory aspects, can reduce stress and facilitate coping.*

If a permanent pacemaker is implanted, provide a comprehensive/holistic plan of care; i.e., involve the patient/significant others in establishing preoperative/postoperative and long-term goals; explain purpose/function of the pacemaker being implanted (e.g., physiologic, rate responsive, single or dual); provide a pacemaker-specific teaching booklet reviewing the concepts with the patient; reassure/explain benefits of pacing related to energy level and dispel misconceptions about restrictions such as sexual activity and noncontact sports. Review

Cardiac output, decreased—cont'd

appropriate precautions (e.g., electrical safety precautions, avoidance of contact sports); reassure patient about cosmetic appearance and self-image in general; introduce concept of ECG telephone transmissions and clinic visits. *Simplify the regimen to meet patient's level of understanding and interest.* Counsel the patient when fears and concerns persist. *The foregoing will maximize patient adherence to therapy and potentially improve patient outcomes.*

Relates positive social interaction

Encourage family/significant others to visit at optimal times for the patient.

Monitor the patient's physiological/emotional response to interactions between the patient, visitors, and staff.

REFERENCES

Bremner SM, McCauley KM, Axtell, KA: A follow-up of patients with implantable cardioverter defibrillators, *J Cardiovasc Nurs* 7(3):40, 1993.

Cavanaugh JA: Overdrive pacing: an approach to terminating ventricular tachycardia, *J Cardiovasc Nurs* 5(3):58, 1991.

Craney J: Radiofrequency catheter ablation of supraventricular tachycardias: clinical consideration and nursing care, *J Cardiovasc Nurs* 7(3):26, 1993.

Guidelines for Cardiopulmonary Resuscitation and Emergency Cardiac Care, *JAMA* 268(16):2171, 1992.

Garvin BJ, Huston GP, Baker CF: Information used by nurses to prepare patients for a stressful event, *Appl Nurs Res* 5(4):158, 1992.

Kern L, Omery A: Decreased cardiac output in the critical care setting, *Nurs Diagn* 3(3):94, 1992.

Lupker BV: Patient adherence: a 'risk factor' for cardiovascular disease, *Cardiovasc Dis* 2(5):418, 1993.

McCloskey JC, Bulechek GM, eds: Dysrhythmia management. In *Nursing interventions classification (NIC)*, St. Louis, 1992, Mosby-Year Book.

Stafford MJ, Kleinschmidt KM: Physiological cardiac pacing: the DDD pacemaker system and rate-responsive modes, *Cardiovasc Nurs* 27(3):13, 1991.

Stewart J, Shrehan A: Permanent pacemakers: the nurse's role in patient education and follow-up care, *J Cardiovasc Nurs* 5(3):32, 1991.

Cardiac output decreased—cont'd

Caregiver role strain

CLINICAL CONDITION/ MEDICAL DIAGNOSIS	RELATED FACTORS
Wife caring for husband with cognitive impairment	Physical/emotional demands of caregiving; perceived isolation of caregiver

Patient goals
Expected outcomes
    Associated nursing/collaborative interventions *and scientific rationale*

Obtain assistance with meeting demands of caregiving role as evidenced by the following:

Verbalizes caregiving tasks that could be delegated
Review/discuss requirements for care with patient and caregiver.
Assist caregiver with identification of caregiving resources, e.g., family members, friends, community agencies.
Develop options for delegation of specific tasks.
Obtains information about costs of home health-care services and respite care
Provide/discuss information about respite care.
Provide caregiver with list of caregiving resources within budgetary limits.
Contracts with health-care providers for specific services
Help caregiver develop a daily schedule that includes pacing direct care activities. *Delegation of specific tasks to formal caregivers may enable patient to remain in home setting despite an expected negative trajectory.*
Explore use of a computer link to supplement in-home services.

Develop support system with friends/neighbors as evidenced by the following:

Identifies social resources that could be mobilized

Caregiver role strain

Requests that neighbors sit/visit with patient while caregiver attends to personal needs
Socializes with a friend on a regular basis

Help caregiver/patient to identify type/source of support that would be most helpful.

Help caregiver negotiate with patient to resume preferred leisure time activity.

Improve caregiver's health status as evidenced by the following:

Develops and implements a plan for daily exercise
Makes and keeps appointments for annual physical/pelvic examinations and mammography

Develop a plan for monitoring caregiver's health status.

Teach and monitor use of daily log for recording caregiver's activities, rest/exercise periods, and hours of sleep.

Help patient/caregiver to develop an alternate plan for patient's care in the event of caregiver's illness. *Demands/stress of caregiving increase vulnerability by depleting energy reserves.*

REFERENCES

Brennan PF, Moore SM, Smyth KA: ComputerLink: Electronic support for the home caregiver. *Adv Nurs Sci* 13(4):14-27, 1991.

Bull MJ: Factors influencing family caregiver burden and health. *West J Nurs Res* 12(6):758, 1990.

Bull MJ: Managing the transition from hospital to home. *Qual Health Res*, 1992, 2(1):27-41.

Bunting SM: Stress on caregivers of the elderly, *Adv Nurs Sci*, 11(2):63, 1990.

Burns C, and others: New diagnosis: caregiver role strain. *Nurs Diagn*, 1993, 4(2):70-76.

Gaynor SE: The long haul: the effects of home care on caregivers. *Image: J Nurs Schol* 22(4):208, 1990.

Given BA, Given CW; Family caregiving for the elderly, *Ann Rev Nurs Res* 9:77, 1991.

Given CW, and others: The caregiver reaction assessment (CRA) for caregivers to persons with chronic physical and mental impairments. *Res Nurs Health*, 1992, 15(4):271-283,

Kuhlman GJ, and others: Alzheimer's disease and family caregiving: critical synthesis of the literature and research agenda. *Nurs Res* 40(6):331-337, 1991.

Langner SR: Ways of managing the experience of caregiving to elderly relatives, *West J Nurs Res*, 1993, 15(5):582-594,

Lindgren CL: Burnout and social support in family caregivers, *West J Nurs Res* 12(4):469, 1990.

Lindgren CL: The caregiver career, *Image: J Nurs Schol*, 1993, 25(3):214.

Stetz KM: Response to caregiving demands: their difficulty and effects on well-being of elderly caregivers. *Schol Inq Nurs Pract*, 1992, 6(2):129-133.

Willhagen I: Caregiving demands: their difficulty and effects on well-being of elderly caregivers. *Schol Inq Nurs Pract*, 1992, 6(2):111-127.

Woods NF, Yates BC, Primomo J: Supporting families during chronic illness. *Image: J Nurs Schol* 21(1):46, 1989.

Caregiver role strain, risk for

CLINICAL CONDITION/ MEDICAL DIAGNOSIS	RISK FACTORS
Diabetic wife, primary wage earner, caring for husband with COPD following hospital discharge	Competing role demands: severity of care recipient's illness

> **Patient goals**
> Expected outcomes
>> Associated nursing/collaborative interventions *and scientific rationale*

Establish a pattern of caregiving that is compatible with role demands as evidenced by the following:

Negotiates with employer for temporary reduction in work hours without loss of benefits

Contracts with health-care provider for specific services

Requests alternating weekend assistance from daughter and son who live within driving distance

> Formulate with caregiver alternatives for decreasing role demands, e.g., temporary reduction in work hours; use of formal health care services.
>
> Plan and facilitate a family conference to negotiate care commitments with caregiver's son and daughter.
>
> Provide caregiver with a list of home health-care providers and other community resources *Early recognition of "at risk" status of caregiver will facilitate realistic planning.*

Provide competent care for spouse as evidenced by the following.

Requests assistance with complex care activities

Keeps appointments to participate in patient care activities before discharge

Verbalizes confidence in ability to provide care

Contracts with health-care providers for specific services

Caregiver role strain, risk for

Help caregiver and patient to develop a written
  plan of care
Determine caregiver's competence to carry out
  required care.
Provide instruction of patient care activities.
Discuss with caregiver the importance of spending
  time with patient when no care is being
  provided. *Patient needs to feel the nurturing aspects
  of the relationship in contrast to "burden" of care.*

**Establish a self-care pattern consistent with role
demands and caregiver's health impairment as
evidenced by the following:**

**Makes appropriate sleeping arrangements
Equips husband's bedroom with electronic communi-
cation device to respond to his needs during night
Continues to follow diabetic regimen**

Negotiate with patient/caregiver for appropriate
  sleeping arrangements with some form of
  electronic communication.
Teach caregiver/recipient to recognize
  signs/symptoms of fatigue.
Teach importance of keeping lights at low level
  during night to prevent difficulty in falling
  asleep after responding to husband's request for
  assistance.
Teach caregiver to use a daily log to monitor own
  health status, e.g., hours of sleep, feelings, loss
  of weight.

REFERENCES

Archbold P and others: Mutuality and preparedness as predictors of caregiver role strain, *Res Nurs Health* 13: 375-384, 1990.
Brennan PF, Moore SM, Smyth KA: ComputerLink: Electronic support for the home caregiver, *Adv Nurs Sci* 13(4):14-27, 1991.
Bull MJ: Factors influencing family caregiver burden and health, *West J Nurs Res* 12(6):758, 1990.
Bull MJ: Managing the transition from hospital to home, *Qual Health Res* 2(1):27-41,1992.
Burns C and others: New diagnosis: caregiver role strain, *Nurs Diag* 4(2):70-76, 1993.
Cossette S, Levesque L: Caregiving tasks as predictors of mental health of wife caregiver of men with chronic obstructive pulmonary disease, *Res Nurs Health* 16, 251-263, 1993.
Gaynor SE: The long haul: the effects of home care on caregivers, *Image: J Nurs Schol* 22(4):208, 1990.

Given BA, Given CW: Family caregiving for the elderly, *Ann Rev Nurs Res* 9·77, 1991.

Given BA and others: Responses of elderly spouse caregivers. *Res Nurs Health* 13:77-85, 1990.

Given CW and others: The caregiver reaction assessment (CRA) for caregivers to persons with chronic physical and mental impairments, *Res Nurs Health* 15:271-283, 1992.

Langner SR: Ways of managing the experience of caregiving to elderly relatives, *West J Nurs Res* 15(5):582-594, 1993.

Lindgren CL: Burnout and social support in family caregivers, *West J Nurs Res* 12(4):469, 1990.

Lindgren CL: The caregiver career, *Image: J Nurs Schol* 5(3):214, 1993.

Stetz KM: Response to caregiving demands: their difficulty and effects on the well-being of elderly caregivers, *Schol Inq Nurs Pract* 6(2):129-133, 1992.

Willhagen MI: Caregiving demands: their difficulty and effects on the well-being of elderly caregivers, *Schol Inq Nurs Pract* 6(2):111-127, 1992.

Woods NF, Yates BC, Primomo J: Supporting families during chronic illness, *Image: J Nurs Schol* 21(1):46, 1989.

Communication, impaired, verbal

CLINICAL CONDITION/ MEDICAL DIAGNOSIS	RELATED FACTORS
Schizophrenia	Psychological barriers

Patient goals
Expected outcomes
> Associated nursing/collaborative interventions *and scientific rationale*

Overcome psychological barriers to increase ability to use or understand language in human interaction as evidenced by the following:

Transmits clear, concise, and understandable messages
> Use facilitative communication techniques while interacting with patient.
> Teach and support use of effective communication techniques. *Use of effective communication techniques, such as reflection, validation, and clarification, results in transmission of understandable messages.*
> Encourage initiation of conversations.
> Encourage expression of feelings.

Attends to appropriate stimuli
> Reduce stimuli to assist patient in attending to pertinent stimuli or increase stimuli to motivate patient.
> Assist in correction of faulty perception.
> Give clear, simple messages using language patient can understand.
> Teach patient to identify and focus on relevant stimuli. *Through manipulation of the environment, teaching, and role modeling, the nurse facilitates the patient's accurate perception of and response to stimuli.*

Uses congruent verbal and nonverbal communication

Match verbal and nonverbal communication during nurse patient interactions.

Validate meaning of nonverbal communication.

Point out discrepancies in verbal and nonverbal communication. *The message component of communication depends on translation of ideas, purpose, and intent into congruent verbal and nonverbal communication.*

Teach and encourage use of stress reduction techniques.

Sends and receives feedback

Increase patient's awareness of strengths and limitations in communication with others

Describe, demonstrate, and encourage use of active listening skills.

Provide feedback to patient.

Teach patient to accept, request, and send both positive and negative feedback. *Communication is modified or corrected through the regulatory process of feedback.*

Support efforts to use feedback.

Experience gratification from communication

Model, teach, and support use of confirming responses when communicating with others.

Teach patient evaluation of own and others' communication.

Demonstrate and support responsibility for communication. *Motivation to communicate is related to the gratification experienced from communication.*

REFERENCES

Boss BJ: Managing communication disorders in stroke, *Nurs Clin North Am* 26(4):985, 1991.

Carter I W: Assessing the emotional status of patients, *Oncol Nurs Forum* 19(3):523, 1992.

Crowther D: Metacommunications: a missed opportunity, *J. Psychosoc Nurs Ment Health Serv* 29:13, 1991.

Lekander BJ, Lehmann S, Lindquist R: Therapeutic listening: key intervention for several nursing diagnoses, *Dimens Crit Care Nurs* (US) 12(1):24, 1993.

Communication, impaired, verbal—cont'd

McFarland GK, Naschinski C: Communication. In Thompson JM, and others: *Mosby's clinical nursing*, ed 3, St Louis, 1993, Mosby-Year Book.

Naschinski C, McFarland GK: Impaired verbal communication. In McFarland GK, McFarlane EA: *Nursing diagnosis and intervention: planning for patient care*, ed 2, St Louis, 1993, Mosby-Year Book.

Putterbaugh S: Communicating when the patient cannot speak English, *Today's OR Nurs* 13(1):31, 1991.

Williams ML: An algorithm for selecting a communication technique with intubated patients, *Dimens Crit Care Nurs* 11(4):222, 1992.

Community coping, potential for enhanced

CLINICAL CONDITION/ MEDICAL DIAGNOSIS	RELATED FACTORS
Health care services not available to meet potential patient needs related to the increasing incidence of HIV-positive cases in a community that provides county public health services through not-for-profit agencies. The nurse, who is the director of the Sexually Transmitted Disease Clinic, initiates and coordinates the planning and intervention.	Lacks a plan for coordinating services between agencies to meet the potential needs of HIV-positive clients.

Patient/Community goals
Expected outcomes
  Associated nursing/collaborative interventions *and*
    scientific rationale

The community will experience enhanced coping by providing and maintaining the necessary health care services for HIV-positive clients as evidenced by the following:

Develops a comprehensive plan in conjunction with the not-for-profit agencies in the county in order to monitor persons with HIV from the time of screening
  Consult with an infectious disease specialist to identify necessary screening and interventions for persons with HIV. *The incubation period between becoming HIV positive and being diagnosed with AIDS may be as long as 10 years.*
  Consult with persons with HIV to identify needs.

Successful programs include consumers during the planning stages.

Identify agencies that have the potential for providing necessary services. *Monitoring of persons with HIV requires numerous services, such as sophisticated laboratory tests, substance abuse counseling and treatment, and home care.*

Identify sources for financing the expansion of existing programs and the development of new ones to meet the emerging needs of persons with HIV. *Funds are available from public and private sources; not-for-profit agencies generally have limited resources.*

Keep state and county health officers apprised of the ongoing efforts to provide services for persons with HIV. *When not-for-profit health care facilities are contractors that provide care for the county or state, it is mandatory that they communicate changing health care delivery needs and potential changes in a timely manner.*

Provide a designated place and time for routine screening specific to HIV-positive clients. *Limiting the clinic to persons with HIV provides an atmosphere where needs specific to these clients (such as social support, education, substance abuse intervention, and grief counseling) can be met.*

Provides resources for continuous and timely monitoring of persons with HIV

Facilitate timely referral to the HIV-positive clinic. *Baseline physical findings are required. Providing emotional support is requisite for coping with the diagnosis.*

Facilitate timely referral of persons with HIV once AIDS is diagnosed. *Care is generally available for patients once AIDS has been diagnosed.*

The community will experience enhanced coping by the coordination of multiagency provision of services to persons with HIV as evidenced by the following:

Identifies strategies for providing care across agencies

Facilitate an ongoing committee composed of community advocates for persons with HIV and a representative from each agency with the potential to provide care to persons with HIV. *Caregivers and advocates can work together to develop and implement a plan that delivers care efficiently.*

Provide a case manager for each person with HIV. *Case managers visit clients in their homes to identify individual needs that may not be recognized in a clinic setting. They monitor changes in health status and arrange for needed care expeditiously.*

Encourage on-site HIV screening of all patients receiving substance abuse treatment. *IV drug users are at increased risk for HIV infection. Making assessment available on site will facilitate early diagnosis and monitoring of HIV-positive cases.*

Provide a substance abuse counselor at all HIV-positive clinics. *Alcohol and drugs are often used by persons with HIV to cope with their diagnosis; these can interfere with immune status.*

Provide education across agencies to keep providers of health care updated with current HIV knowledge. *Research is ongoing that can impact care of HIV-positive clients. For example, screening at-risk pregnant patients is important, because recent studies have shown that treating the mother with acyclovir will decrease chances of the baby's developing AIDS.*

REFERENCES

Flynn B, Wiles D, Rider M: Empowering communities: action research through healthy cities, *Health Educ Q* 21(3):395, 1994.

Israel B, Checkoway B, Schulz A, Zimmerman M: Health education and community empowerment: conceptualizing and measuring perceptions of individual, organizational and community control, *Health Educ Q* 21(2):149, 1994.

Jemmott JB III, Jemmott LS: Alcohol and drug use during sexual activity: predicting the HIV-risk-related behaviors of inner-city black male adolescents, *J Adolesc Res* 8(1):41, 1993.

Swanson JM, Remy L, Chenitz WC, Chastain RL, Trocki KF: Illicit drug use among young adults with genital herpes, *Public Health Nurs* 10(3):197, 1993.

Talashek ML, Tichy A, Salmon M; The AIDS pandemic: a nursing model, *Public Health Nurs* 6(4):182, 1989.

Zidovudine for the prevention of HIV transmission from mother to infant, *MMWR Morb Mortal Wkly Rep* 43(16):285, 1994.

Community coping potential for enhanced—cont d

Community coping, ineffective

CLINICAL CONDITION/
MEDICAL DIAGNOSIS

Inadequate
immunization status
of many children
from a metropolitan
school district's
poorest school,
delaying school entry
which in turn affects
the school budget.
The school nurse
does the community
assessment and
intervention.

RELATED FACTORS

Isolation of families related to fear of
gang violence

Patient/Community goals
Expected outcomes
> Associated nursing/collaborative interventions *and*
> *scientific rationale*

The community will develop a pattern of coping for meeting threats to its health status as evidenced by the following:

Meets the immunization crisis by immunizing all children immediately so they can attend school

> Mobilize the resources of the health department to provide immunizations at the school. *This is resource management to deal with the crisis and is not a method to meet the ongoing needs of the community.*

> Notify parents of the availability of immunizations at the school, with both the mass media and flyers/posters in the community. *Disenfranchised citizens are difficult to reach, so interventions need to be at several levels.*

> Monitor the immunization status of students so that referrals are made in a timely manner. *Families that do not take advantage of available immunizations may be dysfunctional, with a potential for child abuse.*

Meets the well-child needs of all community children in a timely manner rather than in response to a crisis

Collaborate with health department clinic staff to identify issues associated with delivery of well-child services to children from the area with deficits in immunization coverage. *Immunization status is often inadequate for poor, preschool children. One fourth of preschool children and one third of poor children lack recommended immunizations. Organizational readiness is associated with success of programs.*

Identify a cohort of key informants (parents of children whose well-child needs have not been met). *Knowledge of individual perceptions of community problems is requisite to solving deficits in health care. Underuse is often a result of inadequate community involvement during the planning stage.*

Facilitate communication between health care providers of well-child care and community members disenfranchised from care. *Providers and consumers may have different perceptions of the problems associated with nonuse of services by the neediest community members.*

Empower community members to negotiate for needed well-child services. *Transferring power to the community enables members to begin sharing responsibility for their health.*

Mobilize available resources to immunize children in a timely manner. *This will ultimately save the system money by preventing childhood illnesses.*

The community will experience competence for dealing with threats to it as evidenced by the following:

Identifies strategies for reversing the trend toward gang anarchy and violence.

Facilitate formation of a community organizing group. *Community health nurses can be effective in using the social action model to help bring about change for areas with limited resources.*

Arrange for a meeting between area police and the community to develop a plan for better police coverage in this high-crime area. *The school nurse can act as an advocate for the community. There may be fear and resentment of the police, and arranging for them to communicate with community members is necessary for improving neighborhood safety.*

Enhance community competence by indicating community strengths. *Identifying community strengths is one method of capacity building in a community.*

Identify a safe place for children to receive health care. *Services will not be used if they are located in opposing gang territory.*

REFERENCES

Flynn B, Wiles D, Rider M: Empowering communities: action research through healthy cities, *Health Educ Q* 21(3):395, 1994.

Huesman LR, Eron LD, Lefkowitz NM, Walder LO: Stability of aggression over time and generations, *Develop Psychol* 20(6):1120, 1984.

Israel B, Checkoway B, Schulz A, Zimmerman M: Health education and community empowerment: conceptualizing and measuring perceptions of individual, organizational and community control, *Health Educ Q* 21(2):149, 1994.

Martaus TM, Bell ML, Kenyon V, Snow L, Hefty LV: Realities of developing community health orientation programs, *Public Health Nurs* 10(3):173, 1993.

McFarlene J, Fehir J: De madres a madres: a community, primary health care program based on empowerment, *Health Educ Q* 21(3):381, 1994.

Measles—United States, 1990, *MMWR Morb Mortal Wkly Rep* 40(22):369, 1991.

Plaut T, Landis S, Trevor J: Focus group and community mobilization. In Morgan D, ed: *Successful focus group*, Newbury Park, Cal, 1993, Sage.

Report of the Committee on Infectious Diseases of the American Academy of Pediatrics. *Red Book*, 22nd ed, Elk Grove Village, Illinois, 1991, American Academy of Pediatrics.

Rosenberg ML: *Violence in America*, New York, 1993, Oxford University Press.

Community coping, ineffective—cont'd

Confusion, acute

CLINICAL CONDITION/ MEDICAL DIAGNOSIS	RELATED FACTORS
Sixty-seven-year-old patient with history of chronic obstructive pulmonary disease and peripheral vascular disease recovering from abdominal aortic aneurysm surgery and embolectomy for lower extremity emboli and arterial occlusion.	Delirium

---

Patient goals
Expected outcomes
> Associated nursing/collaborative interventions *and scientific rationale*

Resolution of transient cerebral dysfunction as evidenced by the following:

No injury to self or others

Monitor for presence of signs and symptoms of acute confusion (e.g., fluctuation in levels of consciousness, attention, concentration, orientation, psychomotor activity; perceptual disturbances; sleep-wake disturbance that may include daytime somnolence and increased wakefulness at night; disorganization of thoughts and speech). *Patients with acute confusion are at increased risk to impulsively attempt to harm themselves (e.g., pulling out tubes or IV lines, getting out of bed) or others (by striking out).*

Collaborate with patient's physician and other members of multidisciplinary treatment team *to determine underlying causes for delirium (e.g., metabolic disturbances, systemic disease, infection, drug reactions) because delirium can become life-*

Confusion, acute

threatening if untreated and inappropriately managed.

Explain safety mechanisms in patient's immediate environment, such as call light, side rails, equipment alarm systems, surveillance by nurse. *Repeating the information, using short simple sentences, until patient's acute confusion subsides, will assist the patient in understanding the explanations.*

Provide ongoing close surveillance by staff, such as one-to-one around the clock if patient exhibits behaviors that are indicative of self-injury or self-harm.

Ensure close observation by nursing staff if patient becomes highly agitated *to minimize use of soft or leather restraints. Restraints can increase paranoia and agitation, and contribute to additional complications, including pulmonary embolism, deep vein thrombosis, atelectasis, pneumonia, and decubitus ulcers.*

Have a calm family member or friend remain with patient if he/she becomes extremely frightened or agitated *to provide reassurance from a familiar person while minimizing risk for self-harm.*

Achieves satisfactory sleep pattern

Avoid or minimize the use of benzodiazepines and drugs with anticholinergic properties such as diphenhydramine (Benadryl) to promote sleep *because of the propensity of these drugs to potentiate existing acute confusion.*

Collaborate with members of the health team to adhere to patient's scheduled periods of undisturbed rest *to minimize exacerbation of confusion because of sleep deprivation.*

Incorporate patient's usual technique for achieving rest and sleep, (e.g., soothing music, back rub, routine hygiene activities) *to promote satisfactory sleep pattern.*

Eliminate unnecessary environmental stimulation (e.g., staff interactions, excessive TV or radio, monitoring equipment) *to facilitate improved sleep-wake cycle.*

Differentiates between reality and unreality

Ensure that all staff members introduce self by name and call patient by preferred name *to reinforce patient's perception of reality.*

Ensure adequate non-glare lighting in patient's immediate environment, including night light, *to facilitate patient's reorientation to sensory cues and to reduce likelihood of visual distortions, misperceptions.*

Have patient's eyeglasses and hearing aids available (check to be sure that they are in working order) *to maximize accuracy of sensory input and to reduce potential for distortion of reality.*

Place appropriate visual cues within easy viewing of patient (e.g., calendar, clock, familiar photographs).

Do not argue with patient about his/her misinterpretations, and distortions of reality; acknowledge recognition that the experience is real and distressing for the patient.

Meets self-care needs to extent possible

Encourage patient to participate as much as possible in self-care activities, such as hygiene, bathing, grooming.

Provide a reasonable length of time for patient to complete self-care activities *based on assessment of patient's compromised mentation.*

Defer patient's participation in treatment team expectations, such as patient education, specific aspects of discharge planning, and major decision-making, until there is tangible evidence of improved mentation *because cognitive impairments compromise the patient's ability to participate in these activities*

Reduction in patient and family distress associated with mental status changes as evidenced by:

Family experiences reduced distress

Convey assurance to patient and family that the patient is safe in the present environment

171

Encourage family and friends to maintain ongoing contact with patient; keep the patient informed of family activities and plans.

Provide assurance to patient and family that total clearing from the acute confusion may take from several days to several weeks. *This will reduce anxiety associated with recognition of cognitive disturbance and uncertainty about its outcome.*

Conduct an assessment to determine need for debriefing both patient and family after acute confusion has been resolved. *This will reduce undue fear and anxiety about what actually happened and clarify patient's possible distortions of events that transpired during the period of acute confusion.*

REFERENCES

American Psychiatric Association: *Diagnostic and statistical manual of mental disorders*, ed 4, Washington DC., 1994, American Psychiatric Association.

Clark S: Psychiatric and mental health concerns in the patient with sepsis, *Critical Care Clin North Amer*, 6(2):389, 1994.

Evans CA, Kenny PJ, Rizzuto: Caring for the confused geriatric surgical patient, *Geriatric Nurs* 14(5):237, 1993.

Foreman MD: Complexities of acute confusion, *Geriatric Nurs*, 11(3):136, 1990.

Foreman MD: Confusion in the hospitalized elderly: incidence, onset, and associated factors, *Res Nurs Health*, 12:21, 1989.

Inaba-Roland K, Maricle RA: Assessing delirium in the acute care setting, *Heart Lung*, 21(1):48, 1992.

Lipowski ZJ: *Delirium: acute confusional states*, New York, 1990, Oxford University Press.

McFarland GK, Wasli EL, Gerety EK: *Nursing diagnoses and process in psychiatric mental health nursing*, ed 2, Philadelphia, 1992, JB Lippincott.

Sullivan-Marx EM: Delirium and physical restraint in the hospitalized elderly, *Image J Nurs Scholarship* 26(4):295, 1994.

Trzepacz PT: A review of delirium assessment instruments, *Gen Hosp Psychiatry* 16:397, 1994.

Confusion, acute—cont'd

Confusion, chronic

CLINICAL CONDITION/ MEDICAL DIAGNOSIS	RELATED FACTORS
Adult male diagnosed with Alzheimer's type of dementia (moderate) who is attending an adult day health care program.	Cognitive impairment causing inability to function independently on physical and social levels.

Patient goals
Expected outcomes
  Associated nursing/collaborative interventions *and scientific rationale*

Maintain ability to function in a structured adult day care program environment as evidenced by the following:

Participates in individual and group activities

Evaluate baseline health, functional and psychosocial status; i.e., with Mini-Mental State Exam (MMSE), Functional Independence Measure (FIM). *Multidisciplinary use of standard tests can provide common language to discuss change in patient's status.*

Determine previous activities and interests. *Understanding past preferences and activities may facilitate the caregiver's understanding of the context in which the individual is relating.*

Ensure that patient has optimal sensory input; i.e., check for clean eyeglasses, functioning hearing aid, absence of cerumen impaction.

Evaluate patient's stimulation threshold. *Overstimulation may precipitate behavior problems in the cognitively impaired.*

Select activities that the patient can complete successfully.

Engage in highly structured, repetitive group activities.

Provide opportunity for meaningful individual activities; i.e., recycling paper, folding towels, watering plants.

Incorporate rest time between activities. *Fatigue may precipitate behavior problems in the cognitively impaired.*

Use simple one-step commands when providing verbal cues; allow time to respond to command before providing additional instruction.

Observe continually for changes in behavioral and functional status. *Behavior changes often herald a change in health status in the cognitively impaired.*

Collaborate with physician if changes from baseline cognitive status are observed.

Instruct caregiver to report changes and observations to adult day health care program staff. *Caregivers are often the first to recognize subtle changes. Early treatment may prevent hospitalization.*

Maintains sense of self worth

Greet patient by preferred name.

Consistently use a calm approach when interacting with the individual.

Encourage tasks that patient can complete and master. *Mastery of a task contributes to an individual's sense of worth and control.*

Provide positive feedback; i.e., compliment on appearance and for contributions, thank for completing any task.

REFERENCES

Abraham IL, Reel, SJ: Cognitive nursing interventions with long-term care residents: Effects on neurocognitive dimensions, *Psychiatr Nurs* 6(6):356-365, 1992.

Armstrong-Esther CA, Browne KD, McAfee JG: Elderly patients: still clean and sitting quietly, *Advanced Nurs* 19:264-271, 1994.

Burgener SC, Shimer R, Murrell BS: Expressions of individuality in cognitively impaired elders; need for individual assessment and care, *Gerontol Nurs* 19(4):13-22, 1992.

Collins CE, Given BA, Given CW: Interventions with family caregivers of persons with Alzheimer's disease. *Nurs Clin North Amer* 29(1), 1994.

Fisher JE, Fink CM, Loomis CC: Frequency and management difficulty of behavioral problems among dementia patients in long-term care facilities. *Clin Gerontologist* 13(1):3-12, 1993.

Hall GR: Caring for people with Alzheimer's disease using the conceptual model of progressively lowered stress threshold in the clinical setting, *Nurs Clin North Amer* 29(1):129-141, 1994.

Stolley JM, Hall GR, Collins J, Bleuer N, Adrian C, Buckwalter KC: Managing the care of patients with irreversible dementia during hospitalization for comorbidities, *Nurs Clin North Amer* 28(4):767-782, 1993.

Constipation

CLINICAL CONDITION/ MEDICAL DIAGNOSIS	RELATED FACTORS
Chronic depression	Inadequate fluid and fiber in diet; daily ingestion of constipating medications

Patient goals
Expected outcomes
>   Associated nursing/collaborative interventions *and*
>   *scientific rationale*

Experience fewer incidences of constipation as evidenced by the following:

Obtains immediate relief
>   Insert bisacodyl (Dulcolax) suppository within 1 hour of breakfast *to increase stimulation of gastrocolic reflex*; or use lubricated, gloved finger to break up large masses of hard stool. Follow with tap-water enema.
>   Teach patient to exclude fatty acids from breakfast or triggering meal. *Fatty acids delay reflex stimulation and slow digestion.*

Takes fiber supplement once a day
Reports return to usual pattern of elimination: every 2 to 3 days
Verbalizes understanding of constipating effects of selected medications
>   Recommend use of fiber supplement such as psyllium (Metamucil) once a day while on constipating medications with increase to twice a day if needed.
>   Teach patient about constipating effects of medications.

Increase ingestion of fluids and fiber-rich foods as evidenced by the following:

Eats bran muffin or high fiber-bread daily
Eats one high-fiber vegetable daily and gradually increases to two or more
Increase fluid intake to 8 glasses daily

Constipation

Teach patient to record all intake for 48 hours.

Analyze eating pattern with patient.

Recommend diet changes to increase bulk in diet. *Gradual addition of fiber helps to avoid cramping and flatus.*

Recommend intake of 8 glasses of water daily.

REFERENCES

McLane AM, McShane RE: Constipation. In Maas M, Buckwalter KC, Hardy M, eds: *Nursing diagnosis and intervention for the elderly*, Redwood City, Cal, 1991, Addison-Wesley, pp. 147-148.

McLane AM, McShane RE: Empirical validation of defining characteristics of constipation: a study of bowel elimination practices of healthy adults. In Hurley M, ed: *Classification of nursing diagnoses: proceedings of the sixth conference*, St. Louis, 1986, Mosby-Year Book.

McLane AM, McShane RE: Constipation. In Thompson JM, and others: *Mosby's clinical nursing*, ed 3, St. Louis, 1993, Mosby, pp 1474-1477.

McShane RE, McLane AM: Constipation: impact of etiological factors, *J Geront Nurs* 14(4):31, 1988.

Constipation—cont'd

Constipation, colonic

CLINICAL CONDITION/ MEDICAL DIAGNOSIS	RELATED FACTORS
Elderly widower, six weeks after knee replacement	Preference for nonfibrous foods; restricted mobility (uses a walker)

Patient goals
Expected outcomes
    Associated nursing/collaborative interventions *and scientific rationale*

Establish a regular pattern of bowel movements as evidenced by the following:

Has a bowel movement at least every 3 days
Stool passes easily
Experiences sensation of complete passage of stool
Responds immediately to urge to defecate
    Suggest trial of bisacodyl (Dulcolax) suppository instead of oral laxatives within 1 hour of breakfast or triggering meal, *which will elicit gastrocolic reflexes. Reflexes are strongest when stomach is empty.*
    Establish toileting routine without use of suppositories or oral laxative.
    Teach patient importance of immediate response to urge to defecate. *Stool will harden in rectum in the presence of chronic distention.*

Modify dietary intake to increase ratio of high-fiber foods as evidenced by the following:

Eats bran in some form daily
Eats one high-fiber vegetable daily
Substitutes whole grain for white bread
Eats prunes, banana, or preferred fresh fruit daily
    Teach patient to record all intake for 48 hours.
    Analyze eating pattern with patient.

Constipation, colonic

Recommend diet changes to increase bulk in diet,
consistent with financial limitations; substitute
whole grain for white bread.
Recommend gradual addition of dietary fiber; 6 to
10 g of fiber each day. Slow addition of fiber
helps to avoid cramping and flatus

Increase activity level as evidenced by the following:

Increases length of walks 10 ft per week
Engages in active range of motion twice daily
Exercises abdominal muscles daily
**Substitutes 3 point cane for walker as increase in
strength permits**
Encourage outdoor walking (weather permitting).
Increase ambulation distance from 20 ft to 40 ft
and then to tolerance level.
Teach active range of motion and abdominal
strengthening exercises. *Inadequate exercise is a
major contributor to change in stool consistency.*

REFERENCES

Donald IP, and others: A study of constipation in the elderly living at
home *Gerontology* 31:112-118, 1985.
McLane AM, McShane RE: Colonic constipation. In Thompson JM,
and others: *Mosby's clinical nursing*, ed 3, St. Louis, 1993, Mosby, pp
1478-1480.
McLane AM, McShane RE: Bowel management. In Bulechek GM,
McCloskey JC, eds: *Nursing interventions: essential nursing treatments*,
Philadelphia, 1993, Mosby, pp 73-85.
McLane AM, McShane RE: Constipation. In Maas M, Buckwalter KC,
Hardy M, eds: *Nursing diagnosis and intervention for the elderly*,
Redwood City, Cal, 1991, Addison-Wesley, pp. 147-157.
McLane AM, McShane RE: Empirical validation of defining
characteristics of constipation: a study of bowel elimination
practices of healthy adults. In Hurley M, ed: *Classification of nursing
diagnoses: proceedings of the sixth conference*, St. Louis, 1986, Mosby-
Year Book.
McShane RE, McLane AM: Constipation: impact of etiological factors
J Gerontol Nurs 14(4):31, 1988.

Constipation, perceived

CLINICAL CONDITION/ MEDICAL DIAGNOSIS	RELATED FACTORS
Cholecystectomy, day surgery	Cultural health beliefs (expects to have a daily bowel movement; overuse of laxatives)

Patient goals
Expected outcomes
> Associated nursing/collaborative interventions *and scientific rationale*

Modify cultural health beliefs of family with respect for perceived need for having bowel movement as evidenced by the following:

Verbalizes receptivity to suggestion to have a bowel movement every 2 to 3 days

> Explore and acknowledge health beliefs and convictions.
> Confront health beliefs that maintain dysfunctional behavior. *Out-of-date information leads to faulty appraisal of pattern of elimination and need for laxatives.*

Modify toileting routines as evidenced by the following:

Drinks hot liquid before breakfast
Reports use of rectal suppository less than once a week

> Prescribe lemon juice and hot water every morning for 1-week trial.
> Teach patient to recognize and attend to stimulus behaviors, i.e., actions/behaviors that stimulate urge to defecate. *Gastrocolic reflexes are strongest when stomach is empty.*
> Teach patient to use a suppository to stimulate evacuation instead of using laxatives if bowel movements are less frequent than every 2 to 3 days.

Decrease use of laxatives as evidenced by the following:

Substitutes fresh fruit and vegetable sticks for desserts
Gradually increases walking to 1 mile three times a week

Provide instructions about increasing use of bulk and fiber in brown-bag lunches if patient carries a lunch.

Discuss temporary use of psyllium (Metamucil) to supplement gradual increase of natural fiber in diet. *Gradual addition of fiber to diet helps to avoid cramping and flatus.*

Teach patient role of exercise in developing and maintaining acceptable pattern of bowel elimination.

REFERENCES

McLane AM, McShane RE: Perceived constipation. In Thompson JM, and others: *Mosby's clinical nursing*, ed.3, St. Louis, 1993, Mosby, pp. 1477-1478.

McLane AM, McShane RE: Constipation. In Maas M, Buckwalter KC, Hardy M, eds: *Nursing diagnosis and intervention for the elderly*, Redwood City, Cal, 1991, Addison-Wesley, pp. 147-158.

McShane RE, McLane AM: Constipation: impact of etiological factors, *J Gerontol Nurs* 14(4):31, 1988.

Defensive coping

CLINICAL CONDITION/ MEDICAL DIAGNOSIS	RELATED FACTORS
Breast cancer	Stressful event; threat to self-esteem

Patient goals
Expected outcomes
    Associated nursing/collaborative interventions *and scientific rationale*

Experience defenses that are protective against stressful event and threat to self esteem as evidenced by the following:

No further insult to self-esteem
    Support patient's personhood, uniqueness, and right to be involved in decision making.
    Seek to understand patient's perspective of situation and what is stressful or threatening. Specifically, seek to understand patient's sense of self and role expectations of self. *Enhancing an individual's self-esteem involves, as a first step, exploring the discrepancies within his/her self-concept.*
    Gently clarify misconceptions.
    Reduce stressful aspects of life, e.g., encourage expression of emotions.
    Encourage maintenance of social support, including support from family, neighbors, clergy.
    Assist patient in becoming aware of behaviors that are harmful to others, such as ridiculing others, but do not try to push patient from defensive stance.

Demonstrates reduction in use of maladaptive defensive behaviors as evidenced by the following:

Verbalizes a realistic appraisal of the event, its demands, and coping resources available
Verbalizes comfort with ideal and perceived roles and competencies to manage situation
Communicates a sense of personal integrity

Defensive coping

Assist patient in exploring nature and characteristics of demands of breast cancer and coping resources required; identify where discrepancies exist between ideal and perceived roles in the situation. *Pace intervention to patient's readiness for assistance because a period of denial may be present.*

Help patient to identify desired goals in adjusting to breast cancer.

Where possible, reduce stressful aspects of the event and enhance patient's coping abilities through setting realistic, concrete goals with individual; identifying specific strategies for achieving goals; setting realistic time-frames for reaching goals; reviewing capabilities and learning from past experiences; exploring patterns of thinking (especially negative thoughts); teaching necessary knowledge and skills; acknowledging accomplishments toward desired goals; maintaining social networks; and encouraging expression of fears and concerns. *Pacing interventions with the patient's progression helps the patient adapt to the situation.*

REFERENCES

Aguilera D, Messick L: *Crisis intervention,* St. Louis, 1990, Mosby-Year Book.

Crouch MA, Straub V: Enhancement of self-esteem in adults, *Fam Com Health* 6(2):67, 1983.

Curbow B and others: Self concept and cancer in adults, *Soc Sci Med* 31(2):115-128, 1990.

Dean C, Surtees PG: Do psychological factors predict survival in breast cancer? *J Psychosom Res* 33:561 569, 1989.

Hagopian GA: Cognitive strategies used in adapting to a cancer diagnosis, *Oncol Nurs Forum* 20(5):759-763, 1993.

Heidrich SM, Ward SE: The role of the self in adjustment to cancer in elderly women, *Oncol Nurs Forum* 19(10):1491 1496, 1992.

Hoff LA: *People in crisis: understanding and helping,* ed 3, Toronto, 1989, Addison-Wesley.

Lazarus RS, The costs and benefits of denial. In Breznitz S, ed: *The denial of stress,* New York, 1983, International University Press.

Lazarus RS, Folkman S: *Stress, appraisal and coping,* New York, 1986, Springer Publishing.

Ward S, Leventhal H, Easterling D: Social support, self esteem and communication in persons receiving chemotherapy, *J Psychosoc Oncol* 9:98-116, 1991.

Defensive coping—cont'd

Coping, family: potential for growth

CLINICAL CONDITION/ MEDICAL DIAGNOSIS	RELATED FACTORS
Birth of second child	Adaptive tasks effectively addressed; progress toward self-actualization

Patient goals
Expected outcomes
> Associated nursing/collaborative interventions *and scientific rationale*

Actualize growth potential of family as evidenced by:

Verbalizes changes in family roles/relationships
Assist family to identify changes in family dynamics resulting from birth of second child.
Assist family to identify effects of changes on family processes.

Verbalizes changes in individual attitudes, values and goals
Assist family to identify changes in individual family members resulting from birth of second child.
Assist family to identify strengths in coping with changes.

Chooses goals and experiences that foster growth of child
Discuss goals and experiences that maximize growth potential for all family members.
Provide information as needed to enable individuals/family to develop new goals that relate to individuals and total family system.
Facilitate development of new methods of goal attainment.
Collaborate with family members in planning and implementing life style changes. *Most families may be viewed as healthy but in need of temporary support. Intervention should be aimed at promoting family competence.*

Develop broader base of support as evidenced by:

Verbalizes interest in contacting others experiencing a similar situation

Identify family readiness to accept support from additional sources.

Assist family members to identify types of support needed.

Develops additional relationships that provide support during crisis

Inform family members of appropriate health care and community resources.

Refer family to appropriate resources.

Initiate contact with community resources if necessary.

Sustains contact with additional sources

Follow up to assure sustained contact and appropriateness of assistance.

Teach strategies to access and maximize community resources. *Individual/family should be aided in developing a broader base of support in order to maximize growth potential.*

REFERENCES

Bowers JE: Coping, family, potential for growth. In McFarland GK and Thomas MD: *Psychiatric mental health nursing: application of the nursing process,* Philadelphia, 1991, Lippincott.

Craft MJ, Willadsen JA: Interventions related to family, *Nurs Clin North Am* 27(2):517, 1992.

Denehy JA: Interventions related to parent-infant attachment, *Nurs Clin North Am* 27(2):4225, 1992.

Lipman TH: Assessing family strengths to guide plan of care using Hymovich's framework, *J Pediatr Nurs* 4:186, 1989.

Sims SL, Boland DL, O'Neill CA: Decision making in home health care, *West J Nurs Res* 14(2):186, 1992.

Zerwekh JV: Laying the groundwork for family self-help: locating families, building trust, and building strength, *Pub Health Nurs* 9(1):15, 1992.

Coping, ineffective family: compromised

CLINICAL CONDITION/ MEDICAL DIAGNOSIS	RELATED FACTORS
Child with AIDS	Inadequate understanding by family members; temporary family disorganization

> **Patient goals**
> Expected outcomes
>> Associated nursing/collaborative interventions *and scientific rationale*

Develop adequate understanding of situation as evidenced by:

Verbalizes need for more information or clearer understanding relating to the situation

Provide adequate and correct information to patient and family members.

Monitor areas in which knowledge or understanding is inadequate in relation to HIV/AIDS.

Provide coordination of services through a case manager *to prevent failure to meet needs or duplication of services.*

Demonstrates understanding of information given

Encourage family to have realistic perspective based on accurate information.

Discusses changes in patient and family as result of health challenge

Encourage family members to discuss usual reactions to HIV/AIDS, such as anger, anxiety, dependency, and depression.

Verbalizes feelings to health care professionals and other family members

Encourage family members to verbalize feelings such as loss, guilt, or anger.

Use communication techniques that confirm legitimacy of both positive and negative feelings, e.g., reflecting feelings ("You seem frightened") or presenting reality ("Many people feel angry during this situation").

Provide opportunities for patient to discuss need for support with family members.

Encourage patient and family members to discuss expectations with each other. *Supportive and informational family education is essential in helping a family that is experiencing ineffective coping. Family growth can be promoted through fostering a sense of "family" within an educational climate.*

Cope with changes in family processes as evidenced by:

Identifies changes in family processes as a result of the child's illness with AIDS

Help family to appraise the situation, including both strengths and weaknesses.

Help family to identify changes in relationships resulting from child's illness with AIDS.

Assumes new roles as necessary to maintain family integrity

Help family members to recognize role changes needed to maintain family integrity.

Refer family member to appropriate additional sources for help in adjusting to changes in family processes. *Encouragement to use sources outside the family may be appropriate to preserve the supportive capacity of family members in assuming new roles over time.*

Family member participates in care of patient

Involve family member in care of patient as much as possible. *Family competence can be increased by restructuring of role relationships.*

REFERENCES

Boland MG, Conviser R. Nursing care of the child. In Flaskerud JH, Ungvarski PJ, eds: *HIV/AIDS: a guide to nursing care*, Philadelphia, 1992, Saunders.

Brown MA, Powell-Cope GM: AIDS family caregiving: transitions through uncertainty, *Nurs Res* 40(6):338, 1991.

Brown MA, Powell-Cope GM: Themes of loss and dying in caring for a family member with AIDS, *Res Nurs Health* 16(3):179, 1993.

Coping, ineffective family: compromised—cont'd

Flaskerud, JH: Psychosocial aspects, In Flaskerud JH, Ungvarski PJ, eds: *HIV/AIDS: a guide to nursing care*, Philadelphia, 1992, Saunders.

Jansen C, and others: Family problems during cancer chemotherapy, *Oncol Nurs Forum* 20(4):689, 1993.

Panel on Women, Adolescents, and Children with HIV Infections and AIDS: Family-centered comprehensive care for children with HIV infection, Washington, D.C., 1991, US DHHS.

Coping, ineffective family: compromised—cont'd

Coping, ineffective, family: disabling

CLINICAL CONDITION/ MEDICAL DIAGNOSIS	RELATED FACTORS
Parent with senile dementia, Alzheimer's type	Dissonant discrepancy of coping styles; highly ambivalent family relationships

Patient goals
Expected outcomes
    Associated nursing/collaborative interventions *and scientific rationale*

Demonstrate improved coping strategies as evidenced by:

Verbalizes perceptions of coping styles and areas of conflict

Help family members and patient to verbalize own perceptions of coping styles and areas of conflict.

Identify areas of conflict in coping styles among individuals and within family unit.

Monitor individual and family coping styles.

Identifies alternative coping behaviors that may minimize conflict

Help family members and patient to identify alternative coping behaviors to minimize conflict in adapting to health challenge.

Help family members and patient to focus on present feelings.

Incorporates alternative coping behaviors in adapting to health challenge

Assist family members and patient in practicing alternative coping behaviors: relabeling, role playing, contracting, etc. *A family with limited understanding about various coping strategies may need information about alternatives as well as the potential effect of conflict on coping styles.*

Assistance in learning alternative coping behaviors may be essential in aiding the family members and patient in incorporating new behaviors.

Coping, ineffective, family: disabling

Improve level of complementarity in role relationships as evidenced by:

Discusses complementary nature of strengths, needs, and expectations of relationships

Help patient and family members to verbalize individual needs and expectations of relationships as patient's mental status changes.

Help patient and family members to identify individual strengths and weaknesses in adapting to changes in patient's physical and mental health.

Identifies areas where needs and expectations are not being met, leading to feelings of powerlessness

Assist patient and family members to discuss areas where individual strengths, needs, and expectations complement each other in adapting to changes in patient's physical and mental status.

Help patient and family members to identify needs and expectations that are not being met.

Identifies strategies to aid developing complementary relationships which can overcome feelings of powerlessness

Help patient and family members identify additional strategies to develop complementary relationships in adapting to changes in patient's physical and mental status.

Incorporates alternative strategies in relationships

Assist patient and family members in practicing new strategies. *A family experiencing disabling anxiety as a result of inability to cope with the changes in role relationships imposed by a health challenge may be assisted by helping them to identify the changes that have occurred. Once needs and expectations have been explored, specific strategies to develop complementary relationships in the current situation can be identified and practiced.*

REFERENCES

Farren CJ, and others: Finding meaning: an alternative paradigm for Alzheimer's disease family caregivers, *Gerontologist*, 31:483, 1991.

Griffith JL, Griffith ME: Structural family therapy in chronic illness, *Psychosomatics* 28:202, 1987.

Coping, ineffective, family: disabling—cont'd

King S, and others: Institutionalization of an elderly family member: reactions of spouse and nonspouse caregivers, *Arch Psychiatr Nurs* 5(6):323, 1991.

Knafl KA, Deatrick JA: Family management style: concept analysis and development, *J Pediatr Nurs* 5·4, 1990.

McCubbin H, Patterson J, eds: *Systematic assessment of family stress: resources and coping*, St. Paul, 1981, University of Minnesota.

Swearingen PL: *Manual of medical-surgical nursing care: nursing interventions and collaborative management*, ed 3, St. Louis, 1994, Mosby, p. 765.

Weitzman J: Engaging the severely dysfunctional family in treatment: basic considerations, *Fam Process* 24:473, 1985.

Coping, ineffective, family: disabling—cont'd

Coping, ineffective individual

CLINICAL CONDITION/ MEDICAL DIAGNOSIS	RELATED FACTORS
Depressive disorder HIV-infected	Fear of relapse Inadequate social support system

Patient goals
Expected outcomes
  Associated nursing/collaborative interventions *and*
    scientific rationale

Has plan for handling a recurrence of depression and/or appearance of signs of infection as evidenced by:

Identifies two or three scenarios in which depressive thoughts and feelings may return

Assist in recalling knowledge of depression and HIV.

Identify the steps that were taken to deal with problem.

Examine with patient what helped in past and what might be helpful in future. *Identification of stressor, strategies to cope, future stressors, and treatments increases adaptation.*

Identifies two or more actions to take to avoid recurrence of depression

Instruct about ways in which people cope with increased stress.

Teach relaxation techniques.

Discuss usefulness/lack of usefulness of denial of feelings.

Assist in writing down actions to take *in order to enhance appropriate follow-up.*

Identifies signs and symptoms of infections common to HIV-infected patients and the need to take prompt action

Instruct the patient to monitor self for fever, thrush, sore throat, coughing, rashes, etc.

Discuss with patient general medical therapies to treat medical conditions.

Coping, ineffective individual

Identify what preventive actions can be taken to maintain health, i.e., adequate diet, fluids, exercise, rest, medication, etc.

Establishes support system as evidenced by:

Maintains contact with family member by phone, with one or two friends, and with HIV support group

Decrease stress-producing significant other–client relationship by not promoting contact.

Monitor interpersonal problems with friends and assist in resolving problems as they occur.

Promote continued attendance at HIV support group. *Social support provided in groups gives opportunity to learn ways to cope with emotions, thereby reducing anxiety, depression, and other emotional distress.*

Acknowledges the human need for others and the consequences for self when isolation occurs

Provide opportunity to discuss fear of intimacy and rejection by others. *Focusing on interpersonal issues using interpersonal therapy concepts assists patients to solve problems and to use coping resources.*

Instruct about the impact of isolation on thoughts and feelings.

REFERENCES

Anderson BL: Psychological interventions for cancer patients to enhance the quality of life, *J Consult Clin Psychol* 60(4):552, 1992.

Depression Guideline Panel: Depression in primary care, vol 1. Diagnosis and detection. In *Clinical practice guideline*, No. 5 (AHCPR Pub No. 93-0550), Rockville, MD, 1993, USDHHS, PHS, AHCPR.

Depression Guideline Panel: Depression in primary care, vol 2. Treatment of major depression. In *Clinical practice guideline*, No. 5 (AHCPR Pub No. 93-0551), Rockville, MD, 1993, USDHHS, PHS, AHCPR.

Dow MG: Affective disorder. In Bellack AS, Hersen M, eds: *Handbook of behavior therapy in the psychiatric setting*, New York, 1993, Plenum Press.

Kelly JA and others: Outcome of cognitive-behavioral and support group brief therapies for depressed, HIV-infected persons, *Am J Psychiat* 150(11):1679, 1993.

Janis IL: Decision making under stress. In Goldberger L, Breznitz, eds: Handbook of stress: theoretical and clinical aspects, ed 2, New York, 1993, Free Press.

Klerman GJ and others: *Interpersonal psychotherapy of depression*, New York, 1984, Basic Books.

Manderino MA, Brown MC: A practical, step-by-step approach to stress management for women, *Nurs Pract* 17(7):18, 1992.

Markowitz JC, Klerman GL, Perry SW: Interpersonal psychotherapy of depressed HIV-positive outpatients, *Hosp Community Psychiatry* 43(9):885, 1992.

Meichenbaum D, Fitzpatrick D: A constructivist narrative perspective on stress and coping: stress inoculation applications. In *Handbook of stress: theoretical and clinical aspects*, New York, 1993, Free Press.

Wilson PH: Depression. In Wilson PH, ed: *Principles and practice of relapse prevention*, New York, 1992, Guilford Press.

Coping, ineffective individual—cont'd

Decisional conflict (prenatal genetic testing)

CLINICAL CONDITION/ MEDICAL DIAGNOSIS	RELATED FACTORS
Pregnancy	Unclear goals and values; unrealistic expectations

Patient goals
Expected outcomes
    Associated nursing/collaborative interventions *and scientific rationale*

Make and implement an informed choice that is consistent with personal goals and values as evidenced by the following:

Understands what genetic testing can achieve
    Explore patient's goals and clarify alternatives and their possible consequences. *Lack of information or clarity of these items contributes to decisional conflict.*

Expresses realistic consequences of having and not having prenatal testing; values the consequences as positive or negative
    Realign unrealistic expectations. *Distortion in expectations often increases conflict (e.g., anticipating a negative consequence when the likelihood is extremely low) or regret (e.g., anticipating a positive consequence when the likelihood is extremely low).*

Identifies priority of anticipated consequences and implicit tradeoffs in selection process
    With the patient, clarify the patient's views on the desirability of possible consequences and their priority ordering. *Unclear values contribute to decisional conflict.*
    Identify value tradeoffs implicit in making choices. *Having to make tradeoffs often contributes to conflict. Knowing what makes the decision difficult helps in its resolution.*

Selects course of action consistent with personal values

Facilitate alternative selection consistent with personal values. *Value congruence increases satisfaction with the decision and the likelihood the patient will follow through on the choice.*

Uses self-help skills in implementing selected course of action; expresses satisfaction with the decision made

Teach and reinforce self-help skills required to obtain support from others, to deal with unwanted pressure from others, and to implement the choice. *Individuals have difficulty in implementing decisions made without the resources to do so.*

REFERENCES

Janis H, Mann I: *Decision making*, New York, 1977, The Free Press.

Keeney RL: *Value-Focused thinking*, Cambridge Mass, 1992, Harvard University Press.

Pender NJ, Pender AR: *Health promotion in nursing practice*, ed 2, East Norwalk, Conn, 1987, Appleton-Lange.

Rothert ML, Talarczyk GJ: Patient compliance and the decision making process of clinicians and patients, *J Compliance Health Care* 2:55, 1987.

Sjogren B, Vdbenberg N: Decision making during the prenatal diagnostic procedure, *Prenat Diagn* 8:263, 1988.

LINDA O'BRIEN-PALLAS, JANE E. GRAYDON, AND GERTRUDE K. MCFARLAND

Denial, ineffective

CLINICAL CONDITION/ MEDICAL DIAGNOSIS	RELATED FACTORS
Myocardial infarction, MI	Life-threatening event

> **Patient goals**
> **Expected outcomes**
>> Associated nursing/collaborative interventions *and scientific rationale*

Maintain appropriate level of denial in relation to life-threatening event as evidenced by the following:

Remains appropriately defended and expresses low to moderate anxiety

Focus on establishing a trust relationship with patient.

Determine patient's degree of denial and its effectiveness as a coping strategy *because some degree of denial may be necessary for patient functioning.*

If patient is using full denial, make periodic checks as to patient's stage of denial.

Never directly confront patient's denial *because the patient may not be able to handle the resulting anxiety.*

Acknowledges and expresses some reduction of problems and concerns

Provide patient with the opportunity to express any fears or anxieties of which he/she is aware.

Provide patient with specific information about MI and/or reassurance if he/she raises any questions or concerns as appropriate to the stage of denial the patient is experiencing.

Do not push the patient to raise questions or concerns if he/she is not ready. *Working with the patient in terms of his/her particular stage of denial at any point in time is important.*

REFERENCES

Breznitz S: The seven kinds of denial. In Breznitz S, ed. *The denial of stress*, New York, 1983, International University Press.

Forchuck C, Westwall J: Denial, *J Psychosoc Nurs Ment Health*, 25(6):9, 1987.

Forsyth GL, Delaney KD, Gresham ML: Vying for a winning position: management style of the chronically ill, *Res Nurs Health* 7:181, 1984.

Hackett TP, Cassem NH, Wishnic HA: The coronary care unit—an appraisal of its psychological hazards, *N Engl J Med* 279:1365, 1968.

Johnson JL, Morse JM: Regaining control: the process of adjustment after myocardial infarction, *Heart Lung* 19(2):126, 1990.

Keckeison ME, Nyamathi AM: Coping and adjustment to illness in the acute myocardial infarction patient, *J Cardiovasc Nurs* 5(1):25, 1990.

Lazarus RS, The costs and benefits of denial. In Breznitz S, ed: *The denial of stress*, New York, 1983, International University Press.

Lowery BJ: Psychological stress, denial and myocardial infarction outcomes, *Image: J Nurs Schol* 23:51-55, 1991.

Shelp EE, Perl M: Denial in clinical medicine: a reexamination of the concept and its significance, *Arch Intern Med* 145:697, 1985.

Weisman AD: *On dying and denying*, New York, 1982, Behavior Publications.

Denial, ineffective—cont'd

Diarrhea

CLINICAL CONDITION/ MEDICAL DIAGNOSIS	RELATED FACTORS
Malnutrition and dysphagia: enteral tube feeding with infusion pump	Change in enteral feeding; clogged nasogastric tube

Patient goals
Expected outcomes
  Associated nursing/collaborative interventions *and scientific rationale*

Receive enteral feeding, fluids, medications safely as evidenced by the following:

Body weight increases
Number of liquid, nonformed stools decreases
Fluids/electrolytes gradually return to normal

  Consult with physician to replace clogged silicone nasogastric tube with polyurethane nasoduodenal tube, size 10 or 12 Fr. *Polyurethane tubes are coated with a hydrophilic substance that decreases clogging rate.*

  Restart feedings at a slower rate until diarrhea is under control; then gradually increase to desired rate.

  Keep head of bed elevated during feedings and for 1/2 hour after feeding.

  Irrigate tube with 30 ml of water every 2 hours, after every intermittent feeding, and after administration of a medication through tube.

  Provide extra water (0.5 ml of water for every 1 ml of tube feeding) *to help patient excrete the solute load and keep serum sodium within normal range.*

  Check infusion pump every hour.

  Refrigerate opened containers of enteral feedings, discard containers and administration sets every 24 hours.

REFERENCES
Bodkin NL, Hansen BC: Nutritional studies in nursing, *Ann Rev Nurs Res* 9:203-220. 1991.

McCloskey JC, Bulechek GM: *Iowa intervention project: Nursing interventions classification (NIC)*, St. Louis, 1992, Mosby-Year Book, p. 233.

Metheny N, Eisenberg P, McSweeney M: Effect of feeding tube properties and three irrigants on clogging rates. *Nurs Res* 37(3):165-169, 1988.

Metheny N, Eisenberg P, McSweeney M: The effect of three irrigants on clogging rates of feeding tubes. In Funk SG, and others, eds.: *Key aspects of recovery: improving nutrition, rest, and mobility*, 1990, pp. 157-164.

Poyss AS: Fluid therapy. In Bulechek GM, McCloskey JC: *Nursing interventions: essential nursing treatments*, ed 2, Philadelphia, 1992, Saunders, pp. 232-246.

Smith CE and others: Diarrhea associated with tube feeding in mechanically ventilated critically ill patients. *Nurs Res* 39(3):148-152, 1990.

Disuse syndrome, risk for

CLINICAL CONDITION/ MEDICAL DIAGNOSIS	RISK FACTORS
Paralysis, altered level of consciousness	Immobility

Patient goals
Expected outcomes
  Associated nursing/collaborative interventions *and scientific rationale*

Maintain joint movement, muscle size and strength, and bone mineralization as evidenced by the following:

Full ROM in joints
Muscle size and strength within normal limits
Ability to bear weight without discomfort

  Perform active/passive ROM exercises *to maintain functional integrity of muscles and joints through use, prevent disuse atrophy of muscles, and prevent contracture development in muscles and joints through stretching of connective tissue.*

  Maintain anatomic positioning of limbs *to maintain structural integrity of muscles and joints and prevent contracture development.*

  Perform isometric muscle setting exercises *to maintain muscle tone*

  Dangle at bedside as tolerated. Assist patient up to chair as tolerated.

  Ambulate as tolerated. *Weight bearing prevents calcium loss through increased bone deposition.*

Maintain adequate systemic and local tissue perfusion as evidenced by the following:

Blood pressure remains normal and no complaint of dizziness during position changes
Peripheral pulses remain intact
No dependent edema formation
No complaint of weakness/fatigue with activity

Disuse syndrome risk for

Perform bed exercises as tolerated *to promote venous return and CV work capacity.*

Apply antiembolism stockings *to prevent venous pooling in extremities.*

Perform positional change in relation to gravity as tolerated: supine to semi-upright to upright *to prevent decreased orthostatic capacity by enhancing neurovascular tone.*

Actively contract muscles of lower extremities when assuming upright position *to increase muscle pumping of pooled blood to increase venous return and maintain cardiac output.*

Promote feelings of independence and control as evidenced by the following:

Does not verbalize feelings of powerlessness or loss of control

Participates in self-care and ADLs to maximum extent possible

Patient and family/significant others express satisfaction with patient's progress and treatment

Allow opportunity for decision making regarding care *to increase patient's sense of control related to situation and environment.*

Encourage participation in ADLs as tolerated.

Encourage independence in self-care activities.

Introduce and encourage use of assistive devices prn.

Maintain normal skin and tissue integrity as evidenced by the following:

Skin remains dry, pink, warm, and intact, especially over bony prominences and pressure points

Reposition frequently, at least every 1 to 2 hours, *to relieve pressure and promote tissue perfusion.*

Inspect all pressure points at least every 2 hours.

Provide clean, dry, and wrinkle-free bedding.

Use assistive pressure-relief devices as needed (e.g., foam mattress, gel flotation pads, air-fluidized bed).

Consider use of continuous mechanical turning or continuous lateral rotation therapy (CLRT)

(oscillating bed or kinetic treatment table) to provide continuous side-to-side positional changes, *which have been found to decrease incidence of pressure ulcer formation in immobilized patients.*

Maintains normal tissue turgor, elasticity, and strength

Encourage adequate intake of fluid and diet *to provide tissue hydration and nutrient supply.*

Provide adequate protein in diet *to maintain positive nitrogen balance.*

Maintain normal patterns of elimination as evidenced by the following:

Urine output within normal limits
Urine remains clear, light yellow, and without sediment
Urine specific gravity is 1.010 to 1.025
Bowel movement per regular pattern
Stool soft and formed
Absence of discomfort when urinating or defecating
Absence of urinary frequency or urgency

Encourage adequate fluid intake *to increase volume of urine and water volume of stool.*

Assist patient to get up to bathroom or commode as tolerated. *Anatomic position will facilitate complete emptying of bladder and bowel aided by gravity and muscle contraction.*

Reposition frequently *to prevent pooling and stasis of urine in bladder and promote gastric motility.*

Provide adequate roughage (fiber, fruit, vegetables) in diet as tolerated *to provide bulk and stimulate peristalsis.*

Provide acid ash diet *to maintain acidity (lower pH level) of urine.*

Give stool softener/laxatives as indicated.

Provide privacy during acts of voiding/defection.

Maintain appropriate and adequate sensory and perceptual status as evidenced by the following:

Remains oriented to time, person, and place

    Provide access to clock, radio, television, reading materials, and other appropriate diversionary, stimulating activities.

    Encourage visits from others.

    Maintain normal day/night light patterns.

    Avoid monotonous sensory stimuli.

Maintain effective breathing pattern and patent airway as evidenced by the following:

Expectorates secretions

Breath sounds clear

Tidal volume, negative inspiratory force (NIF), and vital capacity within normal limits

Chest excursion is complete and equal bilaterally

    Perform deep breathing and coughing exercises every hour *to promote respiratory muscle excursion and mobilize secretions.*

    Encourage adequate fluid intake *to provide hydration to keep secretions loose and moist.*

    Monitor breath sounds.

    Reposition frequently or consider use of continuous mechanical turning or CLRT (oscillating bed or kinetic treatment table) to prevent pooling of secretions and body fluids. *CLRT has been found to decrease incidence of pulmonary complications in immobilized patients.*

REFERENCES

Dettmer DK, Teasell R: Complications of immobility and bedrest. Part I Musculoskeletal and cardiovascular complications, *Can Fam Physician* 39:1428-32, 1435-37, 1993.

Lentz M: Selected aspects of deconditioning secondary to immobilization, *Nurs Clin North Amer* 16(4):729-737, 1981.

Mobily PR, Kelley LS: Iatrogenesis in the elderly; Factors of immobility, *J Geront Nurs* 17(9):5-11, 1991.

Olson E, ed: The hazards of immobility, *Amer J Nurs* 67(4):780-797, 1967.

Sahn SA: Continuous lateral rotational therapy and nosocomial pneumonia, *Chest* 99(5):1263-7, 1991.

Shekleton ME: Impaired physical mobility. In Shekleton M, Litwack K, ed: *Critical care nursing of the surgical patient*, Philadelphia, 1991, W.B. Saunders

Titler M, and others: Classification of nursing interventions for care of the integument, *Nurs Diagn* 2(2), 45-56, 1991.

GERTRUDE K. MCFARLAND AND KAREN E. INABA

Diversional activity deficit

CLINICAL CONDITION/ MEDICAL DIAGNOSIS	RELATED FACTORS
Elderly patient with a hip replacement	Limited leisure resources; long-term hospitalization

Patient goals
Expected outcomes
    Associated nursing/collaborative interventions *and scientific rationale*

Identify strengths and limitations with respect to engaging in diversional activities as evidenced by the following:

Sets realistic goals for diversional activities

Review patient's usual pattern of diversional activities *to assess activity level, tolerance, and preferences.*

Assist patient in describing desired or required activity level changes needed because of altered health status.

Encourage discussion of limitations in usual pattern of diversional activities *to assess impact of stressors and level of adjustment.*

Seeks out realistic opportunities within limited resources for involvement in diversional activities

Provide opportunities to continue meaningful diversional activities that are realistic within current environment *to support patient's sense of self-worth and productivity.*

Assist patient in adapting diversional activities to changed health status.

Include patient in making decisions about varying the daily routine *to promote a sense of control and recognition of personal preferences.*

Facilitate opportunities for visits from friends and family *to stimulate social interaction and contact with the outside world.*

Diversional activity deficit

Identifies strategies for dealing with limited leisure resources and obtains needed resources as evidenced by the following:

Assumes responsibility for choosing and participating in diversional activities in current environment

Assist patient in identifying realistic resources and energy expenditures required to participate in meaningful activities. *Discussion provides opportunities for mutual goal setting and problem-solving.*

Inform patient about options for diversional activities available in current setting (e.g., recreational therapy, occupational therapy, art/music therapy, remotivation therapy, support groups) *to assist in structuring free time and decreasing boredom.*

Support patient's perceptions of resources needed to participate in satisfying diversional activity in individual situation (e.g., confinement).

Engages in satisfactory diversional activities during long-term hospitalization as evidenced by the following:

Initiates participation and demonstrates ongoing interest in diversional activities available in current environment

Help patient assess changes in ability to engage in preferred diversional activities and assist with problem-solving.

Provide feedback to patient about observed level of participation and self-structuring of free time. *Social reinforcement encourages continued efforts by the patient.*

Expresses pleasure and satisfaction with diversional activities in current setting

Integrate diversional activity into patient's daily schedule of care whenever possible.

Adapt daily routine and environment to provide physical and mental stimulation and variety (e.g., change of scenery, creative activities) *to enhance socialization, coping, and involvement in the milieu.*

Encourage patient to provide feedback about satisfaction with choice of activities.

REFERENCES

Abraham IL and others: Therapeutic work with depressed elderly, *Nurs Clin North Am* 26(3):635, 1991.

Badry E, Robins M, Forestier M: Diversional therapy, *Can Nurs* 86(2):33, 1990.

Chin-Sang V, Allen KR: Leisure and the older black woman, *J Gerontol Nurs* 17:30, 1991.

Hutchinson SA, Bondy E: The pals program intergenerational remotivation, *J Gerontol Nurs* 16(12):19, 1990.

Janssen JA, Gilberson DL: Remotivation therapy, *J Gerontol Nurs* 14(6):31, 1988.

Jongbloed L, Morgan D: An investigation of involvement in leisure activities after a stroke, *Am J Occupat Ther* 45(5):420, 1991.

Radziewicz RM, Schneider SM: Using diversional activity to enhance coping, *Cancer Nurs* 15(4):293, 1992.

Reed PG: Mental health of older adults, *West J Nurs Res* 11(2):143, 1989.

Rubenfeld MG: Diversional activity deficit. In McFarland GK, McFarlane EA, eds: *Nursing diagnosis and intervention*, ed 2, St. Louis, 1993, Mosby-Year Book

Dysreflexia

CLINICAL CONDITION/ MEDICAL DIAGNOSIS	RELATED FACTORS
Patient has a spinal cord injury (T7 or above) with afferent stimulation below the level of the injury	Distended bladder Cutaneous stimuli below T7

Patient goals
Expected outcomes
> Associated nursing/collaborative interventions *and scientific rationale*

Prevent episodes of dysreflexia as evidenced by the following:

Recognizes the signs and symptoms of autonomic dysreflexia

> Teach signs and symptoms of dysreflexia (e.g., elevation of blood pressure >20 mm Hg above patient baseline, pounding headache, visual changes, pallor below level of injury, bradycardia, sweating, piloerection, facial flushing, flushed warm skin above the injury, nasal stuffiness).

Demonstrates understanding of effects of bladder and bowel distention on dysreflexia.

> Teach methods to prevent bladder distention (e.g., Foley care, intermittent catheterization). *Bladder distention is the most common cause of autonomic dysreflexia.*

> Maintain adequate fluid intake. *Adequate fluid intake will help to prevent bladder infection.*

> Adhere to bowel training program. *Bowel distention is the second most common cause of autonomic dysreflexia.*

Recover from episode of dysreflexia without residual effects as evidenced by:

Skin dry and without red splotches above the level of the lesion

Dysreflexia

Absence of pallor below lesion
Remove stimuli for dysreflexia by the following:

Examine urinary drainage system for obstruction; eliminate obstruction or remove catheter.

Avoid performing Credé maneuver.

Catheterize if on intermittent catheterization program.

Assess signs and symptoms of UTI.

Loosen tight clothing or restrictive appliances.

Apply topical anesthetic around anus and in rectum; check for and manually remove fecal impaction.

Inspect skin for evidence of pressure sore or rashes. *Sympathetic stimulation below T7 can stimulate an exaggerated, unopposed autonomic nervous system response. The response is exaggerated because the response cannot cross the injured area of the cord and is therefore unopposed by the parasympathetic nervous system.*

Blood pressure and pulse within normal limits for patient

Elevate head of the bed or place patient in sitting position. *Elevation of the head can create orthostatic hypotension and lower the blood pressure.*

Monitor the blood pressure and pulse every 5 minutes during acute episode.

Prepare to administer an antihypertensive agent if bowel and bladder interventions fail.

REFERENCES

Geron GE, Rakowski-Reinhardt AC: Action stat! Autonomic dysreflexia, *Nursing 91* February: 33, 1991.

Dunn, KL: Autonomic dysreflexia: a nursing challenge in the care of the patient with a spinal cord injury, *J Cardiovasc Nurs* 5(4): 57, 1991.

Finocchiaro DN, Herzfeld ST: Understanding autonomic dysreflexia, *Am J Nurs* 90(9):56, 1990.

Trop CS, Bennett CJ: Autonomic dysreflexia and its urological implications: a review, *J Urol* 146:1461, 1991.

Trop CS, Bennett CJ: The evaluation of autonomic dysreflexia, *Semin Urol* 10(2):95, 1992.

Energy field disturbance

CLINICAL CONDITION/ MEDICAL DIAGNOSIS	RELATED FACTORS
Elderly male with congestive heart failure and recent hip replacement	Substitute caregiver from home health agency is unfamiliar with complexities of care; care recipient experiences difficulty in responding verbally to caregiver queries

> **Patient goals**
> Expected outcomes
>> Associated nursing/collaborative interventions *and scientific rationale*

Participate in daily care activities without placing undue burden on caretaker as evidenced by the following:

Follows caretaker's directions

Relate reason for substitution and provide information about when previous caretaker will resume care. *Meaning of the event is known only to individual undergoing experience.*

Sit with care recipient; use physical touch to reassure him of your concern and willingness to follow care plan. *Reviewing plan of care with recipient will help restore balance in energy field.*

Wait for some sign from individual that he is ready to begin daily routine. *It takes time for individual to separate from care expectations and to reconnect with new caregiver.*

Regain verbal ability to communicate fully as evidenced by the following:

Answers telephone and speaks with daughter who visits daily

Carries on conversation with neighbor who brings daily meal

Expresses appreciation to caregiver for attention to needs.

Attend to individual's verbal and nonverbal expressions of concerns, and be cognizant of what is not said. *Presence, how the nurse is with the patient, is respecting the other's human dignity and freedom to choose in a situation.*

Collaborate with individual in preparation of written report for next caregiver. *Mutuality in nurse-patient relationship helps to restore energy field. To keep energy field in balance, individual assists with construction of report of event.*

REFERENCES

Cowling WR III: Unitary knowing in nursing practice, *Nurs Sci Quart*, 1993, 6(4):201-207.

Eisenhauer LA: A typology of nursing therapeutics, *Image*: 1994, 26(4):261-264.

Gardner DL. Presence. In Bulechek GM, McCloskey JC (eds): *Nursing interventions: essential nursing treatments*, Philadelphia, 1992, WB Saunders Co.

Morse JM, Miles MW, Clark DA, Doberneck BM: "Sensing" patient needs: exploring concepts of nursing insight and receptivity used in nursing assessment. *Scholarly Inquiry for Nursing Practice*, 1994, 8(3):233-254.

Parse RR. Quality of life: sciencing and living the art of human becoming. *Nurs Sci Quart*, 1994, 7(1):16-21.

Environmental interpretation syndrome: impaired

CLINICAL CONDITION/ MEDICAL DIAGNOSIS	RELATED FACTORS
Adult male diagnosed with multi-infarct dementia	Ongoing incidents of disorientation and cognitive impairment

Patient goals
Expected outcomes
  Associated nursing/collaborative interventions *and scientific rationale*

Experience a consistent, structured environment as evidenced by the following:

Returns to own room that he/she identifies as "home."

  Collaborate with family to determine usual patterns of predementia home life. *Previous life patterns often remain intact in cognitively impaired individuals.*

  Collaborate with family to determine meaningful personal items.

  Incorporate personal items that patient recognizes as his/her own into current room environment. *Meaningful personal items provide a familiar context to the environment.*

  Modify room environment, for example, bed placement, hygiene items, and room lighting, to personal preference. *Visual interpretation of the environment is enhanced by sufficient lighting to distinguish boundaries and contrasting colors.*

  Adjust the pattern of daily activities, such as bath time and bedtime rituals, to match predementia life patterns. *Previous life patterns often remain intact in cognitively impaired individuals.*

  Select meaningful personal items, such as self-photo selected by the patient, to identify the room. *Self-image may be from a perspective in long-term memory.*

Provide consistency in staff and care provider to
the extent possible. *Predictable and familiar
environmental elements support feelings of comfort
and safety in the cognitively impaired.*

Refer to and treat room as patient's home.

Does not attempt to leave foster home

Select room away from usual exit areas. *Cognitively
impaired individuals may follow others out of the
environment and become lost.*

Plan activities according to the stimulus tolerance
of the patient. *With increased stimulation there is
increased risk for agitated behavior.*

Redirect patient activities when he or she attempts
to go home.

Use diversion strategies including walking with
patient, folding washcloths, arranging books
and magazines.

Reminisce about what home was like. *Agenda
behavior technique is more effective with the
cognitively impaired; reality orientation results in
high levels of frustration.*

Role-model agenda behavior techniques for less
experienced staff.

Prepare a plan to use in the event that patient
elopes. identify community resources available
in the event that patient elopes; ensure
identification bracelet with current information
is on patient; keep recent photograph on file;
develop a search process.

REFERENCES

Abraham IL, Reel SJ: Cognitive nursing interventions with long-term
care residents: effects on neurocognitive dimensions, *Arch Psychiatr
Nurs*, 6(6):366-365, 1992.

Armstrong-Esther CA, Browne KD, McAfee JG: Elderly patients: still
clean and sitting quietly. *Advanced Nurs*, 19;264-271, 1994.

Burgener SC, Shimer R, Murrell BS: Expressions of individuality in
cognitively impaired elders: need for individual assessment and
care. *Gerontol Nurs*, 19(4):13-22, 1992.

Collins CE, Given BA, Given CW: Interventions with family
caregivers of persons with Alzheimer's disease, *Nurs Clin North
Amer*, 29(1), 1994.

Fisher JE, Fink CM, Loomis CC: Frequency and management
difficulty of behavioral problems among dementia patients in long-
term care facilities, *Clin Gerontolog*, 13(1):3-12, 1993.

Environmental interpretation syndrome: impaired—cont'd

Hall GR: Caring for people with Alzheimer's disease using the conceptual model of progressively lowered stress threshold in the clinical setting. *Nurs Clin North Amer*, 29(1):129-141, 1994.

Stolley JM, Hall GR, Collins J, Bleuer N, Adrian C, Buckwalter KC: Managing the care of patients with irreversible dementia during hospitalization for comorbidities, *Nurs Clin North Amer*, 28(4):767-782, 1993.

Environmental interpretation syndrome: impaired—cont'd

Family processes, altered: alcoholism

CLINICAL CONDITION/ MEDICAL DIAGNOSIS	RELATED FACTORS
Wife of a public figure admitted to acute hospital with alcoholic liver disease	Resistance to treatment; strained relationships between wife and nondrinking husband and between husband and children age 10 and 12.

Patient goals
Expected outcomes
 Associated nursing/collaborative interventions *and scientific rationale*

Family to create conditions that enable drinking family member to enter substance abuse treatment program as evidenced by the following:

Recognizes and acknowledges that family problem is alcoholism
Makes decision to enter alcohol abuse treatment program
Locates and accesses needed child care services

 Challenge family to use the acute illness as impetus to deal with the real problem.

 Explore willingness to recognize and acknowledge the problem as alcoholism. *Since alcoholism is a stigma, family may masquerade situation as another health problem.*

 Confront patient and family when denial is evident.

 Provide information about medical and social resources. *Knowing that a solution to a problem exists makes it easier to acknowledge.*

 Alert family to the possibility of emergence of alcohol related interpersonal problems during the transition to recovery. *Transition to recovery is a long process and a series of related difficulties may require identification and problem solving.*

 Discuss importance of accessing reliable child care services to facilitate continuing in treatment program. *Lack of child care facilities is one of main reasons for not entering or staying in treatment.*

215

Family processes, altered: alcoholism

Family to acquire insight into the association among family functioning, role demands, role expectations, and alcoholism as evidenced by the following:

Participates in long-term family counseling
Reports improved family relationships

Assist family to identify specific areas of needed emotional and social support.

Encourage expression of feelings about specific areas of need.

Refer to family therapist and/or recovered alcoholism counselor with experience in dealing with alcoholic families. *An experienced family therapist or counselor will be alert to emergence of alcohol-related difficulties and will assist with problematization and interventions.*

Help family to focus on improving problem-solving skills using nonthreatening example, such as planning a family vacation.

REFERENCES

Hall JM: How lesbians recognize and respond to alcohol problems: a theoretical model of problematization, *Adv Nurs Sci*, 1994, 16(3):46-63.

Hughes TL: Research on alcohol and drug use among women: a review and update. In McElmurry BJ, Parker RS (eds): *Annual review of women's health*, New York, 1993, National League for Nursing, 245-285.

Lindeman M, Hawks JH, Bartek JK: The alcoholic family: a nursing diagnosis validation study, *Nurs Diagnosis*, 1994, 5(2):65-73.

Rosenfield SN, Stevenson JS: Perception of daily stress and oral coping behaviors in normal, overweight and recovering alcoholic women. *Res Nurs Health*, 1988, 11:166-174.

Sullivan EJ, Handley SM: Alcohol and drug abuse, *Annual Review of Nursing Research*, 1993, 11:166-174.

Watson WL: Family therapy. In Bulechek GM, McCloskey JC: *Nursing interventions: essential nursing treatments*, (2nd ed), Philadelphia, 1992, WB Saunders, 379-391.

Whall AL, Loveland-Cheery CJ: Family unit-focused research: 1984-1991. *Annual Review of Nursing Research*, 1993, 11:227-247.

Family processes, altered

CLINICAL CONDITION/ MEDICAL DIAGNOSIS	RELATED FACTORS
Anorexia nervosa	Situational transition
	Health problem of family member (wife)

Patient goals
Expected outcomes
  Associated nursing/collaborative interventions *and scientific rationale*

Family will achieve stabilized functioning after situational transition as evidenced by:

Views problem as having meaning for members of family unit

  Help family redefine situation in terms that lead to increased options and possibilities for change and not labeling the "patient" as "bad" or faulting another system. *Redefinition assists family to reexamine the situation as a response to multiple stressors (e.g., new culture, loss of extended family, need to find new job, adjustment to illness) rather than blaming wife for refusing to adjust to new situation.*

  Assist in clarification of the new cultural environment of the family. *Accurate information on conditions in environment help prevent negative perceptions of situation which impede adaptation.*

Demonstrates problem-solving skills from the identification of problem to the evaluation of the action taken and affective responsiveness to members

  Support efforts of family to clarify the who, what, when, where, and how of the stress, and to identify their responses as a family unit. *Consensus of problems and actions to be taken can result in creative, helpful solutions to health problems.*

  Assist family in problem solving by providing information, raising questions, assisting to summarize progress, helping to reallocate

Family processes, altered

important functions of family during crisis period.

Model and validate ways to express emotions in a supportive, nonthreatening, less critical manner.

Family will use knowledge about anorexia nervosa, wife's health problem, in order to promote wellness of its member as evidenced by:

Attempts to understand how weight loss represents a way to feel better, to be in control

Refer family to life-style group which discusses western culture, thinness, self-control, etc.

Support family involvement in treatment.

Avoids giving messages about value of thinness or having lengthy conversations about fashion, diets, placing scale in bathroom, or asking family member to model new bathing suit

Identify situations, public attitudes, nonverbal messages which increase stress for family member.

Encourage ways for family members to express appropriate concern and support for each other.

REFERENCES

Anderson AE: Analysis of treatment experience and outcome from the Johns Hopkins Eating Disorders Program 1975-1990. In Halmi KA, ed: *Psychobiology and treatment of anorexia nervosa and bulimia nervosa*, Wash, DC, 1992, American Psychiatric Press.

Casper RC: Integration of psychodynamic concepts into psychotherapy. In Halmi KA, ed: *Psychobiology and treatment of anorexia nervosa and bulimia nervosa*, Wash, DC, 1992, American Psychiatric Press.

Cox RP, Davis LL: Social constructivist approaches for brief, episodic, problem-focused family encounters, *Nurse Pract* 18(8):45, 1993.

Cravener P: Establishing therapeutic alliance across cultural barriers, *J Psychosoc Nurs Ment Health Serv* 30(12):10, 1992.

Orimoto L, Vitouser KB: Anorexia nervosa and bulimia nervosa. In Wilson PH, ed: *Principles and practice of relapse prevention*, New York, 1992, Guilford Press.

Practice guideline for eating disorders, *Am J Psychiatry* 150(2):212, 1993.

Shuval JT: Migration and stress. In Goldberger L, Breznitz S, eds: *Handbook of stress: theoretical and clinical aspects*, ed 2, New York, 1993, Free Press.

Strachan A: Family management. In Liberman RP, ed: *Handbook of psychiatric rehabilitation*, New York, 1992, Macmillan Pub.

Wilson GT, Fairburn CG: Cognitive treatments for eating disorders, *J Consult Clin Psychol* 61(2):261, 1993.

Family processes, altered—cont'd

Fatigue

CLINICAL CONDITION/ MEDICAL DIAGNOSIS	RELATED FACTORS
Business executive with lung cancer	Role demands; increased metabolic demands

Patient goals
Expected outcomes
> Associated nursing/collaborative interventions *and*
> *scientific rationale*

Establish a pattern of rest/activity that enables fulfillment of role demands as evidenced by the following:

Negotiates realistic goal expectations
> Help patient to identify excessive demands of
> various role obligations.
> Instruct patient to maintain a fatigue diary for a 1-
> week period.

Exercises 3 times a week within own tolerance
Engages in preferred leisure 2 to 3 times a week
Verbalizes decreased sense of fatigue
> Monitor level of fatigue using Rhoden Fatigue Scale
> and Fatigue Severity Scale. *Analysis of the*
> *relationship between activities and levels of fatigue*
> *will help define areas in which to reduce role*
> *demands and energy losses.*
> Formulate with patient options for decreasing work
> demands (e.g., reduction in work hours,
> delegation of selected tasks).
> Help patient to plan a daily schedule that includes
> pacing leisure activities, rest, and exercise.

Verbalizes feeling well-rested on arising
> Monitor sleep pattern.
> Teach patient to eliminate/reduce physical
> activities 1 hour before bedtime. *A function of*
> *sleep is to restore both mental and physical energy.*

Improve nutritional status as evidenced by the following:

Stabilizes body weight

Consumes well-balanced diet based on individual needs

Teach use of food diary to monitor eating habits.

Review food diary/food preferences with patient.

Help patient to identify foods high in protein and complex carbohydrate.

Provide information on use of high-calorie food supplements.

Teach patient/significant other short-cuts to meal planning/preparation. *Role demands and coping with the effects of illness increase energy demand and requirement for nutrients.*

Restore mental energy as evidenced by the following:

Uses a relaxation technique at least once a day

Verbalizes an increased sense of control

Teach and monitor relaxation techniques agreeable to patient, e.g., progressive music relaxation, creative imagery, and music.

Negotiate use of meditation or prayer. *Stress depletes energy, which contributes to fatigue. Relaxation techniques can be effective in stress management.*

REFERENCES

Alstars J: Fatigue in the cancer patient: a conceptual approach to a clinical problem, *Oncol Nurs Forum* 14:(6):25, 1987.

Basia LB and others: Correlates of fatigue in older adults with rheumatoid arthritis, *Nurs Res* 42(2):93-99, 1993.

Blesch KS and others: Correlates of fatigue in people with breast or lung cancer, *Oncol Nurs Forum* 18(1):81-87.

Chen M: The epidemiology of self-perceived fatigue among adults, *Prev Med* 15:74-81, 1986.

Fryback PB: Health for people with a terminal diagnosis, *Nurs Sci Quarterly* 6(3):147-159, 1993.

Grandjean E: Fatigue: its physiological and psychological significance, *Ergonomics* 11(5):427, 1988.

Hegyvary ST: Patient care outcomes related to management of symptoms, *Ann Rev Nurs Res* 11:145-168, 1993.

Kobashi-Schoot JAM and others: Assessment of malaise in cancer patients treated with chemotherapy, *Cancer Nurs* 8(6):3, 1985.

Mason DJ, Redeker N: Measurement of activity, *Nurs Res* 42(2):87-92, 1993.

Morris M: Tiredness and fatigue. In Norris C, ed: *Concept clarification in nursing* pp 263-275, Rockville, Md, 1982, Aspen.

Piper BF, Lindsey AM, Dodd MJ: Fatigue mechanisms in cancer patients: developing nursing theory, *Oncol Nurs Forum* 14(6):17-23.

Fatigue—cont'd

Potempa KM: Chronic fatigue, *Ann Rev Nurs Res* 11:57-76, 1993.

Sheppard KC: The relationships among nursing diagnoses in discharge planning for patients with lung cancer, *Nurs Diagnosis* 4(4):148-155, 1993.

Sheppard KC: The relationships among nursing diagnoses and community agencies and services required for lung cancer patients at discharge. In Carroll-Johnson RM, Paquette M, eds: *Classification of nursing diagnoses: proceedings of the tenth conference* pp 257-259, Philadelphia, 1994, Lippincott.

Fear

CLINICAL CONDITION/ MEDICAL DIAGNOSIS	RELATED FACTORS
Bowel cancer	Impending surgery with possible pain, loss of control, and disfigurement

Patient goals
Expected outcomes
    Associated nursing/collaborative interventions *and scientific rationale*

Identify specific aspects of impending surgery that are sources of fear as evidenced by the following:

Verbalizes specific fears relating to surgery, such as possible pain, realistic perception of danger, own coping ability, and need for assistance; *specificity in identifying the causes of fear facilitates specificity in intervention strategies*

    Using techniques of therapeutic communication, encourage patient to verbalize feelings such as those related to potential personal perception of danger, perception of own coping skills or limitations, and need for assistance from nursing staff. *Verbalizing feelings can lessen the intensity and duration of fear.*

Acquire knowledge/skills for dealing with specific fears as evidenced by the following:

Verbalizes perceptions which are consistent with reality

    Provide information to reduce distorted perceptions. Encourage specifics rather than generalizations. *A realistic appraisal promotes effective problem solving to decrease danger.*

Verbalizes and displays comfort with unit environment, procedure, and staff

    Initiate teaching about surgery, including colostomy. For unfamiliar environment, orient patient to unit and staff.

Fear

Demonstrates effective coughing, deep breathing, and leg exercises

Teach rationale and procedure for turning, coughing, deep breathing, and leg exercises; allow time for practice and return demonstration.

Explains events expected to occur before and after surgery

Teach specifics for type of surgery, as appropriate for patient.

Verbalizes realistic expectations for postoperative period

Teach what to expect after surgery, especially sensations that will be experienced (e.g., recovery room, wound dressings, pain, colostomy, irrigation). *Knowledge of what to expect, particularly on a sensory level, decreases fear of the unknown.*

Identify and teach specifics of the surgical experience that the patient would like to know.

Teach about postoperative analgesia, and encourage patient to request analgesic when needed *in order to cope with fear of pain.*

Teach ways of enhancing control (e.g., include patient in planning care; share test results as appropriate) *in order to deal with loss of control.*

Consider visit by someone who has successfully experienced and is well adjusted to the surgery (e.g., colostomy) *in order to deal with fear of disfigurement. Fear decreases when one identifies with someone who has successfully dealt with a similar fearful situation.*

Engage in adaptive coping as evidenced by the following:

Verbalizes increased psychological comfort and coping skills

Use available support system to increase comfort and relaxation.

Include family and significant others in teaching *so that they are supportive and knowledgeable, rather than fearful.*

Encourage comforting measures (e.g., music, religious objects, own pajamas, pillow). *Familiar sources of comfort can alleviate the distress that accompanies fear.*

Arrange a visit with clergy, if desired by patient.

Verbalizes positive attitude toward outcome of surgery and adjustment to disfigurement

Adopt a positive attitude that patient can cope and have a positive surgical experience.

Experiences a restful sleep

Facilitate a good night's sleep preoperatively.

Experience reduced fear as evidenced by the following:

Has normal pulse and respiration rates
Has normal blood pressure
Verbalizes decreased fear

Continually monitor level of fear (many surgeons will cancel surgery if patient is especially fearful). *The neuroendocrine physiologic response to fear may precipitate life-threatening arrhythmias during stressful situations.*

REFERENCES

Caldwell LM: The influence of preference for information on preoperative stress and coping in surgical outpatients, *Appl Nurs Res* 4(4):177, 1991.

Grainger RD: Conquering fears and phobias, *Am J Nurs* 91(5):15, 1991.

McFarland GK, Thomas MD: *Psychiatric mental health nursing: application of the nursing process,* Philadelphia, 1991, Lippincott.

Mock VL: Fear. In McFarland GK and McFarlane EA: *Nursing diagnoses and intervention: planning for patient care,* ed 2, St Louis, 1993, Mosby-Year Book.

Salmon P: Psychological factors in surgical stress: implications for management, *Clin Psych Rev* 12:681, 1992.

Tarsitano BP: Structured preoperative teaching. In Bulecheck GM, McCloskey JC: *Nursing interventions: essential nursing treatments,* ed 2, pp 168-178, Philadelphia, 1992, WB Saunders.

Taylor-Loughran AE, O'Brien ME, LaChapelle R, Rangel S: Defining characteristics of the nursing diagnoses fear and anxiety: a validation study, *Appl Nurs Res* 2(4):178, 1989.

Teasdale K: Information and anxiety: critical reappraisal, *J Adv Nurs* 18:1125, 1993.

Whitney GG: Concept analysis of fear, *Nurs Diag* 3(4):155, 1992.

Fluid volume deficit (1)

CLINICAL CONDITION/ MEDICAL DIAGNOSIS	RELATED FACTORS
Hyperglycemic hyperosmotic nonketotic coma	Failure of regulatory mechanism

Patient goals
Expected outcomes
  Associated nursing/collaborative interventions *and scientific rationale*

Achieve fluid volume and electrolyte balance as evidenced by the following:

Has vital signs and lab values within normal limits
  Monitor vital signs every 15 minutes until stable; monitor level of consciousness.
  Administer insulin per order according to blood glucose levels; *insulin is required to reverse hyperglycemia.*

Has balanced intake and output, stable weight
  Monitor intake and output every hour and weigh patient daily; *these provide a good measure of body fluid balance.*
  Maintain IV therapy for replacement of fluid per order.
  Monitor for circulatory overload during fluid replacement (e.g., neck vein distention, rales, dyspnea, S_3, increase in CVP or PAP, and tachycardia).
  Administer replacement K^+ therapy for hypokalemia as appropriate; *osmotic diuresis causes K^+ depletion and insulin administration causes K^+ to shift intracellularly.*
  Continue to monitor and report to physician worsening fluid volume deficit/electrolyte imbalance signs and symptoms (e.g., dilute urine, increased urine output, hypotension, increased pulse rate, decreased skin turgor, increased body temperature, weakness).

Fluid volume deficit (1)

REFERENCES

Cullen L: Interventions related to fluid and electrolyte balance, *Nurs Clin North Am* 27(2):569, 1992.

Graves L: Diabetic ketoacidosis and hyperosmolar hyperglycemic nonketotic coma, *Crit Care Nurse Quarterly* 13(3):50, 1990.

Leske JS: Hyperglycemic hyperosmolar nonketotic coma: a nursing-care plan, *Crit Care Nurse* 5(5):49, 1985.

Pflaum S: Investigation of intake-output as a means of assessing body fluid balance, *Heart Lung* 8(3):495, 1979.

Fluid volume deficit (1)—cont'd

Fluid volume deficit (2)

CLINICAL CONDITION/ MEDICAL DIAGNOSIS	RELATED FACTORS
Hypovolemic shock	Active loss of body fluid

Patient goals
Expected outcomes
   Associated nursing/collaborative interventions *and scientific rationale*

Maintain fluid volume and electrolyte balance as evidenced by:

Has blood pressure and pulse within his/her normal limits

Monitor vital signs every hour; monitor level of consciousness; monitor hemodynamic status, including CVP, MAP, PAP, and PCWP if available.

Determine cause of active loss and use nursing actions to prevent further loss.

Has balanced Intake and output, stable weight

Monitor intake and output every hour and report urine output of less than 30 to 60 ml/hr. *Urine volume decreases in hypovolemia because decreased plasma volume results in decreased renal blood flow.*

Weigh patient at the same time daily. *Weights with intake and output provide a good measure of body fluid balance.*

Maintain IV therapy for replacement of fluid using colloids, crystalloids, or blood products per order. *Colloids hydrate the intravascular space and pull fluids from the interstitium into the blood stream; crystalloids replace intracellular fluid and are distributed to the interstitium and intravascular space, and blood replacement must be given to provide oxygen-carrying capacity if hemoglobin is significantly decreased.*

Push oral fluids to 2600 ml/day if appropriate.

Monitor skin condition: color, moisture, turgor.

Monitor circulatory overload during fluid replacement (e.g., neck vein distention, rales,

227

dyspnea, S$_3$ increase in CVP or PAP, and tachycardia).

Has urine specific gravity and lab results within normal limits

Monitor urine specific gravity every 2 hours; *concentrated urine (specific gravity >1.030) is response to water deficit as ADH is released in response to increased osmolarity of body fluids).*

Monitor lab results relevant to fluid balance (Hct, BUN, albumin, total protein, serum osmolarity).

Monitor and report worsening fluid volume deficit and/or electrolyte imbalance including signs and symptoms of decreased urine output, concentrated urine, output greater than intake, hypotension, increased pulse rate, increased body temperature, weakness, and change in mental status.

REFERENCES

Cullen L: Interventions related to fluid and electrolyte balance, *Nurs Clin North Am* 27(2):569, 1992.

Meyers K, Hickey MK: Nursing management of hypovolemic shock, *Crit Care Nurse Quarterly* 11(1):57, 1988.

Pflaum S: Investigation of intake-output as a means of assessing body fluid balance, *Heart Lung* 8(3):495, 1979.

Fluid volume deficit (2)—cont'd

Fluid volume deficit, risk for

CLINICAL CONDITION/ MEDICAL DIAGNOSIS	RISK FACTORS
Congestive heart failure and hypertension	Daily use of diuretics

Patient goals
Expected outcomes
  Associated nursing/collaborative interventions *and scientific rationale*

Maintain adequate fluid volume and electrolyte balance as evidenced by:

Patient/family verbalizes knowledge of monitoring fluid status

  Teach patient/significant other the following:

  Monitor weights and intake and output; *these provide a good measure of body fluid balance.*

  Record blood pressure.

  Teach maintaining of regular schedule for taking diuretics, K^+ supplements, and eating K^+ rich foods, such as bananas, oranges, and raisins; *thiazide diuretics may result in potassium depletion.*

  Monitor side effects of diuretics as necessary.

  Teach about importance of good nutrition and fluid intake; *adequate fluid intake is important to prevent dehydration, in elderly patients thirst is decreased and drinking is less.*

  Change positions slowly *to minimize orthostatic hypotension.*

  Monitor skin turgor and avoid excessive dryness; *poor skin turgor and dryness may indicate dehydration.*

  Avoid very hot environments; *heat may cause excessive water loss.*

  Teach importance of calling physician with weight loss/gain or signs and symptoms of electrolyte imbalance.

Fluid volume defi=it, risk for

REFERENCES

Andreoli K and others: *Comprehensive cardiac care*, ed 7, St Louis, 1991, Mosby.

Cullen L: Interventions related to fluid and electrolyte balance, *Nurs Clin North Am* 27(2):569, 1992.

Lapinski ML: Cardiovascular drugs and the elderly population, *Heart Lung* 11(5):430, 1982.

Mendyka B: Fluid and electrolyte disorders caused by diuretic therapy, *AACN Clinical Issues* 3(3):672, 1992.

Pflaum S: Investigation of intake-output as a means of assessing body fluid balance, *Heart Lung* 8(3):495, 1979.

Porth C, Erickson M: Physiology of thirst and drinking: implication for nursing practice, *Heart Lung* 21(3):273, 1992.

Fluid volume deficit, risk for—cont'd

KRISTIN M. KLEINSCHMIDT, MARGARET J. STAFFORD, AND MI JA KIM

Fluid volume excess

CLINICAL CONDITION/ MEDICAL DIAGNOSIS	RELATED FACTORS
Congestive heart failure (CHF)	Impaired myocardial contractility, decreased cardiac output

Patient goals
Expected outcomes
  Associated nursing/collaborative interventions *and scientific rationale*

Achieve normal level of fluid volume as evidenced by the following:

Has body weight within his/her normal range

Weigh patient daily and consult physician to adjust diuretic dosage as necessary.

Monitor intake and output.

Restrict fluid intake in presence of dilutional hyponatremia with serum Na^+ level below 130 mEq/L and monitor intake and output daily; *excessive water intake will cause further dilution of Na^+ in the blood.*

Signs of fluid volume excess are eliminated; the risks of further complications (e.g., pulmonary edema/shock) are reduced

Assess neck veins for jugular venous distension (JVD); auscultate lungs for presence of crackles; assess liver for increased size and hepatojugular reflux (HJR); assess legs and dependant areas for symmetrical bilateral swelling. *Patients with CHF may have an increase in intravascular and extravascular fluid volume.*

Auscultate heart for presence of S_3 and S_4 sounds. *An S_3 may indicate decreased compliance or increased ventricular diastolic volume; an S_4 may indicate decreased compliance or increased volume of filling.*

Hemodynamic status is restored to normal/acceptable range for this patient

Monitor mean arterial pressure (MAP) and pulse pressure (via arterial line if available) to determine hemodynamic status. *MAP indicates overall perfusion of tissues/organs. Pulse pressure provides an estimate of the heart's stroke volume or pumping ability and is an index of the resistance to left ventricular emptying (afterload).*

Monitor pulmonary artery (PA) pressures (via PA catheter if available). *Central venous pressure (CVP) detects hemodynamic changes in the right side of the heart; pulmonary artery diastolic pressure (PAD) and pulmonary capillary wedge pressure (PCWP) secure an accurate evaluation of the volume of blood in the left ventricle before contraction (preload); cardiac output (CO) (indirect determination via the PA catheter) serves as a means to evaluate therapy; systemic vascular resistance (SVR) is an index of afterload or the pressure of blood in the arterial circulation against which blood in the heart must be ejected.* Consult physician if values exceed acceptable ranges and discuss therapeutic options.

Administer diuretics (e.g., furosemide, bumetanide) as ordered. *These drugs are effective and fast acting "loop" diuretics blocking Na^+ and Cl^- absorption in the ascending limb. Diuretics increase the effective circulating blood volume to normal/acceptable range, thus decreasing preload.*

Administer inotropic agents (e.g., digitalis, dobutamine, amrinone, milrinone) as ordered. *Inotropic agents increase myocardial contractility, decrease preload, and therefore increase cardiac output.*

Administer vasopressor agents (e.g., dopamine) as ordered. Dopamine at low dosages (1 to 2 mcg/kg/min) increases renal blood flow, promoting diuresis.

Administer vasodilator agents (e.g., sodium nitroprusside, hydralazine, nitrates) if ordered. *Sodium nitroprusside has a dual action, dilating both arterioles and veins, with a dramatic decrease in preload and afterload. Vasodilators, in general, reduce peripheral resistance (afterload) and secondarily augment cardiac output and renal blood flow.*

Administer angiotensin converting enzyme (ACE) inhibitors (captopril, enalapril, lisinopril) as ordered. *ACE inhibitors effectively block angiotensin II production which reduces Na^+ and water retention by the kidneys, therefore reducing preload.*

Monitor response to drug therapy, report untoward reactions, and discuss with the physician alternative therapies.

Electrolyte levels are within normal range for this patient

Monitor serum level of electrolytes, particularly K^+ and Mg^{++}. *Hypokalemia and hypomagnesemia predispose the patient to the development of arrhythmias. If patient's heart rate and rhythm are being monitored, observe for PVCs, flat or inverted T wave, or a prominent U wave. These ECG changes are warning signs of hypokalemia.* The nurse may need to provide a K^+ rich diet as appropriate; consult physician for K^+ or Mg^{++} supplement as necessary.

Monitor laboratory results (e.g., increased specific gravity, increased urine osmolality; presence of protein, urea, and granular casts in urine; increased BUN; increased mean corpuscle volume (MCV); and decreased hematocrit) *relevant to fluid retention.*

Provide reduced Na^+ diet (2 g or less, if indicated).

Experience less discomfort due to excessive fluid volume as evidenced by the following:

Verbalizes less dyspnea and experiences more comfort

Provide position that will promote venous return and allow fluid shift (e.g., semi-Fowler's position).

Provide support to edematous areas (e.g., pillow under arms and scrotal support).

Teach passive and active ROM exercises as appropriate. Advance activity to patient's individual tolerance level.

Assist with activities of daily living, as indicated, and have patient's personal items within easy reach *to preserve energy level.*

Provide high-protein and high-calorie diet *to improve nutritional status and enhance the healing of waterlogged body tissue, if present.*

Monitor serum albumin level. *Patients with chronic CHF may have low albumin levels secondary to a malnourished and/or dilutional state. Adequate serum albumin levels are necessary to maintain plasma oncotic pressure and maintain fluid in the intravascular spaces.*

Counsel patient if concerns are expressed about body image and self-esteem as a result of excessive fluid retention.

Provide appropriate skin care if edematous and monitor potential for infection.

Maintain an acceptable level of fluid volume as evidenced by the following:

Sets realistic goals for maintaining optimal fluid level
Collaborate with patient/significant other to determine mutually agreeable goals of therapy if feasible.

Complies with prescribed therapy, appropriate referrals for therapy related to personal fears/concerns as indicated, scheduled clinic appointments
Provide information about disease process and prescribed therapy.

Initiate psychological, dietary, and spiritual counseling as indicated.

Reinforce importance of regular follow-up.

Provide individualized patient teaching appropriate to age, reading level, and cultural background.

Teach patient the purpose of prescribed medications, medication schedule, and common side effects.

Keeps written record of fluctuations of weight and reports abnormal excess

Teach patient the importance of continuing daily weight measurement after discharge.

Encourage patient to report a weight gain in excess of 4 pounds to physician or nurse.

Lists foods to avoid

Teach patient that high Na^+ level induces fluid retention.

Teach patient the importance of eliminating table salt and offer alternatives to salt (e.g., herbs/spices).

Sleeps 6 hours or more a night

Discuss measures to promote uninterrupted sleep (e.g., use of additional pillows, recliner chair, taking of diuretics more than 6 hours before bedtime).

Discuss alternative patterns of sleep times.

REFERENCES

Bousquet GL: Congestive heart failure: a review of non-pharmacologic therapies, *J Cardiovasc Nurs* 4(3):35, 1990.

Gulanick M, Ruback C: Shock management. In Bulechek GM, McCloskey JC, eds: *Nursing interventions: essential nursing treatments*, ed 2, Philadelphia, 1992, WB Saunders.

Kern L, Omery A: Decreased cardiac output in the critical care setting, *Nurs Diagn* 3(3):94, 1992.

Navas JP, Martinez-Maldonado M: Pathophysiology of edema in congestive heart failure, *Heart Dis and Stroke* 2(4):325, 1993.

Poyss AS: Fluid therapy. In Bulechek GM, McCloskey JC, eds: *Nursing interventions: essential nursing treatments*, ed 2, Philadelphia, 1992, WB Saunders.

Prizant-Weston M, Castiglia K: Hemodynamic regulation in nursing interventions. In Bulechek GM, McCloskey JC, eds: *Nursing interventions: essential nursing treatments*, ed 2, Philadelphia, 1992, WB Saunders.

Schaefer KM: Care of the patient with congestive heart failure. In Schaefer KM, Benson PJ, eds: *Levine's conservation model: a framework for nursing practice*, Philadelphia, 1991, FA Davis.

Schwertz DW, Piano MR: New inotropic drugs for treatment of congestive heart failure, *Cardiovasc Nurs* 26(2):7, 1990.

Wight SM: Pathophysiology of congestive heart failure, *J Cardiovasc Nurs* 4(3):1, 1990.

Yusef S: Clinical experience in protecting the failing heart, *Clin Cardiol* 6:(Suppl. II):25, 1993.

Fluid volume excess—cont'd

Gas exchange, impaired

CLINICAL CONDITION/ MEDICAL DIAGNOSIS	RELATED FACTORS
Acute respiratory failure, after anesthesia	Altered oxygen supply, alveolar hypoventilation

> **Patient goals**
> **Expected outcomes**
> > Associated nursing/collaborative interventions *and scientific rationale*

Maintain adequate oxygen supply and alveolar ventilation as evidenced by the following:

Hypoxemia is resolved or improved with or without oxygen supplement or mechanical ventilation
Eucapnia or usual compensated $PaCO_2$ and pH levels
Impairment of mental status and restlessness are absent or reduced

> Maintain patent airway while patient is both awake and asleep.
>
> Encourage patient to take deep breaths (see Airway Clearance, Ineffective).
>
> Position patient to facilitate ventilation/perfusion matching ("good side down"). *Positioning affects distribution of pulmonary circulation and ventilation. Position patient so that most normal area of lung is dependent.*
>
> Remove secretions by coughing or suctioning (see Airway Clearance, Ineffective).
>
> Consult physician regarding supplementary oxygen during rest, activity and/or sleep. If ordered, select devices that enable the patient to perform ADLs.
>
> If hypoxemia persists, consult physician for possible mechanical assistance or ventilation.
>
> If mechanical ventilation is prescribed, monitor ventilator settings, endotracheal and tracheal tube function, and function of ventilator and breathing circuits. Assess patient's ability to wean daily.

Gas exchange, impaired

Initiate weaning and support oxygenation requirements as described above. *Weaning is the titration of the intervention of mechanical ventilation. A patient's ability to wean depends on a number of physiological and psychological variables, e.g., control of breathing, respiratory muscle strength and endurance, lung mechanics, gas exchange, as well as the patient's psychological readiness to be separated from the ventilator.*

If mechanical ventilation becomes long-term, assess for home management by self or significant other. (see Ventilation, inability to sustain spontaneous).

Performs techniques that maximize ventilation and perfusion matching

Teach patient and significant other about treatments, medications, oxygen therapy, and equipment.

Counsel patient who has chronic hypoxemia to obtain supplementary oxygen prescription from physician before air travel or trips to high altitude.

REFERENCES

American Association of Critical-Care Nurses: *AACN outcome standards for nursing care of the critically ill*, California, 1990, AACN.

American Thoracic Society: Research priorities in respiratory nursing, *Am Rev Respir Dis* 142:1459-1464, 1990.

American Thoracic Society: Standards of nursing care for adult patients with pulmonary dysfunction, *Am Rev Respir Dis* 143:231-236, 1991.

Glauser F, Polatty R, Sessler C: State of the art: worsening oxygenation in the mechanically ventilated patient-causes, mechanisms and early detection, *Am Rev Respir Dis* 138(2):458-465, 1988.

Hoffman C and others: Effect of transport time and FiO_2 on SpO_2 during transport from the OR to the PACU, *Nurse Anesth* 2(3):119-125, 1991.

Hoffman LA and others: Transtracheal delivery of oxygen: efficacy and safety for long-term continuous therapy, *Ann Otol Rhinol Laryngol* 100(2):108-115, 1991.

Hoffman LA and others: Nasal cannula and transtracheal oxygen delivery. A comparison after 6 months of each technique, *Am Rev Respir Dis* 145(4 pt 1):827-831, 1992.

Knebel AR: Weaning from mechanical ventilation: current controversies, *Heart Lung* 20(4):321-31, 1991.

Slutsky AS and others: American College of Chest Physicians' Consensus Conference—Mechanical ventilation, *Chest* 104:1833-1859, 1993.

Tobin MJ, Jung K, Weaning from mechanical ventilation, *Crit Care Clin* 6(3):725-747, 1990.

Gas exchange, impaired—cont'd

Grieving, anticipatory

CLINICAL CONDITION/ MEDICAL DIAGNOSIS	RELATED FACTORS
Wife of spouse with non-Hodgkin's lymphoma	Perceived potential loss of spouse

Patient goals
Expected outcomes
Associated nursing/collaborative interventions *and scientific rationale*

Wife participates in constructive anticipatory grief work as evidenced by the following:

Discusses thoughts and feelings related to potential loss of spouse

Encourage wife to describe perceptions of potential loss *to identify specific aspect of grieving process wife is experiencing.*

Encourage verbalization of fears, concerns, and other emotions; *recognize that the expression of intense emotions, such as anger, is common, and should not be taken as a personal attack; verbalization of thoughts and feelings facilitates the grieving process.*

Provide assurance that experiencing intense, chaotic feelings and reactions is normal *to minimize wife's concerns that she is experiencing abnormal reactions.*

Avoid judgmental and defensive responses to criticisms of health care providers. *It is important to keep in mind the difference between criticism generated as a result of displaced anger related to potential loss of spouse and valid criticism of providers.*

Provide wife with ongoing information of husband's diagnosis, prognosis, progress, and plan of care for husband's diagnosis of non-Hodgkin's lymphoma.

Meets ongoing self-care needs

Determine current sources of social support, such as family, friends, and church, and disruptions in current life-style related to potential loss of spouse, such as finances, living arrangements, and transportation. *Social support is an important resource to assist wife/patient/children during this health crisis, and it can influence the extent to which wife is able to meet self-care needs.*

Encourage wife to attend to her own self-care needs, such as rest, sleep, nutrition, leisure activities, and time away from patient. *This will help her maintain her own health, have the ability to devote time to the children, if any, and continue to provide support to patient.*

Maintains constructive family functioning as a family unit

Help wife, spouse, and children to share mutual fears, concerns, plans, and hopes with each other.

Evaluate need for referral to resources, such as mental health professional for wife, husband, and/or children; referral to school counselor, Social Security representative, legal consultant, or grief support groups. *Parents' preoccupation with their own grief may affect their ability to recognize their children's distress; uncertainties about finances and legal worries can have an adverse effect on family closeness. Early intervention can reduce the likelihood of dysfunctional grieving.*

Enlist support from others, such as family, friends, and clergy.

Encourage wife to describe desires and information needs in caring for patient.

Facilitate wife's assistance with patient's physical care; include children as appropriate.

Facilitate flexible visiting hours that include the children.

Discuss indicators of change in physical condition of patient with wife and children, *to minimize undue anxiety and to help prepare them for the loss of their loved one.*

Provide comforting measures for patient; encourage wife, children, additional significant others to assist if they wish.

Demonstrate competence by meeting patient's psychosocial and physical needs promptly and with empathy.

Encourage wife, children, and additional significant others to maintain verbal communication and touch with their loved one during times when he may be unable to respond, *to maintain closeness for the patient and to decrease family's sense of helplessness.*

Provide as much privacy as possible for wife, children, and others to be alone with patient *for them to share freely.*

REFERENCES

Cowles KV, Rodgers BL: The concept of grief: a foundation for nursing research and practice, *Res Nurs Health* 14:119, 1991.

Curry LC, Stone JG: The grief process: a preparation for death, *Clin Nurse Specialist* 5(1):17, 1991.

Dobratz MC: Causal influences of psychological adaptation in dying, *Western J Nurs Res* 15(6):708, 1993.

Dracup KA, Breu CS: Using nursing research findings to meet the needs of grieving spouses, *Nurs Res* 27(4):212, 1978.

Hampe SO: Needs of the grieving spouse in a hospital setting, *Nurs Res* 24:113, 1975.

Rosenheim E, Reicher R: Children in anticipatory grief: the lonely predicament, *J Clin Child Psychol* 15(2):115, 1986.

Siegel K and others: Perceptions of parental competence while facing the death of a spouse, *Am J Orthopsychiatry* 60(4):567, 1990.

Welch D: Anticipatory grief reactions in family members of adult patients, *Issues Ment Health Nurs* 4:149, 1982.

Grieving, dysfunctional

CLINICAL CONDITION/ MEDICAL DIAGNOSIS	RELATED FACTORS
Elderly widower whose wife recently died from cancer; exacerbation of chronic obstructive pulmonary disease (COPD)	Absence of anticipatory grieving, loss of health

---

Patient goals
Expected outcomes
    Associated nursing/collaborative interventions *and scientific rationale*

Experience resolution of dysfunctional grieving as evidenced by the following:

Acknowledges awareness of losses

Encourage verbalization of thoughts and feelings related to death of spouse and loss of health. *Aging survivors have an increased tendency to deny their own feelings as well as deny the death of a loved one.*

Monitor for suicidal ideation/intent. *Initial known risk factors include age, marital status, and health problems.*

Encourage description of current and anticipated problems related to loss of spouse and loss of health.

Evaluate need for referral to resources, such as brief psychotherapy, spiritual counseling.

Differentiate between helpful and maladaptive use of denial associated with wife's death as well as own health. *Initial denial protects from emotional pain; prolonged denial inhibits grief recovery.*

Gradually present patient with more facts *to facilitate awareness of losses and to lay groundwork for adaptive behaviors.*

Facilitate working through feelings by demonstrating tolerance for expression of negative feelings, supporting verbalizations of ambivalence, and helping patient to understand reasons for feelings. *Working through intense feelings facilitates resolution of grief and allows for engagement in problem solving.*

Point out universality of need for normal grieving.

Develops appropriate goals for COPD management

Monitor patient's current level and pattern of mood, energy, concentration, appetite, sleep. *Newly bereaved may experience a diminished immune response; there is a higher incidence of chronic disease among this population. It is important to differentiate from signs and symptoms of dysfunctional grieving and COPD exacerbation.*

Encourage description of current and anticipated problems related to loss of health.

Clarify and offer factual information about COPD exacerbation.

Offer realistic hope for positive coping in the present, as well as the future.

Facilitate patient's developing a daily schedule that addresses dietary management, exercise, sleep and rest periods, diversional and recreational activities. *Dysfunctional grieving may result in inadequate attention to health maintenance activities.*

Make referral to Behavioral Medicine Clinic Better Breathers Club.

Identifies alternate plans for meeting goals that were significant before loss of spouse

Assist patient to develop realistic goals and life-style changes.

Promote patient's recognition of past and present strengths that can be used for coping with current losses *to reinforce confidence in grief recovery.*

Monitor patient's perception of current adaptation to loss of spouse and loss of health, patient's perception of use of coping skills/problem-solving abilities, and perception of available social support. *Perception of the existence of social support is a positive indicator for successful grief recovery.*

Encourage family and friends to offer support by visiting patient frequently on a regular basis. *Weekly visits by family have been found to be related to constructive grief resolution.*

Provide guidance about available community resources (e.g., senior citizens activity center, grief recovery groups). *Facilitating, encouraging, and teaching patient about use of resources will assist adjustment to changes resulting from current losses.*

REFERENCES

Curry LC, Stone JG: Moving on: recovering from the death of a spouse, *Clin Nurs Specialist* 6(4):180, 1992.

Gabriel RM, Kirschling JM: Assessing grief among the bereaved elderly: a review of existing measures, *Hosp J* 5(1):29, 1989.

Herth K: Relationship of hope, coping styles, concurrent losses, and setting to grief resolution in the elderly widow(er), *Res Nurs Health* 13(2):109, 1990.

Kallenberg K, Soderfelt B: Three years later: grief, view of life, and personal crisis after death of a family member, *J Pallia Care* 8(4):13, 1992.

Lazare A: Bereavement and unresolved grief. In Lazare A, ed: *Outpatient psychiatry: diagnosis and treatment*, ed 2, Baltimore, 1989, Williams and Wilkins.

Steele L: Risk factor profile for bereaved spouses, *Death Studies* 16(5):387, 1992.

Steele LL: The death surround: factors influencing the grief experience of survivors, *Oncol Nurs Forum* 17(2):235, 1990.

Worden JW: *Grief counseling and grief therapy*, ed 2, New York, 1991, Springer.

Growth and development, altered

CLINICAL CONDITION/ MEDICAL DIAGNOSIS	RELATED FACTORS
Fetal alcohol syndrome	Inadequate caretaking, poor support system

---

Patient goals
Expected outcomes
    Associated nursing/collaborative interventions *and scientific rationale*

Reach maximal potential in mental and physical development as evidenced by the following:

Physical and emotional needs will be met as a result of adequate maternal caretaking

At regular intervals, monitor child's cognitive, social and psychomotor development; monitor height and weight. *Diagnosis of fetal alcohol syndrome (FAS) requires manifestations in three categories: prenatal or postnatal growth retardation (below tenth percentile for gestational age); CNS dysfunction (neurological impairment; cognitive or developmental delay); and presence of at least two characteristic dysmorphic facial features.*

Assist mother in providing adequate care; and support her with praise for each accomplishment. *Nurturing of mother increases self-esteem and promotes nurturing of infant.*

Involve significant others in the care of the infant. *Addictive mothers have limited coping skills and may need help to care adequately for their baby.*

Facilitate access to well-child care, monitor compliance.

Monitor the child's safety within the home environment; involve Child Protective Services as necessary. *Use of alcohol lowers inhibitions and impairs judgment. This results in compromised parenting abilities which places the child at greater risk of physical and sexual abuse and neglect.*

Growth and development, altered

Provide support and reinforce appropriate
parenting activities; suggest ways to provide
appropriate environment and stimulation based
on infant's cues. *FAS infants have a higher
incidence of irritability, abnormal sleep patterns,
agitation, increased crying, and resistance to
cuddling or holding. This behavior may frustrate
mother, causing her to withdraw, or result in abuse
or child's failure to thrive.*

Monitor nutritional status: in collaboration with
nutritionist, assess mother's feeding technique,
provide guidance related to feeding problems,
and assist/encourage mother to select foods that
will provide calories and nutrition. *Although FAS
infants have normal patterns of oral motor function,
they have delays in the development of oral feeding.
Many breastfeed poorly, have difficulty coordinating
sucking and swallowing with breathing, have
persistent vomiting and difficulty adjusting to solid
foods, and show little interest in food.*

Achieve adequate support system as evidenced by the following:

Obtains and uses appropriate supportive services

Make appropriate referrals to Alcoholics
Anonymous for help with alcohol addiction,
early intervention program/physical therapist to
support motor and cognitive development,
nutritionist to ensure adequate caloric intake,
and day-care or respite-care agency for special-
needs children.

Collaborate with professionals involved in care.
*Care for FAS child is similar to other chronic
conditions requiring multi-disciplinary approach;
needs are long-term; neurological problems continue
through life-span and can include: delays in fine and
gross motor development, cognitive functioning,
expressive and receptive language; vision deficits;
learning disabilities; psychosocial problems;
difficulties in adaptive functioning.*

REFERENCES

Bays J.: The care of alcohol and drug-affected infants, *Pediatr Ann* 21(8), 1992.

Coles CD: Impact of prenatal alcohol exposure on the newborn and the child, *Clin Obstet Gynecol* 36(2), 1993.

Day NL and Richardson GA: Prenatal alcohol exposure: a continuum of effects, *Semin Perinatol* 15(4), 1991.

Harris SR and others: Effects of prenatal alcohol exposure on neuromotor and cognitive development during early childhood: a series of case reports, *Phys Therapy* 73(9), 1993.

Olson HC: The effects of prenatal alcohol exposure on child development, *Infants and Young Children* 6(3):10, 1994.

Spohr HL, Willms J, Steinhausen HC: Prenatal alcohol exposure and long-term consequences, *Lancet* 341(8850), 1993.

Streissguth AP and others: Fetal alcohol syndrome in adolescents and adults, *J Am Med Assoc* 265(15), 1991.

Streissguth AP: Fetal alcohol syndrome: early and long-term consequences, *NIDA Res Monogr* 119, 1992.

Growth and development, altered—cont'd

Health maintenance, altered

CLINICAL CONDITION/ MEDICAL DIAGNOSIS	RELATED FACTORS
Diabetes mellitus	Impaired ability to make deliberate and thoughtful judgments; insufficient material resources

Patient goals
Expected outcomes
   Associated nursing/collaborative interventions *and scientific rationale*

Seek help as needed to maintain diabetic control as evidenced by the following:

Clarifies needs related to maintaining diabetic control
Assist patient in identifying and clarifying needs related to maintaining diabetic control including meal planning, exercise and medication regimen. *The primary purpose of diabetes care is preventing complications.*

Provide opportunity for discussion of health alteration and related self-care needs. *Adult learning principles guide practice including assessing readiness to learn and using experiential learning.*

Assist patient in understanding how choice of health care practices will affect diabetic control. *Educational plans should include current, relevant information and be geared to patient's educational level, interest level, and cultural practices. Ethnicity affects food choices, health beliefs, and health behaviors.*

Defines type of help needed for diabetic control
Assist patient in defining what help is needed to maintain diabetic control by monitoring blood glucose levels. *Patients should establish individual blood glucose goals with health care team.*

Help patient identify potential risk factors including hypoglycemia and cardiovascular changes. *Assessment of patient's perceived risk can enhance relevant health maintenance behaviors.*

Consult with significant others in defining diabetic control needs.

Discuss with patient how significant others may be helpful. *Family and caregivers' involvement will support control maintenance activities.*

Assist patient in determining approaches to obtaining help from significant others.

Support significant others with their role in helping patient maintain diabetic control. *Involving significant others can enhance and reinforce the practice of health maintenance behaviors.*

Describes resources available to facilitate diabetic control behaviors

Teach patient/significant others about helpful resources available in the family and community. *Knowledge of resources facilitates action.*

Facilitate patient and family contact with relevant resources; initiate referrals as necessary. *Diabetes control may be better if patient and support persons are actively involved in care decisions.*

Selects helping resources based on evaluation in relation to needs

Discuss with patient perceived needs and aim to match with available resources.

Help patient evaluate potential of helpfulness of available resources. *To be useful resources must be readily accessible, economical, and responsive to specific needs.*

Contacts resources as appropriate

Assist patient in determining ways to make contact and discuss needs.

Reinforce patient's contact with appropriate resources.

Reports use of help as needed to maintain diabetic control

Discuss with patient outcomes of resource contacts.

Assist patient to evaluate usefulness of resources.

Help patient to identify factors affecting the maintenance of diabetic control. *Active learning leads to more effective interpretation and integration of knowledge.*

Establish ability to maintain diabetic control as evidenced by the following:

Identifies factors affecting present altered health maintenance ability

>   Help patient to evaluate personal strengths and weaknesses that affect ability to maintain diabetic control. *Helping the patient make adjustments needed will depend on where the patient started and how he/she moves along in identified tasks.*

>   Support patient in organizing and using strengths to maintain diabetic control. *Individuals all have unique strengths that can be used to maintain health. Individual values will affect decision making.*

>   Teach patient about safety precautions related to diabetes (Medic-alert ID, foot care, response to hypoglycemia).

Uses community resources appropriately

>   Assist patient to evaluate the effectiveness of use of community resources.

Monitor and identify future diabetic control needs as evidenced by the following:

Develops effective behavior to support maintaining diabetic control

>   Monitor patient's progress in establishing diabetic control and maintaining health. *Individuals can be helped to modify life-style and control health behaviors.*

>   Continue to educate patient to recognize altered health state including signs and symptoms to report to health professionals.

>   Help patient to develop behaviors that support continued diabetic control. *A person's perspective of health, loss of control, self-esteem, and health status influence health prevention behavior.*

>   Recommend regular follow-up with health professional.

Health maintenance, altered—cont'd

Participates actively in diabetic control behaviors

Discuss with patient and provide positive feedback on behaviors that are effective in maintaining diabetic control. *Increased commitment and participation by patient will enhance effectiveness of behavior.*

Assist patient to evaluate effectiveness of behaviors selected to maintain diabetic control at specific intervals.

Collaborate with patient to determine additional behaviors needed to maintain diabetic control. *Interpersonal interactions support a person's tendency to be self-actualizing.*

REFERENCES

Boynton P: Health maintenance alteration: a nursing diagnosis of the elderly, *Clin Nurs Spec* 3(1):5, 1989.

Carlson SL: Altered health maintenance. In McFarland GK, McFarlane EA: *Nursing diagnosis and intervention*, ed 2, St Louis, 1993, Mosby-Year Book.

Cox CL, Miller EH, Mull CS: Motivation in health behavior: measurement, antecedents and correlates, *Adv Nurs Sci* 9(4):1, 1987.

Duffy ME: Determinants of health promotion, *Nurs Res* 37(6):358, 1988.

Fleury JD: Empowering potential: a theory of wellness motivation, *Nurs Res* 40(5):286, 1991.

Funnell MM, Merritt JH: The challenges of diabetes in older adults, *NCNA* 28(1):45, 1993.

Hinnen D: Issues in diabetes education, *NCNA* 28(1):113, 1993.

Pender NJ, Pender AR: Attitudes, subjective norms and intentions to engage in health behaviors, *Nurs Res* 35(1):15, 1986.

Peret KK, Stachowiak B: Alteration in health maintenance: conceptual bases, etiology, and defining characteristics. In Kim MJ, McFarland GK, McLane AM, eds: *Classification of nursing diagnoses: proceedings of the fifth national conference*, St Louis, 1984, Mosby-Year Book.

Tripp SL, Stachowiak B: Health maintenance, health promotion: is there a difference? *Pub Hlth Nurs* 9(3):155-161, 1992.

Health seeking behaviors
(stress management)

CLINICAL CONDITION/ MEDICAL DIAGNOSIS	RELATED FACTORS
History of irritable bowel syndrome	Desire for improved quality of life

Patient goals
Expected outcomes
  Associated nursing/collaborative interventions *and scientific rationale*

Experience a trusting relationship as evidenced by the following:

Identifies present state of wellness and areas in lifestyle that require attention
  Introduce client to Travis Wellness Inventory and Crumbaugh and Maholick's Purpose in Life Test.
  Promote client's interest in completing Inventory and Life Test.
  Assist client in interpreting findings.
  Help client to identify factors that threaten personal wellness and action that can be taken.
  Discuss with client the interdependent and interactive relationship of present state of well-being to daily behaviors, thinking, attitudes, and beliefs.
Identifies realistic goals and plans for enhancing health
  Facilitate verbalization of desire for change, fears, excitement, priorities, goals, and possible action.

Experience enhanced self awareness as evidenced by the following:

Verbalizes present patterns of response to stress and use of coping strategies
  Assist client in identifying present stressors: internal processes and external events.
  Assist client in identifying behavioral responses to stress. *The immune system weakens under*

conditions of chronic stress, increasing susceptibility to illness.

Explore client's use of coping strategies and degree of effectiveness.

Assist client in assessing quality of dietary intake and physical activity program. Share with client the relationship of nutritional status, exercise, and stress management.

Examine with client the feasibility of using conscious relaxation as a means of taking positive personal control. *Learning internally-oriented relaxation techniques (e.g., autogenic training or meditation) helps patient gain/maintain a sense of control.*

Consistently engages in one self-training approach
Communicates outcomes of engaging in program(s) of choice and modifies approach as desired

Elicit client's willingness and interest in expanding self-awareness through self-training programs: self-hypnosis, creative visualization, meditation, sound therapy, etc.

Share with client the process of integrating selected/desired programs. Provide client with follow-up resource material.

Emphasize importance of consistency, patience, working within unique capacity in carrying out self-training program.

REFERENCES

Crumbaugh JC, Maholick LT: *Purpose in life test.* Available from Psychometric Affiliates, PO Box 3167, Munster, Ind 46231.

Duffy ME: Determinants of health promoting lifestyles in older persons, *Image* 25(1):23-28, 1993.

Manderino MA, Brown MC: A practical, step-by-step approach to stress management for women, *Nurs Practit* 17(7):18, 21, 24, 1991.

Scandrett-Hibdon S, Uecker S: Relaxation training. In Bulechek GM, McCloskey JC, eds: *Nursing interventions: essential nursing treatments,* ed 2, Philadelphia, 1992, WB Saunders.

Travis J, Ryan R: *Wellness workbook: a guide to attaining high level wellness,* Berkeley, Calif, 1986, Ten Speed Press.

Health seeking behaviors (stress management)—cont'd

Home maintenance management, impaired

CLINICAL CONDITION/ MEDICAL DIAGNOSIS	RELATED FACTORS
Total hip replacement	Inadequate knowledge about postoperative home management; impaired functional status

---

Patient goals
Expected outcomes
    Associated nursing/collaborative interventions *and scientific rationale*

Integrate hip precautions into ADLs as evidenced by the following:

Maintains proper hip alignment (i.e., avoid extreme flexion, abduction and internal rotation)
    Collaborate with physical therapist about hip precaution teaching. *An interdisciplinary approach enhances teaching.*
    Provide written instructions to reinforce learning about hip precautions. *Written instructions ensure a consistent resource.*
    Encourage use of adaptive equipment (e.g., elevated toilet seat, abduction wedge, or pillows).
    Monitor integration of hip precautions into performance of ADLs as independence progressively increases. *This ensures that patient incorporates teaching into practice.*
    Instruct patient about signs and symptoms of dislocation. *Ensure that patient has knowledge of potential complications*

Progress toward independence in ADLs as evidenced by the following:

Uses assistive devices correctly and consistently to facilitate ADLs
    Monitor patient's use of assistive devices and correct performance as indicated.

Participates actively in performance of ADLs with less assistance over time

Promote gradual independence in ADLs. *Attaining maximal independence fosters successful reintegration into home environment.*

Encourage use of analgesics before activities. *Comfort is conducive to compliance with medical regime.*

Teach patient to pace activities. *This enhances healing of involved hip joint and muscle.*

Encourage progressive increase in activities inside/outside the home, with physician approval. *Progressive activity increase allows for healing and strengthening.*

Verbalizes knowledge of treatment plan and community resources

Collaborate with patient/significant other to arrange for home health services (e.g., home health aide and/or registered nurse). *Such services promote return to independent living situation.*

Collaborate with patient/significant other or household member to arrange for continuing rehabilitative services (e.g., physical therapy provided in outpatient department or in the home setting). *These services promote return to independent living situation.*

Plan for adapting home environment to promote maximal safety as evidenced by the following:

Begins adaptation of environment to promote safety

Collaborate with patient/significant other to plan for a safe home environment (e.g., move furniture to clear pathway for walker, remove loose scatter rugs). *Mutual planning enhances compliance.*

Instruct patient to keep environment well lighted. *This enhances safe mobility.*

Encourage use of cordless telephone *to ensure ability to summon emergency assistance.*

Encourage patient to wear non-skid shoes. *This enhances safe mobility.*

Provide patient/significant other or household member with 24 hour emergency number for health services *to ensure ability to summon emergency assistance.*

Begins adaptation of environment for optimal daily functioning

Instruct patient to use chair with firm seat and armrests. *This maintains correct hip alignment at no more than 90 degrees flexion and facilitates safe transfer activities.*

Assist patient in negotiating rental/purchase and installation of bathtub rails, tub bench, elevated toilet seat, and grab bars *to promote independence and safety with ADLs.*

REFERENCES

Brown JS, Furstenberg AL: Restoring control: empowering older patients and their families during health crises, *Soc Work Health Care* 17(4):81-97, 1992.

Browning MA: Discharge planning. In Hogstel MO: *Clin Manag Gerontol Nurs*, St Louis, 1992, Mosby-Year Book p 253-269.

Hough D, Crossat S, Nye P: Patient education for total hip replacement, *Nurs Manag* 22(3):80I-J, 80N-80P, 1991.

Orr P: An educational program for total hip and knee replacement patients as part of a total arthritis center program, *Orthop Nurs* 9(5):61-69,89, 1990.

Wong J and others: Affects of an experimental program in post hospital adjustment of early discharged patients, *International J Nurs Studies* 26(1):7-20, 1990.

Hopelessness

CLINICAL CONDITION/ MEDICAL DIAGNOSIS	RELATED FACTORS
Chronic obstructive pulmonary disease	Isolation from prolonged activity restriction

Patient goals
Expected outcomes
    Associated nursing/collaborative interventions *and scientific rationale*

Identify choices available to mobilize energy on own behalf as evidenced by the following:

Reduces isolation from the environment
    Establish contact and rapport with patient.
    Assist patient in identifying enjoyable diversional activities.
    Provide opportunities for patient to spend time with one other person; gradually increase amount of time and number of persons.
    Discuss with patient options for increasing support network. *Hope depends on interaction with significant others and thrives in an atmosphere of trust.*

Expresses feelings
    Provide opportunity for patient to express feelings verbally and nonverbally (e.g., writing or drawing).
    Facilitate expression of feelings by active listening, open-ended questions, and reflection.
    Provide opportunity for physical expression of feelings (e.g., punching bag or exercise), when possible, and within physical capabilities.
    Express empathy while communicating belief that patient can act contrary to the way he/she feels.
    Offer realistic hope through communicating belief that patient has or can learn skills needed to cope with problems and physical limitations.

Hopelessness

Assist patient in identifying person(s) with whom he/she is comfortable expressing feelings. *Expressing feelings abates hopelessness.*

Observe for signs of suicidal intent (e.g., sudden behavior or mood change, conversations about the futility of life).

Reports increased feelings of self-confidence

Demonstrate unconditional positive regard for patient.

Assist patient in identifying those roles that can consistently be carried out successfully within physical limitations.

Assist patient in developing self-care skills that contribute to mastery of the environment.

Encourage patient to identify and participate in satisfying experiences. *Developing self-confidence depends on repetitive positive interactions and mastery of the environment.*

Encourage positive self-statements by patient.

Provide honest praise about patient's accomplishments.

Verbalizes ability to control or influence self and environment

Involve patient in decisions about ADLs and health care.

Teach patient how to discriminate between controllable and uncontrollable events. *The perception of control over self and environment is enhanced through expanding the patient's ability to cope, problem-solve, and communicate.*

Assist patient in determining realistic goals.

Assist patient in identifying alternative ways to cope.

Assist patient in identifying consequences of implementing identified alternatives.

Teach patient new coping strategies.

Demonstrate and teach effective communication techniques (e.g., active listening).

REFERENCES

Keane SM, Sells S: Recognizing depression in the elderly, *J Gerontol Nurs* 16(1):21, 1990.

Naschinski C: Hopelessness. In Thompson JM, McFarland G, Hirsch J, Tucker S: *Mosby's manual of clinical nursing,* ed 3, St Louis, 1992, Mosby-Year Book.

O'Brien ME, Pheifer W: Physical and psychosocial nursing care for patients with HIV infection, *Nurs Clin North Amer* 28(2):303, 1993.

Wake M, Fehring R, Fadden T: Multination validation of anxiety, hopelessness and ineffective airway clearance, *Nurs Diagnos* 2:57, 1991.

Wurzbach ME: Assessment and intervention for certainty and uncertainty, *Nurs Forum* 27(2):29, 1992.

Hopelessness—cont'd

Hyperthermia

CLINICAL CONDITION/ MEDICAL DIAGNOSIS	RELATED FACTORS
Heat stroke	Exposure to a hot environment

Patient goals
Expected outcomes
    Associated nursing/collaborative interventions *and scientific rationale*

Establish normothermia as evidenced by:

Maintains temperature within normal range
    Monitor temperature by continuous rectal or pulmonary artery method.

Respiration, pulse, and blood pressure within normal limits for patient
    Monitor vital signs every 15 minutes until stable.

Absence of hyperthermia signs and symptoms, such as tachycardia, hyperventilation, flushed skin, and seizures
    Apply external cooling measures.

    Apply cooling blankets at a temperature of 23.9° C; *this temperature causes less shivering and is effective in reducing febrile temperatures.*

    Apply ice packs in axillae and groin; *axillae and groin are close to large blood vessels that will lose heat readily by conduction.*

    Wrap hands and feet in terry-cloth toweling to prevent shivering; *hands and feet have many nerve endings sensitive to heat loss; shivering should be avoided as it causes increases in metabolic rate, CO_2 production, oxygen consumption, and myocardial work and decreases in O_2 saturation and glycogen stores.*

    Provide IV fluid therapy per order.

    Provide fluids, 3000 ml/day or as ordered; *dehydration may be present due to loss of fluid from diaphoresis and increased ventilation.*

Administer antipyretics as ordered and note response; *antipyretics reduce fever by affecting hypothalamic response to pyrogens.*

REFERENCES

Bruce J, Grove S: Fever: pathology and treatment, *Crit Care Nurse* 12(1):40, 1992.

Caruso C and others: Cooling effects and comfort of four cooling blanket temperatures in humans with fever, *Nurs Res* 41(2):68, 1992.

Holtzclaw B: Shivering, *Nurs Clin North Am* 25(4):977, 1990.

Holtzclaw B: The febrile response in critical care: state of the science, *Heart and Lung* 21(5):482, 1992.

Stevens T: Managing postoperative hypothermia, rewarming and its complications, *Crit Care Nurs Quarterly* 16(1):60, 1993.

Hyperthermia—cont'd

Hypothermia

CLINICAL CONDITION/ MEDICAL DIAGNOSIS	RELATED FACTORS
Cold injury	Exposure to a cold environment

Patient goals
Expected outcomes
    Associated nursing/collaborative interventions *and*
      scientific rationale

Establish normothermia as evidenced by:

Maintains temperature within normal range
    Monitor temperature using low reading
      thermometer; rectal or pulmonary artery core
      continuous for very low temperatures.

Maintains pulse, respiration, and blood pressure
within normal limits for patient
    Monitor vital signs every 15 minutes until stable;
      monitor ECG continuously; report arrhythmias,
      such as bradycardia, and treat per order; *during*
      hypothermia, circulating volume decreases causing
      decreased cardiac output and resulting in decreased
      oxygen delivery and arrhythmias.
    Monitor for hypotension; *if rapid rewarming occurs*
      sudden vasodilitation may cause severe hypotension.

Absence of signs and symptoms of hypothermia:
shivering, cool skin, pallor, decreased level of
consciousness
    Warm body slowly with passive techniques; i.e.,
      increase environmental temperature to 27° to
      30° C.
    Use warmed blankets *in order to prevent convective*
      heat loss and transfer heat to peripheral tissues.
    Cover the head; *60% of total body heat loss occurs*
      through top of head.
    Use active techniques, such as fluid
      circulating/forced warm air blankets.
    Use heat lamps; *patients report comfort and shivering*
      may be reduced.

Warm crystalloids at 37° to 39° C and use blood warmer for blood transfusions.

Use morphine sulfate or meperidine per order to control shivering; *shivering causes increases in metabolic rate, CO_2 production and decreases in O_2 saturation and glycogen stores.*

Monitor arterial blood gas levels; *because of medullary respiratory depression, respiratory acidosis may result.*

REFERENCES

Augustine S: Hypothermia therapy in the postanesthesia unit: a review, *J Postanesthes Nurs* 5(4):254, 1990.

Danzi D, Ghezzi K: Hot tips on handling hypothermia, *Patient Care* 25(20):89, 1991.

Erickson R, Yount S: Effect of aluminized covers on body temperature in patients having abdominal surgery, *Heart Lung* 20(3):255, 1991.

Giuffre M and others: Rewarming postoperative patients: lights, blankets or forced warm air, *J Postanesthesia Nurs* 6(6):387, 1991.

Heffline M: A comparative study of pharmacological versus nursing interventions in the treatment of postanesthesia shivering, *J Postanesthesia Nurs* 6(5):311, 1991.

Heidenreich T and others: Temperature and temperature measurement after induced hypothermia, *Nurs Res* 41(5):296, 1992.

Holtzclaw B: Shivering, *Nurs Clin North Am* 25(4):977, 1990.

Lawson L: Hypothermia and trauma injury; temperature monitoring and rewarming strategies, *Crit Care Nurse Quarterly* 15(1):21, 1992.

Oliver S, Fuessel E: Control of postoperative hypothermia in cardiovascular surgery patients, *Crit Care Nurse Quarterly* 12(4):63, 1990.

Stevens T: Managing postoperative hypothermia, rewarming and its complications, *Crit Care Nurse Quarterly* 16(1):60, 1993.

Whitman G: Hypertension and hypothermia in the acute postoperative period, *Crit Care Nurs Clin North Am* 3(4):661, 1991.

Hypothermia—cont'd

Incontinence, functional

CLINICAL CONDITION/ MEDICAL DIAGNOSIS	RELATED FACTORS
Congestive heart failure	No established toileting regimen; impaired mobility requiring use of a walker

Patient goals
Expected outcomes
>   Associated nursing/collaborative interventions *and scientific rationale*

Establish/adhere to toileting routine as evidenced by the following:

Attempts voiding every hour; gradually increases to every 3 to 4 hours
Voids before retiring
Uses voiding log to record voiding and attempts to void
>   Collaborate with patient to establish a 1-hour prompted voiding schedule; gradually increase to 3 to 4 hours if tolerated.
>   Teach and monitor use of voiding record *to identify changes in pattern of urination.*

Achieve continence as evidenced by the following:

Reports gradual decrease in episodes of incontinence
Records episodes of involuntary loss of urine
Performs pelvic floor exercises (PFEs) 3 times a day
Takes afternoon diuretic 4 to 5 hours before bedtime
>   Teach progressive use of PFEs. Provide written instructions. Sit or stand without tensing muscles of legs, buttocks, or abdomen. Contract and relax circumvaginal muscles and urinary and anal sphincters for 3 to 4 seconds and repeat in a staccato fashion. Do PFEs 25 to 30 times, 3 times daily. *PFEs strengthen the circumvaginal muscles, urinary sphincter, and external anal sphincter.*

Incontinence, functional

Develop with patient a schedule for taking diuretic.
Monitor medications for drugs that influence bladder tone, e.g., *low K+ level decreases bladder tone.*

Modify environment to facilitate continence as evidenced by the following:

Accepts use of commode on a temporary basis
Keeps walker, supplies, and telephone nearby
Wears clothing easy to manage for toileting
Uses continence aids to protect skin and clothing

Collaborate with patient to establish a self-care system for managing urinary incontinence.

Assist patient with selection and creation of a private area for commode and supplies. *Private area for commode will facilitate patient-initiated voiding attempts.*

Demonstrate sensitivity to patient's feelings about incontinence.

Provide information about continence aids. *Use of continence aids helps to alleviate patient's anxiety and contributes to continence.*

REFERENCES

Agency for Health Care Policy and Research: *Clinical practice guidelines for urinary incontinence in adults* (AHCPR 92-0038), Rockville, Md: US Department of Health and Human Services, 1992.

Brink CA and others: A digital test for pelvic muscle strength in older women with urinary incontinence, *Nurs Res* 38(4):196-199, 1989.

Dowd TT: Discovering older women's experience of urinary incontinence, *Res Nurs Health* 14(3):179-186, 1991.

Ouellet LL, Ruch KL: A synthesis of selected literature on mobility: a basis for studying impaired mobility, *Nurs Diagnosis* 3(2):72-80, 1992.

Palmer MH and others: Detecting urinary incontinence in older adults during hospitalization, *Appl Nurs Res* 5(4):174-180, 1992.

Palmer MH, German PS, Ouslander JG: Risk factors for urinary incontinence one year after nursing home admission, *Res Nurs Health* 14(6):405-412, 1991.

Pieper B and others: Inventing urine incontinence devices for women, *Image: J Nurs Sch* 21(4):205-209, 1989.

Sampselle CM, DeLancey JO: The urine stream interruption test and pelvic muscle function, *Nurs Res* 41(2):73-77, 1992.

Wyman JF and others: Influence of functional, urological, and environmental characteristics on urinary incontinence in community-dwelling older women, *Nurs Res* 42(5):270-275, 1993.

Incontinence, reflex

CLINICAL CONDITION/ MEDICAL DIAGNOSIS	RELATED FACTORS
Spinal cord lesion above the level of the reflex arc	No sensation of voiding; incomplete emptying of the bladder

> **Patient goals**
> **Expected outcomes**
>   Associated nursing/collaborative interventions *and scientific rationale*

Achieve continence as evidenced by the following:

Expresses willingness to try manual voiding techniques
Participates in selection of reminders to void
Episodes of incontinence are rare

   Assist in selection, teaching, and trial of manual voiding facilitation techniques (e.g., stimulation of anus, tapping lower abdomen, doing push-ups on commode). *A reflex bladder contraction occurs in response to perineal or lower abdominal stimulation.*

   Establish reminders to void.

   Monitor amount of residual urine.

Participates in learning clean intermittent catheterization (CIC)
Participates in development of manual voiding on schedule
Monitors signs and symptoms for evidence of bladder and/or urinary tract infection

   Demonstrate and have patient/significant other return demonstrate CIC. *Patient/significant other must learn CIC to monitor residual urine; knowing CIC gives patient greater sense of control.*

   Teach and monitor use of appropriate hygienic measures, cleaning and storage of catheters.

   Teach patient/significant other signs and symptoms of bladder urinary tract infection.

Determine need for use of urinary containment device at night.

Establish a manual voiding and/or catheterization schedule, usually every 4 to 6 hours.

REFERENCES

Agency for Health Care Policy and Research: *Clinical practice guidelines for urinary incontinence in adults* (AHCPR 92-0038), Rockville, Md: US Department of Health and Human Services, 1992.

Brink CA and others: A digital test of pelvic muscle strength in older women with urinary incontinence, *Nurs Res* 38(4):196-199, 1989.

Dowd TT: Discovering older women's experience of urinary incontinence, *Res Nurs Health* 14(3):179-186, 1991.

McCormick KA, Palmer MH: Urinary incontinence in older adults, *Ann Rev Nurs Res* 10:25-53, 1992.

Palmer MH and others: Detecting urinary incontinence in older adults during hospitalization, *App Nurs Res* 5(4):174-180, 1992.

Pieper B and others: Inventing urinary incontinence devices for women, *Image: J Nurs Sch* 21(4):205-209, 1989.

Specht J and others: Urinary incontinence. In Maas M, Buckwalter KC, Hardy M, eds: *Nursing diagnosis and interventions for the elderly*, pp 181-204, Redwood City, Calif, 1991, Addison-Wesley.

Voith AM: Alterations in urinary elimination: concepts, research, and practice, *Rehab Nurs* 13(3):122, 1988.

Incontinence, reflex—cont'd

Incontinence, stress

CLINICAL CONDITION/ MEDICAL DIAGNOSIS	RELATED FACTORS
Postpartum 5 weeks with 5 children	Weak pelvic muscles with sphincter incompetence; displacement of urethra and bladder neck during exertion

Patient goals
Expected outcomes
> Associated nursing/collaborative interventions *and scientific rationale*

Increase pelvic floor muscle tone and sphincter function as evidenced by the following:

Performs pelvic floor exercises (PFEs) 3 times a day for 6 months

> Teach patient a method for doing PFEs and provide written instructions. Sit or stand without tensing muscles of legs, buttocks, or abdomen. Contract and relax circumvaginal muscles and urinary and anal sphincters for 3 to 4 seconds and repeat in a staccato fashion. Do PFEs 25 to 30 times, 3 times daily. *PFEs strengthen the circumvaginal muscles, urinary sphincter, and external anal sphincter.*

Implement a voiding routine as evidenced by the following:

Keeps a voiding record
Uses timer to provide cue to void every 2 hours
Reduces episodes of incontinence
Drinks 6 to 8 glasses of water a day
Uses continence aids

> Teach patient to keep a voiding log.
> Instruct patient to void by the clock, beginning with 2-hour intervals; gradually lengthen interval between attempts to void.
> Collaborate with patient to establish a fluid intake pattern to maintain hydration, e.g., 200 ml every 2 hours during day.

Incontinence, stress

Teach use of incontinence aids. *Use of incontinence aids will help decrease anxiety.*

REFERENCES

Agency for Health Care Policy and Research: *Clinical practice guidelines for urinary incontinence in adults* (AHCPR 92-0038), Rockville, Md: US Department of Health and Human Services, 1992.

Brink CA and others: A digital test for pelvic muscle strength in older women with urinary incontinence, *Nurs Res* 38(4):196-199, 1989.

McCormick KA, Palmer MH: Urinary incontinence in older adults, *Ann Rev Nurs Res* 10:25-53, 1992.

Sampselle CM, Delancey JO: The urine stream interruption test and pelvic muscle function, *Nurs Res* 41(2):73-77, 1992.

Specht J and others: Urinary incontinence. In Maas M, Buckwalter KC, Hardy M, eds: Nursing diagnoses and interventions for the elderly, Redwood City, Calif, 1991, Addison-Wesley.

Voith AM: Alteration in urinary elimination concepts, research and practice, *Rehab Nurs* 13(3):122, 1988.

Incontinence, stress—cont'd

Incontinence, total

CLINICAL CONDITION/ MEDICAL DIAGNOSIS	RELATED FACTORS
Pelvic trauma/fistula	No established toileting regimen; self-care limitations (functional level 3)

Patient goals
Expected outcomes
    Associated nursing/collaborative interventions *and scientific rationale*

Achieve a complete, regular bladder evacuation as evidenced by the following:

Incontinent episodes are contained
Residual urine is less than 50 ml
    Provide urinary containment device for immediate use because *most routine treatment modalities are ineffective.*
    Develop with patient/caregiver strategies for coping with use of urinary containment devices.
    Monitor residual urine.

Avoid urological complications as evidenced by the following:

Makes and keeps appointment with urologist for fistula closing
Returns demonstration of intermittent catheterization
    Refer patient for medical evaluation.
    Monitor color, odor, and amount of urine.
    Demonstrate/monitor clean intermittent catheterization *to prevent urinary infection.*
    Implement written plan for fluid intake, e.g., 200 ml every 2 hours from 8 AM to 6 PM.

Achieve desired level of independence in self-care as evidenced by the following:

Establishes a plan to gain independence in self-care consistent with limitation

Monitors own fluid intake/voiding patterns and
makes adjustments
Sets goals for increase in self-care activities
Identifies problems/potential problems related to use
of urinary containment devices

**Maintain skin integrity as evidenced by the
following:**

Skin remains intact
Uses continence aids to keep self dry
>Implement written plan for keeping skin clean/dry.
>Monitor skin for signs of redness, abrasions, etc.
>Demonstrate use of easy-to-remove protective
>clothing.

**Maintain patient's/caregiver's dignity and feelings
of self-worth as evidenced by the following:**

Increases number of positive self-statements
>Monitor nurse/patient interactions for negative
>self-statements.
>Teach patient thought-stopping and thought-
>substitution techniques.
>Use behavioral approaches acceptable to patient
>and caregiver.

Primary caregiver participates in outside
recreational/social activities weekly
>Evaluate caregiver's perceived health, sense of well-
>being, and feelings of burden.
>Discuss with patient/caregiver importance of
>planning for caregiver's participation in desired
>recreational/social activities.

REFERENCES

Agency for Health Care Policy and Research: *Clinical practice guidelines
for urinary incontinence in adults*, 1992 (AHCPR 92-0038).
Dowd TT: Discovering older women's experience of urinary
incontinence, *Res Nurs Health* 14(3):179-186, 1991.
McCormick KA, Palmer MH: Urinary incontinence in older adults,
Ann Rev Nurs Res 10:25-53, 1992.
Specht J and others: Urinary incontinence. In Maas M, Buckwalter
KC, Hardy M, eds: *Nursing diagnoses and interventions for the elderly*
pp 181-204, Redwood City, Calif, 1991, Addison-Wesley.
Wyman JF and others: Influence of functional, urological, and
environmental characteristics on urinary incontinence in
community-dwelling older women, *Nurs Res* 42(5):270-275, 1993.

Incontinence, urge

CLINICAL CONDITION/ MEDICAL DIAGNOSIS	RELATED FACTORS
Interstitial cystitis	No established toileting routine; inadequate intake of noncaffeine liquids

Patient goals
Expected outcomes
> Associated nursing/collaborative interventions *and scientific rationale*

Establish and adhere to toileting routine as evidenced by the following:

Attempts voiding every 2 hours; gradual increase to every 3 to 4 hours
Exercises pelvic floor muscles regularly
Records voiding attempts, pelvic floor exercises, and episodes of incontinence in voiding log
Voids before going to bed
> Collaborate with patient to develop and implement toileting regime.
> Teach and monitor use of voiding record.
> Teach pelvic floor exercises (PFEs) to *strengthen circumvaginal muscles.*
> Monitor change in voiding pattern

Alter pattern of response to urge to void as evidenced by the following:

Avoids rushing to the toilet
Responds to urge to void by pausing and relaxing abdominal muscles, then proceeding at a normal pace
> Teach patient to alter pattern of response to urge to void, including avoiding rushing to toilet; responding to urge to void by pausing to relax abdominal muscles; and proceeding at a normal pace. *Relaxation of abdominal muscles decreases sense of urgency and helps patient remain continent.*

Modify fluid intake to maintain acid urine as evidenced by the following:

Drinks concentrated cranberry juice daily
Takes superphysiological amounts of vitamin C, at least 1000 mg per day
Substitutes herbal tea for caffeine-containing liquids
Drinks 8 oz of water with meals, between meals, and in early evening

Teach patient to drink concentrated cranberry juice and/or take superphysiological doses of vitamin C. *In very large doses some vitamin C is excreted in urine as ascorbic acid. The acidity of urine helps to prevent bacterial growth.*

Teach patient to drink 8 oz of water with and between meals and in early evening.

Provide patient with written information about caffeine-containing liquids; teach to substitute caffeine-free liquids.

REFERENCES

Agency for Health Care Policy and Research: *Clinical practice guidelines for urinary incontinence in adults* (AHCPR 92-0038), Rockville, Md, 1992, US Department of Health and Human Services.

Dowd TT: Discovering older women's experience of urinary incontinence, *Res Nurs Health* 14(3):179-186, 1991.

Kinney AB, Blount M: Effect of cranberry juice on urinary pH, *Nurs Res* 28:287, 1979.

McCormick KA, Scheve AAS, Leahy E: Nursing management of urinary incontinence in geriatric patients, *Nurs Clin North Am* 23(1):231, 1988.

McCormick KA, Palmer MH: Urinary incontinence in older adults, *Ann Rev Nurs Res* 10:25-53, 1992.

Specht J and others: Urinary incontinence. In Maas M, Buckwalter KC, Hardy M, eds: *Nursing diagnoses and interventions for the elderly*, pp 181-204. Redwood City, Calif, 1991, Addison-Wesley.

Voith AM: Alteration in urinary elimination concepts, research and practice, *Rehab Nurs* 13(3):122, 1988.

Wyman JF and others: Influence of functional, urological, and environmental characteristics on urinary incontinence in community-dwelling older women, *Nurs Res* 42(5):270-275, 1993.

Infant behavior, disorganized

CLINICAL CONDITION/ MEDICAL DIAGNOSIS	RELATED FACTORS
Painful procedures for the premature infant	Excessive environmental stimulation; long-term hospitalization requiring painful procedures

---

Patient goals
Expected outcomes
>Associated nursing/collaborative interventions *and scientific rationale*

Experience less pain as evidenced by the following:

Fewer, less intense episodes of crying

Assess infant's responses, on a routine basis, to painful stimuli and pharmacologic and nonpharmacologic soothing techniques.

Premedicate infant before painful procedures. *Reducing pain level will reduce physiologic and behavioral stress in the infant.*

Reduce number of routine blood drawing events; group blood drawing episodes and conduct on a once daily or weekly basis as indicated by health status.

Create one long-term access route when frequent blood drawing is indicated.

Allow only precertified and experienced personnel to perform painful procedures, including insertion of IVs, PCVC, or central lines

Apply minimal amount—and the least irritating type—of tape; remove tape carefully for all equipment requiring tape for stabilization.

Administer pharmacologic agents as indicated.

Use nonpharmacologic techniques to enhance the therapeutic effects of pharmacologic agents. *Employing soothing techniques may comfort and/or distract the infant and reduce irritability.*

Swaddle the infant.

Place hands on the infant to contain the infant's extremities.

Decrease the excessive environmental stimulation.

Reposition the infant to maximize infant comfort.

Help the infant to console itself by freeing hands so the infant may put hands to mouth.

Provide pacifier. *Sucking on the pacifier may decrease irritability and improve oxygenation.*

Hold the infant and provide soothing verbal cues.

Soothe the infant by lightly stroking the infant on the back, abdomen, or extremities.

Experience less distress during procedures as evidenced by the following:

Fewer and less intense episodes of crying and other nonverbal cues of distress such as body language.

Facilitate motor stability and function by the following strategies:

- Provide pacifier. *Sucking on the pacifier may console the infant and reduces irritability.*
- Contain the infant by placing two hands on the infant and holding extremities close to the infant.
- Swaddle the infant. *Swaddling may comfort the infant and reduce irritability.*
- Position infant prone or side-lying with hands and extremities in flexion. *Positioning with proper body alignment will promote motor development.*
- Free infant's hands when swaddling so that the infant may put hands to mouth. *Allowing the infant access to his/her hands will assist the infant to learn how to console self and reduce level of stress.*
- *Providing motor stability reduces stress and irritability and promotes motor development.*

Facilitate autonomic stability and function by the following strategies:

- Monitor physiologic responses to procedures.
- Allow time for the infant to recover physiologically between procedures.
- Swaddle the infant.

- Position infant prone or side-lying with hands and extremities in flexion.
- Provide soft verbal cues to the infant by talking softly to the infant.
- Reduce sound and light to lowest levels.

REFERENCES

Als H, Lawhon G, Brown E, Gibes R, Duffy FH, McAnulty G, Blickman JG: Individualized behavioral and environmental care for very low birth weight infants at high risk for bronchopulmonary dysplasia: neonatal intensive care unit and developmental outcome, *Pediatrics* 1986, 78(6), 1123.

Field TM, Goldson E: Pacifying effects of nonnutritive sucking on term and preterm neonates during heelstick procedures, *Pediatrics* 1984, 74(6):1012.

Franck LS: A new method to quantitatively describe pain behavior in infants, *Nurs Res* 1986, 35:28.

OGN Nursing practice resource: Prevention, recognition and management of neonatal pain. Washington, DC, NAACOG:3, 1991.

VandenBerg K, Franck LS: Bronchopulmonary dysplasia: strategies for total patient care, Petaluma, Cal, 1990, Neonatal Network.

Infant behavior, disorganized: risk for

CLINICAL CONDITION/ MEDICAL DIAGNOSIS	RELATED FACTORS
Prematurity; intraventricular hemorrhage	Excessive environmental stimulation; autonomic instability

Patient goals
Expected outcomes
> Associated nursing/collaborative interventions *and scientific rationale*

Experience reduction in environmental stimuli as evidenced by the following:

Sleeps for appropriate periods of time

Demonstrate fewer episodes of irritability.

Regulate the nursery environment by the following strategies:

- Maintain low noise levels in the nursery, not greater than 60 decibel, 40 decibel optimal. *Elevated sound levels may induce stress in the premature infant and effect physiologic function.*
- Decrease movement of personnel around incubator.
- Train ancillary support hospital staff to decrease noise levels during their work.
- Conduct rounds away from the incubator.
- Remove sources of noise, such as garbage cans, hospital tube system, ancillary equipment.
- Lower the sound levels of the intercom and the telephone within the unit.
- Keep all objects such as thermometers or glass bottles off the top of the incubator.
- Close incubator portholes quietly.
- Cover the open bassinet or incubator with an adult bath blanket to absorb sound.
- Evaluate potential equipment purchases for sound levels.
- Decrease light levels in the nursery. *Excessive light levels may affect the development of vision.*

- Reduce overhead lighting to no greater than 25 footcandles.
- Provide day/night rotation of light.
- Cover the incubator with a receiving blanket during sleep.

Experience less distress during procedures as evidenced by the following:

Fewer and less intense episodes of crying and other nonverbal cues of distress such as body language.

Cluster nursing care around feedings and divide procedures over the 24 hour period to distribute them evenly.

Procedures such as suctioning or chest physical therapy should not be routine; infants should be carefully assessed for need and response to these procedures.

Facilitate motor stability and function by the following strategies:

- Provide pacifier *to assist with modulation of state and reduce irritability.*
- Contain the infant by placing two hands on the infant and holding extremities close to the infant.
- Swaddle the infant. *Swaddling may comfort the infant and reduce irritability.*
- Position infant prone or side-lying with hands and extremities in flexion. *Positioning with proper body alignment will promote motor development.*
- *Providing motor stability reduces stress and promotes motor development.*

Facilitate autonomic stability and function by the following strategies:

- Monitor physiologic responses to procedures.
- Allow time for the infant to recover physiologically between procedures.
- Swaddle the infant.
- Free infant's hands when swaddling so that the infant may put hands to mouth. *Allowing the infant access to his or her hands will assist the*

infant to learn how to console self and reduce level of stress.

- Position infant prone or sidelying with hands and extremities in flexion. *Prone or sidelying position improves oxygenation.*
- Provide soft verbal cues to the infant by talking softly to him or her.
- Further reduce sound levels and light levels.

Experience complete sleep cycles as evidenced by the following:

Sleeps for appropriate periods of time

Facilitate complete sleep cycles by the following strategies:

- Do not allow the infant's sleep to be disrupted for routine physical examinations, radiographs, or blood drawing.
- Construct boundaries (nesting) around the infant during sleep.
- Administer oral tactile stimulation by a lemon glycerine swab when central apnea occurs during sleep. *Administration of the lemon glycerine swab during central apnea will promote reinitiation of respiratory effort without altering the infant's sleep state.*
- *Completion of sleep cycles promotes growth, including brain growth.*

Experience social interaction as evidenced by the following:

Demonstrates responsive body language
Cries less frequently

Promote parental visits by including parents in the planning and implementation of their infant's care.

Promote opportunities for social interaction by the following strategies:

- Modulate behavioral state to the quiet alert state after feeding by administering verbal stimulation (soft human voice), eye-to-eye contact (when the infant is alert), touch (light

stroking or skin-to-skin contact), and
vestibular stimulation (rocking) as tolerated by
the infant. *Modulating the behavioral state will
promote alertness and behavioral responsiveness in
the infant while providing the opportunity for
interaction between parent (or caregiver) and
infant.*
- Stroke infant and talk to infant softly during
  routine assessments.
- Swaddle and hold infant outside incubator or
  bassinet during feeding and talk to the infant
  with eye-to-eye contact during feeding.

Progress with oral feeding as evidenced by the following:

Demonstrates tolerance for more breastfeeding sessions

Demonstrates more effective sucking reflex
Facilitate progression of oral feeding by providing
nonnutritive sucking before oral feeding and
during gavage feeding; support mother in
frequent breast-feeding sessions.

Modulate behavioral state from sleep to active alert
before feeding by administering verbal
stimulation (soft human voice), eye-to-eye
contact (when the infant is alert), touch (light
stroking or skin-to-skin contact), and vestibular
stimulation (rocking). *Modulating behavioral state
to the active alert state just prior to feeding may
enhance feeding behaviors.*

Experience age-appropriate sensory stimulation as evidenced by the following:

Demonstrates appropriate sensory responses.
Provide age-appropriate infant sensory stimulation
by the following strategies:
- Select sensory intervention based on the
  infant's health status, postconception age,
  extent of perinatal injury, and individual
  response patterns. *Providing appropriate sensory
  interventions in a nursery that has a stress*

reduction program in place will promote optimal development.

- Initiate constant vestibular stimulation at birth for infants less than 34 weeks' gestation at birth and wean to intermittent vestibular stimulation at 32 to 34 postconception weeks.
- Maintain boundaries (nesting) for infants during sleep and alertness.
- Teach parents about their infant's responses to environmental stimuli and promote parental provision of age-appropriate sensory stimuli.
- Place visual stimuli more than 8 inches away from the infant's face. *Placing visual stimuli more than 8 inches away from the infant's face will promote optimal visual development.*

REFERENCES

Als H, Lawhon G, Duffy FH, McAnulty GB, Gibes-Grossman R, Blickman JG: Individualized developmental care for the very-low-birth-weight preterm infant: medical and neurofunctional effects, *JAMA*, 21(11):853, 1994.

Becker PT, Grunwald PC, Moorman J, Stuhr S: Effects of developmental care on behavioral organization in very-low-birth-weight infants, *Nurs Res* 42(4):214, 1993.

Burns KC, Cunningham NA, White-Traut RC, Silvestri JM, Nelson MN: Infant stimulation: modification of an intervention based on physiologic and behavioral cues, *JOGNN* 23(7):581, 1994.

Garcia AP, White-Traut RC: Preterm infants' responses to taste/smell and tactile stimulation during an apneic episode, *J Ped Nurs* 8(4):245, 1993.

Gill NE, Behnke ML, Conlon M, McNeely JB, Anderson GC: Effect of nonnutritive sucking on behavioral state in preterm infants before feeding, *Nurs Res* 37(6):347, 1992.

Holditch-Davis D: The development of sleeping and waking states in high risk preterm infants, *Inf Beh Dev* 13(513), 1990.

Mann NP, Haddow R, Stokes L, Goodley S, Rutter N: Effect of night and day on preterm infants in a newborn nursery: randomized trial, *Br Med J* 293(15):1265, 1986.

White-Traut RC, Nelson MN, Burns KC, Cunningham NA: Environmental influences on the developing premature infant: theoretical issues and applications to practice, *JOGNN* 23(5):393, 1994.

White-Traut RC, Nelson MN, Silvestri JM, Patel M, Kilgallon D: Patterns of physiologic and behavioral response of intermediate care preterm infants to intervention, *Ped Nurs* 19(6):625, 1993.

White-Traut RC, Pate CH: Modulating infant state in premature infants, *J Ped Nurs* 2(2):96, 1987.

Infant behavior, disorganized: risk for—cont'd

Infant behavior, organized: potential for enhanced

CLINICAL CONDITION/ MEDICAL DIAGNOSIS	RELATED FACTORS
Prematurity; periventricular leukomalacia	Excessive environmental stimulation; long-term hospitalization

Patient goals
Expected outcomes
    Associated nursing/collaborative interventions *and scientific rationale*

Experience reduction in environmental stimuli as evidenced by the following:

Sleeps for appropriate periods of time
Demonstrates fewer episodes of irritability
    Regulate the nursery environment by the following strategies:

- Maintain low noise levels in the nursery, not greater than 60 decibel, less than 40 decibel optimal. *Elevated sound levels may induce stress in the premature infant and affect physiologic function.*
- Decrease movement of personnel around incubator.
- Train ancillary support hospital staff to decrease noise levels during their work.
- Conduct rounds away from the incubator.
- Remove sources of noise, such as garbage cans, hospital tube system, ancillary equipment.
- Lower the sound levels of the intercom and the telephone within the unit.
- Keep all objects such as thermometers or glass bottles off the top of the incubator.
- Close incubator portholes quietly.
- Close the open bassinet or incubator with an adult bath blanket to absorb sound.
- Evaluate potential equipment purchases for sound levels.
- Decrease light levels in the nursery. *Excessive light levels may affect the development of vision.*

- Reduce overhead lighting to no greater than 25 footcandles.
- Provide day/night rotation of light.
- Cover the incubator or open bassinet with a receiving blanket during sleep.

Experience complete sleep cycles as evidenced by the following:

Sleeps for appropriate periods of time
Facilitates complete sleep cycles.
- Do not allow the infant's sleep to be disrupted for routine physical examinations, radiographs, blood drawing.
- Construct boundaries (nesting) around the infant during sleep.
- Administer oral tactile stimulation with a lemon glycerine swab when central apnea occurs during sleep. *Administration of the lemon glycerine swab during central apnea will promote reinitiation of respiratory effort without altering the infant's sleep state.*
- *Completion of sleep cycles promotes growth, including brain growth.*

Experience social interaction as evidenced by the following:

Demonstrates responsive body language
Cries less frequently
Promote parental visits by including parents in the planning and implementing of their infant's care.

Promote opportunities for social interaction.
Modulate behavioral state to the quiet alert state after feeding by administering verbal stimulation (soft human voice), eye-to-eye contact (when the infant is alert), touch (light stroking or skin-to-skin contact), and vestibular stimulation (rocking) as tolerated by the infant. *Modulating the behavioral state will promote*

alertness and behavioral responsiveness in the infant while providing the opportunity for interaction between parent (or caregiver) and infant.

Progress with oral feeding as evidenced by the following:

Demonstrates tolerance for more breastfeeding sessions
Demonstrates more effective sucking reflex

Facilitate progression of oral feeding by providing nonnutritive sucking before oral feeding and during gavage feeding; support mother in frequent breastfeeding sessions.

Modulate the behavioral state from sleep to active alert prior to feeding by administering verbal stimulation (soft human voice), eye-to-eye contact (when the infant is alert), touch (light stroking or skin-to-skin contact), and vestibular stimulation (rocking). *Modulating the behavioral state to the active alert state just prior to feeding may enhance feeding behavior.*

Experience age-appropriate sensory stimulation as evidenced by the following:

Demonstrates appropriate sensory responses

Promote opportunities for social interaction by the following strategies:

- Modulate the behavioral state to quiet alert state after feeding by administering verbal stimulation (soft human voice), eye-to-eye contact (when the infant is alert), touch (light stroking or skin-to-skin contact), and vestibular stimulation (rocking) as tolerated by the infant. *Modulating the behavioral state will promote alertness and behavioral responsiveness in the infant while providing the opportunity for interaction between parent (or caregiver) and infant.*
- Stroke infant and talk to infant softly during routine assessments.

Infant behavior, organized: potential for enhanced—cont'd

- Swaddle and hold infant outside incubator or bassinet during feeding and talk to the infant with eye-to-eye contact during feeding.

Provide age-appropriate infant sensory stimulation.

- Select sensory interventions based on the infant's health status, postconception age, extent of perinatal injury, and individual response patterns. *Providing appropriate sensory interventions in a nursery that has a stress-reduction program in place will promote optimal development.*
- Initiate constant vestibular stimulation at birth for infants less than 34 weeks' gestation at birth and wean to intermittent vestibular stimulation at 32 to 34 postconception weeks.
- Maintain boundaries (nesting) for infants during sleep and alertness.
- Teach parents about their infant's responses to environmental stimuli and promote parental provision of age-appropriate sensory stimuli.
- Place visual stimuli more than 8 inches away from the infant's face. *Placing visual stimuli more than 8 inches away from the infant's face will promote optimal visual development.*

Experience less distress during procedures as evidenced by the following:

Fewer and less intense episodes of crying and other nonverbal cues of distress such as body language

Cluster nursing care around feedings and divide procedures over the 24 hour period to evenly distribute them.

Procedures such as suctioning or chest physical therapy should not be routine; infants should be carefully assessed for need and response to these procedures.

Facilitate motor stability and function by the following strategies:

- Provide a pacifier.

- Contain the infant by placing two hands on the infant and holding extremities close to the infant.
- Swaddle the infant. *Swaddling may comfort the infant and reduce irritability.*
- Position infant prone or side-lying with hands and extremities in flexion. *Positioning with proper body alignment will promote motor development.*
- Free infant's hands when swaddling so that the infant may put hands to mouth. *Allowing the infant access to his or her hands will assist the infant to learn how to console self.*
- *Providing motor stability reduces stress and promotes motor development.*

Facilitate autonomic stability and function by the following strategies:

- Monitor physiologic responses to procedures.
- Allow time for the infant to recover physiologically between procedures.
- Swaddle the infant. *Swaddling may comfort the infant and reduce irritability.*
- Position infant prone or side-lying with hands and extremities in flexion. *Positioning with proper body alignment will promote motor development.*
- Provide soft verbal cues to the infant by talking softly to him or her.
- Further reduce sound levels and light levels.

REFERENCES

Als H, Lawhon G, Duffy FH, McAnulty GB, Gibes-Grossman R, Blickman JG: Individualized developmental care for the very low-birth weight preterm infant: medical and neurofunctional effects, *JAMA* 21(11):853, 1994.

Becker PT, Grunwald PC, Moorman J, Stuhr S: Outcomes of developmentally supportive nursing care for very low birth weight infants, *Nurs Res* 40(3):150, 1991.

Burns KC, Cunningham NA, White-Traut RC, Silvestri JM, Nelson MN: Infant stimulation: modification of an intervention based on physiologic and behavioral cues, *JOGNN* 23(7), 581, 1994.

Garcia AP, White-Traut RC: Preterm infants' responses to taste/smell and tactile stimulation during an apneic episode, *J Ped Nurs* 8(4):245, 1993.

Gill NE, Behnke ML, Conlon M, McNeely JB, Anderson GC: Effect of nonnutritive sucking on behavioral state in preterm infants before feeding, *Nurs Res* 37(6):347, 1992.

Holditch-Davis D: The development of sleeping and waking states in high risk preterm infants, *Inf Beh Dev* 13:513, 1990.

Mann NP, Haddow R, Stokes L, Goodley S, Rutter N: Effect of night and day on preterm infants in a newborn nursery: randomized trial, *Br Med J* 293(15):1265, 1986.

White-Traut RC, Nelson MN, Burns KC, Cunningham NA: Environmental influences on the developing premature infant: theoretical issues and applications to practice, *JOGNN* 23(5):393, 1994.

White-Traut RC, Nelson MN, Silvestri JM, Patel M, Kilgallon D: Patterns of physiologic and behavioral response of intermediate care preterm infants to intervention, *Ped Nurs* 19(6):625, 1993.

White-Traut RC, Pate CH: Modulating infant state in premature infants, *J Ped Nurs* 2(2):96, 1987.

Infant feeding pattern, ineffective

CLINICAL CONDITION/ MEDICAL DIAGNOSIS	RELATED FACTORS
Prematurity	Uncoordinated sucking, swallowing, and breathing mechanisms

---

Patient goals
Expected outcomes
    Associated nursing/collaborative interventions *and scientific rationale*

Recognize the methods to deliver expressed mother's milk (EMM) to the high-risk preterm infant as evidenced by the following:

Knows why gavage method is to be used
Provide information to the mother that most small, preterm infants cannot be breastfed directly. Therefore they receive EMM by artificial feeding such as gavage infusion until they have demonstrated the ability to feed orally. *Preterm infant's ability to coordinate sucking, swallowing, and breathing varies from 32 to 36 weeks of gestation, depending on feeding method.*

Knows the types of gavage feeding
Discuss possible adverse, short-term, physiological, and biochemical responses to intermittent bolus gavage feeding, such as apnea, bradycardia, and hypoxemia *to determine whether to use continuous or intermittent gavage feeding.*
Use intermittent bolus gavage infusion of EMM at a slow rate for all preterm infants whenever possible *to minimize or prevent adverse sequelae of rapid gastric filling.*

Achieve adequate nutritional state as evidenced by the following:

Infant gains weight and grows within expected limits
Administer EMM by continuous nasogastric (CNG) infusion, if needed, by using following safeguards:

Infant feeding pattern, ineffective

Perform routine bacteriologic surveillance of EMM so that EMM contains only skin flora in concentration not exceeding 10^3 colony-forming units (cfu) per ml.

Infuse the EMM at the highest possible rate that is safe for the infant, *to minimize the bacterial growth and nutrient loss.*

Use syringe pump placed at 45-degree angle and small-lumen infusion tubing *to minimize nutrient loss.*

Measure lipid content of EMM by creamatocrit at the distal end of the infusion system. *If lipid adheres to the infusion syringe and tubing, infant may receive a more dilute, low-calorie milk and subsequently demonstrate suboptimal growth.*

Change syringe and tubing every 4 hours *to minimize bacterial growth.*

REFERENCES

Brennan-Behm M and others: Caloric loss from expressed mother's milk during continuous gavage infusion, *Neonatal Network* 13(2):26-33, 1994.

Churella HR, Bachhuber WL, MacLean WC: Survey: methods of feeding low-birth-weight infants, *Pediatrics* 76:243, 1985.

Heldt G: The effect of gavage feeding on the mechanics of the lung, chest wall, and diaphragm of preterm infants, *Pediatr Res* 24:55, 1988.

McCoy R and others: Nursing management of breast feeding for preterm infants, *J Perinat Neonat Nurs* 2:42, 1988.

Meier PP: Bottle and breast feeding: effects on transcutaneous oxygen pressure and temperature in preterm infants, *Nurs Res* 37:36, 1988.

Meier PP, Pugh EJ: Breast feeding behavior of small preterm infants, *MCN* 10:396, 1985.

Meier PP, Wilks SO: The bacteria in expressed mother's milk, *MCN* 12:420, 1987.

Meier PP and others: Bottle and breastfeeding: physiologic effects on preterm infants (abstract), *Neonatal Network* 10:78, 1991.

Infant feeding pattern, ineffective—cont'd

Infection, risk for

CLINICAL CONDITION/ MEDICAL DIAGNOSIS	RELATED FACTORS
Cancer chemotherapy-induced immunosuppression; neutropenia	Suppressed immune system

---

Patient goals
Expected outcomes
    Associated nursing/collaborative interventions *and scientific rationale*

Experience no infection as evidenced by the following:

Has no signs and symptoms of infection

Monitor temperature every 4 hours; report elevation.

Auscultate lungs daily; have patient report sore throat or peri-anal tenderness. *Typical signs of inflammation may be absent in neutropenia.*

Weigh patient daily.

Check body fluids for alterations in color, odor, or consistency.

Limit use of aspirin/acetaminophen, *because these can mask a fever.*

Obtain cultures per order and report abnormalities.

Wash hands before each contact with patient.

Use gloves as necessary.

Discontinue invasive lines as soon as possible.

Avoid invasive procedures.

Use strict aseptic technique when performing invasive procedures.

Prevent patient exposure to infected visitors/staff.

Avoid fresh flowers and plants in room and raw vegetables/fruits in diet; *organisms in these may cause a problem in neutropenia.*

Monitor results of CBC and report WBC abnormalities. Use reverse isolation if indicated;

neutropenia of 500 to 1000 increases risk of infection.

Patient/significant other verbalizes knowledge of infection prevention

Teach patient to choose high-calorie, high-protein, high-vitamin foods; *such foods will promote cellular repair and regeneration and help produce lymphocytes.*

Teach patient to follow steps for prevention of impaired skin integrity.

Teach patient to shower daily and use good oral hygiene.

Teach patient to drink fluids, 2600 ml/day, *because this helps avoid UTI/constipation.*

Administer and teach patient about colony-stimulating factors.

REFERENCES

Camp-Sorrell D: Controlling adverse effects of chemotherapy, *Nursing* 21(4):34, 1991.

Fazio MT, Glaspy JA: The impact of granulocyte colony-stimulating factor on quality of life in patients with severe chronic neutropenia, *Oncol Nurs Forum* 18(8):1411, 1991.

Flyge HA: Meeting the challenge of neutropenia, *Nursing 93* 23(7):60, 1993.

Griffin J: Nursing care of the critically ill immunocompromised patient, *Crit Care Quarterly* 9(1):25, 1986.

Gurevich I, Tafuro P: Nursing measures for the prevention of infection in the compromised host, *Nurs Clin North Am* 20(1):257, 1985.

Reheis C: Neutropenia, *Nurs Clin North Am* 20(1):219, 1985.

Injury, perioperative positioning: risk for

CLINICAL CONDITION/ MEDICAL DIAGNOSIS	RELATED FACTORS
General surgery	Neuromuscular deficits; immobilization

Patient goals
Expected outcomes
> Associated nursing/collaborative interventions *and scientific rationale*

Become mobile and maintain tissue perfusion as evidenced by the following:

Moves all extremities without complaints of paresthesia

Pad neuromuscular junctions pertinent to each surgical position by the following strategies:
- Pad ulnar site when patient is in supine, Trendelenburg, and reverse Trendelenburg positions. *Compression of ulnar nerves will cause intermittent to continuous paresthesia.*
- Pad ulnar site when patient is in sitting position; provide pillow across abdomen to rest forearms.
- Pad brachial plexus site when patient is in prone and lateral positions; place axillary rolls bilaterally to eliminate compression upon plexus.

Avoid acutely hyperextending or abducting extremities.
- Avoid abducting the upper extremities more than 90 degrees when patient is in the following positions: supine, Trendelenburg, reverse Trendelenburg, lithotomy, and prone. *This causes compression of the cervical plexus between the scapula and the first rib.*
- Avoid acute flexion of the patient's thigh because it *causes compression of the peroneal nerve in the lithotomy position.*

Place safety strap 2 inches above the patella to negate the incidence of falls.

Specific anatomic tissue sites exhibit decreased erythema

Pad and protect all bony prominences pertinent to each surgical position by the following techniques:

- Pad occiput, scapula, olecranon and ulna, sacrum, and ischial tuberosities when patient is in supine, Trendelenburg and reverse Trendelenburg positions. *After short periods of vascular occlusion, erythema will occur. This is reactive hyperemia, which is a sudden increase of blood flow as a result of a sudden release of compression.*

- Elevate and lower extremities simultaneously while in patient lithotomy position in order to *facilitate venous return and eliminate back strain.*

- Avoid strapping the popliteal spaces tightly when knee-padded stirrups are used, to avoid compressing the popliteal artery, or the osseofascial compartment. *After prolonged pressure, damaged tissue liberates large quantities of histamine into the surrounding fluid. This increases capillary permeability, thereby causing more fluid to leak into surrounding tissues. This increase in pressure within the small osseofascial compartment causes additional compression of nerves and blood vessels, leading to obliteration of blood flow, neuromuscular dysfunction, and tissue ischemia.*

- Pad the occiput, scapula, olecranon, ulna, sacrum, ischial tuberosity, and calcaneus when patient is in sitting position.

- Pad the eyes, ear, and cheeks when patient is in prone position, using a Mayfield headrest or doughnut; place long rolls parallel with the torso from the nipples to the iliac crests in order to protect the breasts; check the male genitals for pressure and anatomic alignment; use pillows to pad patellas and toes; place arms alongside the body, tucked in with palmar surfaces up or on armboards alongside the head, flexed at the elbow.

- Pad the ear, acromion process, iliac crest, greater trochanter, and malleoli when patient is in lateral position; place a pillow between the legs to decrease skin surfaces' pressure upon one another; flex the leg that comes in contact with the table *for stability*; place 4- to 6-inch wide adhesive across the hips *for stability*, but do not have the tape in direct contact with skin because this can cause abrasions or allergic reactions.
- Pad the footboard to decrease shearing force of the patient's posterior surface caused by sliding when patient is in reverse Trendelenburg position.
- Pad the tissue extending past or in direct contact with the metal table surface for obese patients. *Adipose tissue has little or no vascularity.*

REFERENCES

Agency for Health Care Policy and Research: Clinical practice guideline number 3, Pressure ulcers in adults, Publication no. 92-0047, May, 1992.

Agency for Health Care Policy and Research: Clinical practice guideline number 3, Pressure ulcers in adults: Prediction and prevention, Publication no. 92-0050, May, 1992.

Association of Operating Room Nurses: *Standards, recommended practices*, Denver, 1994.

Guyton: *Medical Physiology*, (3rd ed.), Philadelphia, 1994, WB Saunders.

Hagisawa, Fergusonpell M, Cardi M, Miller SD: Assessment of skin blood content and oxygenation in spinal cord injury subjects during reactive hyperemia, *J Rehab Research and Develop* 31(1):1-14, 1994.

Kneedler: *Perioperative nursing care*, (3rd ed.), Boston, 1994, Blackwell Scientific.

Phippen ML, Wells MP: *Perioperative Nursing Practice*, Philadelphia, 1994, Saunders.

Rothrock M, Meeker M: *Alexander's care of the patient in surgery*, (10th ed.), St. Louis, 1994, Mosby.

Sabisten DC: *Textbook of surgery*, Philadelphia, 1991, WB Saunders.

Schubert V, Heraud J: The effects of pressure and shear on skin microcirculation in elderly stroke patients lying in supine or semirecumbent positions, *Age and Aging* 23(5):405-410, 1994.

Slater RR, Weiner TM, Karuda MJ: Bilateral leg compartment syndrome complications from prolonged lithotomy position, *Orthopedic* 17(10):954-959, 1994.

Spector WD: Correlates of pressure sores in nursing homes—evidence from the National Expenditure Survey, *J Invest Dermatol* 102(6):542-545, 1994.

Injury, perioperative positioning risk for—cont'd

Injury, risk for

CLINICAL CONDITION/ MEDICAL DIAGNOSIS	RISK FACTORS
Borderline personality disorder	Emotional lability

> **Patient goals**
> **Expected outcomes**
> > Associated nursing/collaborative interventions *and scientific rationale*

Experience no self-destructive impulses and maintain appropriate judgment, as evidenced by the following:

Demonstrates decreased emotional lability along with appropriate impulse control

Foster interpersonal trust with patient.

Identify personal or environmental risk factors *to assess and quantify safety needs and level of vulnerability for self-injury.*

Monitor emotional state (e.g., depression, anxiety, anger, suspiciousness) *to determine level of arousal and early signs of escalation.*

Monitor mental status to assess for the possibility of cognitive impairment and *decreased impulse control related to organic mental disorders.*

Examine physical environment for possible risks and remove hazardous objects or make modifications in setting *to promote safety.*

Assess suicidal risk *to determine the need for increased surveillance.*

Contract with patient about desired responses to stressors and acceptable behaviors (e.g., "no-harm" contract) *to facilitate consistency, set limits, and identify therapeutic goals.*

Avoid power struggles with patient by allowing opportunities for reasonable choices.

Administer medications to calm patient, if appropriate.

Plan for unpredictable behaviors toward self or
others.

**Recognizes stressors that may increase risk of self-
injury**

Assist patient in identifying specific stressors
within self or the environment that may
increase risk of injury *to obtain patient's
perception of threat and to assess coping capacity.*

Encourage patient to seek a protective environment
when needed.

Monitor stress level of patient (observation and
patient self-report).

Reduce environmental overstimulation (e.g.,
excessive noise, crowding, invasion of personal
space, frustrating situations) *to minimize sense of
threat.*

Determine appropriate interpersonal boundaries
and nonverbal communication *to minimize
anxiety, dependence, and patient's fear of
abandonment by staff.*

Evaluate social network and role of significant
others in affecting patient's behavior. *Social
pressure and support may facilitate positive coping
and reinforce appropriate responses.*

**Learns new strategies to cope with stress and
experiences no self-destructive impulses**

Encourage patient to express feelings *to decrease
escalation and build-up of negative emotions.*

Teach patient about self-monitoring emotional
state *to promote greater awareness of personal
threshold for stress.*

Teach patient constructive physical and mental
strategies to channel emotions *to provide
appropriate outlets for tensions.*

Assist patient in planning and rehearsing coping
strategies *to reduce stress and maintain control
during crises.*

Refer patient to individual or group psychotherapy,
or other resources as appropriate.

REFERENCES

Burgess JW: Relationship of depression and cognitive impairment to self-injury in borderline personality disorder, major depressions, and schizophrenia, *Psychiatry Res* 38(1):77, 1991.

Fine M, Sansone R: Dilemmas in the management of suicidal behavior in individuals with borderline personality disorder, *Am J Psychother* 44(2):160-171, 1990.

Gainer MJ, Torem MS: Ego-state therapy for self-injurious behavior, *Am J Clin Hypnosis* 35(4):257, 1993.

Gallop R: Self-destructive and impulsive behavior in the patient with a borderline personality disorder: rethinking hospital treatment and management, *Arch Psychiatr Nurs* 6(3):178, 1992.

Hemkendreis M: Increase in self-injuries on an inpatient psychiatric unit during evening hours, *Hosp Community Psychiatry* 43(4):394, 1992.

Katz SE, Levendusky PG: Cognitive-behavioral approaches to treating borderline and self-mutilating patients, *Bull Menninger Clin* 54(3):398, 1990.

Kerr NJ: The ego competency model of psychiatric nursing: theoretical overview and clinical application, *Persp Psych Care* 26(1):13, 1990.

Piccinimo S: The nursing care challenge: borderline patients, *J Psychosoc Nurs* 28(4):22, 1990.

Sebree R, Popkess-Vawter S: Self-injury concept formation: nursing diagnosis development, *Persp Psych Care* 27(2):27, 1991.

Winchel RM, Stanley M: Self-injurious behavior: a review of the behavior and biology of mutilation, *Am J Psychiatry* 148(3)306, 1991.

Knowledge deficit (home IV therapy)

CLINICAL CONDITION/ MEDICAL DIAGNOSIS	RELATED FACTORS
Pancreatic cancer	New treatment experience
	Delayed readiness for learning.

Patient goals
Expected outcomes
  Associated nursing/collaborative interventions *and scientific rationale*

Develop trusting relationship as evidenced by the following:

Discusses with caregiver fears and concerns about health state, previous experiences with health care delivery, and therapeutic regimen
  Allow sufficient time during each visit for one-to-one interaction.
  Engage in active listening.
  Inform patient about time of each scheduled visit.
Seeks assistance for financial insecurities
  Instruct patient as to caregiver's availability via phone and between visits and types of concerns/questions that could be discussed.
  Leave contact person's name for patient to call about financial information.
  Document patient's phone calls: time, date, content, and action taken.
  Capitalize on opportunities to compliment and/or praise.

Develop readiness for learning as evidenced by the following:

Identifies past pattern of effective learning
  Determine competency and comprehension regarding home IV therapy.
Seeks information through active dialogue
  Monitor readiness to learn and determine best methods for teaching/learning. *Certain aspects of*

Knowledge deficit (home IV therapy)

current/ongoing health situation may alter a patient's ability to learn and retain information.

Uses printed information pieces as reinforcement to learning

Provide specific instructions including pictures for home IV therapy.

Establish best approach for teaching: structured, unstructured, or both.

Use patient teaching flow sheet.

Increase knowledge and skill of basic IV therapy as evidenced by the following:

Demonstrates handwashing procedure and use of aseptic technique

Demonstrate and have patient return demonstration on handwashing technique and aseptic technique.

Inspect site of IV puncture at each visit.

Demonstrates correct preparation of IV fluids (i.e., attaching tubing and cleaning the line)

Evaluate home setting for an area to store supplies and for preparing solutions.

Label needle device with data, time, size, and length of catheter.

Change tubing and give complete site care in keeping with standard.

Give complete site care every 48 hours.

Demonstrate and have patient return demonstration of how to add IV solution.

Demonstrate and have patient return demonstration of use of infusion pump.

Demonstrates correct discontinuance of IV fluid

Demonstrates correct method of capping line

Demonstrate and have patient return demonstration of discontinuance of IV solution and capping of line.

Disposes of equipment as demonstrated

Evaluate patient's disposal of IV equipment.

Demonstrate disposal of IV equipment in home setting.

Knowledge deficit (home IV therapy)—cont'd

Demonstrates correct recording on IV sheet

Demonstrate method for recording IV therapy.

Evaluate entries made by patient on IV record.

Teaching/learning effectiveness is enhanced when patient becomes actively engaged in the learning process.

Offset potential complications as evidenced by the following:

Identifies signs and symptoms of infiltration and phlebitis

Describe signs and symptoms of infiltration and how it occurs.

Describe signs and symptoms of phlebitis and basis of its occurrence.

Verbalizes action to take if evidence of infiltration or phlebitis is noted

Instruct actions to be taken if evidence of either infiltration or phlebitis is noted.

Checks IV site and flow rate at designated intervals during infusion
Verbalizes rationale for regulation of flow
Verbalizes action to take of uncertain about events

Instruct patient to check IV site and flow rate at regular intervals.

REFERENCES

Christman NJ, Kirchoff KT, Oakley MG: Concrete objective information. In Bulechek GM, McCloskey JC, eds: *Nursing interventions—essential nursing treatment*, ed 2, Philadelphia, 1992, WB Saunders.

Gardner G: Home IV therapy, I, *Nat Intraven Ther Assoc* 9:95, 1986.

Gardner GI: Home IV therapy, II, *Nat Intraven Ther Assoc* 9:193, 1986.

Rakel B: Knowledge deficit. In Maas M, Buckwalter KC, Hardy M, eds: *Nursing diagnoses and interventions for the elderly*, Redwood City, Cal, 1991, Addison-Wesley.

Redman BK: *The process of patient education*, ed 6, St. Louis, 1988, Mosby Year Book.

Reed-Ash C, Gianella A: Patient education, *Cancer Nurs* 5:261, 1982.

Rountree D: the PIC catheter: a different approach. *AJN* 21(91); August, 1991.

Loneliness, risk for

CLINICAL CONDITION/ MEDICAL DIAGNOSIS	RISK FACTORS
Transition to widowhood after recent move to retirement area of the country	Lives alone in own home in semirural area; retired recently after 30 years of teaching.

Patient goals
Expected outcomes
> Associated nursing/collaborative interventions *and scientific rationale*

Learn to accept and enjoy living alone as evidenced by the following:

Searches for meaning in sudden transition to widowhood

Monitors tasks required to continue living in own home

Paces daily activities to decrease risks such as falling and fatigue

Negotiates reliance on others for tasks beyond physical capability

Exercises three times a week to increase or maintain body strength

> Refer patient to counselor for help in searching for meaning in sudden loss of spouse. *Finding meaning enables individuals to seek new opportunities for personal growth.*

> Provide information about process of transition. *Knowing what to expect helps to decrease stress. Stress and emotional distress can be expected during the transition.*

> Monitor transition to see if expectations are congruent with reality. *Development of a timeline that shows process of transition may help validate a healthy transition.*

> Determine need for new knowledge and skill, and for resources in the community.

Develop a network of friends and companions, as evidenced by the following:

Volunteers to assist teacher in local school two mornings a week
Participates in church-related activities; for example, plays bridge, joins guild
Invites new acquaintances to attend a concert or other activity
Attends class at community college to learn a new craft, such as quilting
Verbalizes subjective sense of well-being

Assist patient to create conditions conducive to a healthy transition.

Provide opportunities for development of new relationships; for example, discuss local needs for volunteers in schools, libraries, and hospitals. *New relationships help to prevent bouts of loneliness that accompany widowhood.*

Provide information about educational institutions in the community. *Attending classes together helps individuals make new friends with common interests.*

Monitor indicators of a healthy transition and provide feedback to client; examples are mastery of new behaviors and well-being that comes with making new friends.

REFERENCES

Elsen J, Blegen M: Social isolation. In Maas M, Buckwalter KC, Hardy M (eds): *Nursing diagnoses and interventions for the elderly,* Redwood City, Cal, 1991, Addison-Wesley Nursing, pp. 519-529.

Lien-Gieschen T: Validation of social isolation related to maturational age: elderly. *Nursing Diagnosis,* 1993, 4(1):37-44.

Lopata HZ, Heinemann GD, Baum J: Loneliness: antecedents and coping strategies in the lives of widows. In Peplau LA, Perlman D: *Loneliness: a sourcebook of current theory, research and therapy,* New York: 1982, John Wiley and Sons, pp. 310-326

Peplau LA, Bikson TK, Rook KS, Goodchilds JD: Being old and living alone. In Peplau LA, Perlman D: *Loneliness: a sourcebook of current theory, research and therapy,* New York, 1982, John Wiley and Sons, pp. 327-347.

Porter EJ: Older widows' experience of living alone at home. *Image J of Nsg Scholarship,* 1994, 26(1):19-24.

Porter EJ: "Reducing my risks:" a phenomenon of older widows' lived experience. *Adv Nurs Sci,* 1994, 17(2):54-65.

Russel D: The measurement of loneliness. In Peplau LA, Perlman D: *Loneliness: a sourcebook of current theory, research and therapy,* New York, 1982, John Wiley and Sons, pp. 81-104.

Schultz NR, Moore D: Loneliness: differences across three age levels, *Soc Personal Relationships*, 1988, 5:275-284.

Schumacher KL, Meleis AI: Transitions: a central concept in nursing. *Image*, 1994, 26(2):119-127.

Weiss RS. Issues in the study of loneliness. In Peplau LA, Perlman D: *Loneliness: sourcebook of current theory, research and therapy*, New York, 1982, John Wiley and Sons, pp. 71-80.

Management of therapeutic regimen, community: ineffective

CLINICAL CONDITION/ MEDICAL DIAGNOSIS	RELATED FACTORS
Cognitively impaired older adults living with family members in rural communities	Limited personal and community resources; increasing evidence of neglect and abuse of elderly.

Patient goals
Expected outcomes
    Associated nursing/collaborative interventions *and scientific rationale*

Community will experience increased awareness of the extent of the problems as evidenced by the following:

Establishes a task force of representatives of health care and social agencies concerned with the problem
Gathers data from community agencies to determine the extent of the problems and inventory of resources
Disseminates Information about findings through public service announcements (PSAs) and other media

    Collaborate with regional council on aging to obtain funding from regional agencies and foundations to support appointment of an ombudsman and work of task force. *Staff of council will have access to funding sources and could serve as liaison to funding agencies.*

    Recruit applicants for position of ombudsman and make a recommendation to the task force.

    Recruit task force members from health and social agencies; include representatives from funding sources when possible. *Funding sources like to know status of ongoing work and may be more generous when included.*

    Prepare bulletins and informational pamphlets for PSAs, newspapers, and other media. *Keeping the public informed of progress of task force will help ensure citizens' support for additional resources.*

Community will mobilize existing resources to provide immediate assistance to any families in a crisis situation as evidenced by the following:

Recruits volunteers from local service organizations to provide respite time for caregivers.
Makes discretionary funds from the departments of social services (DSSs) available.
Publicizes emergency assistance numbers.
Urges caregivers to report families needing immediate assistance.

Contact service organizations and offer to provide information about needs of families. *A personal contact will meet with success more often than a letter, especially when that contact is made by a recognized leader, such as a community health nurse.*

Meet with personnel in DSS to review known cases of need and obtain information about financial resources.

Work with task force to provide accurate PSAs that include a reminder to respect an individual's right to privacy. *Some individuals and families do not want any assistance from a social agency regardless of the situation.*

Weigh privacy issues with the need to expedite services.

Assist the informal support systems in the community: neighbors, friends, and family members. *In rural communities caregivers receive most of their support from informal networking.*

Community will develop a long-term plan for dealing with care of cognitively impaired adults and with issues of neglect and abuse as evidenced by the following:

Collaborates with regional council on aging to prepare grant proposals to obtain funds from community block grants to meet needs of the rural cognitively impaired elderly

Reviews policies for adult protection in each
community and identifies need for adult protection
teams where none exist
Develops an elder abuse training program
Offers training to formal and informal caregivers

Serve as patients' advocate on task force, regional
council, and with DSSs. *Providing patients with
information about their rights in particular
situations enables them to make informed decisions.*

Inform individuals and family members about
adult protection services available in the local
community.

Provide consultation and assistance with
development of elder abuse training program.
*The professional expertise of the nurse is valued by
colleagues.*

REFERENCES

Bull MJ: Factors influencing family caregiver burden and health, *West
Nurs Res*, 1990, 12:758-776.

Fulmer TT: Elder mistreatment, *Annual Review of Nursing Research*,
1994, 12:51-64.

Given BA, Given CW: Family caregiving for the elderly, *Annual Review
of Nursing Research*, 1991, 9:77-101.

Magilvy JK, Congdon JAG, Martinez R: Circles of care: home care and
community support for rural older adults, *Adv Nurs Sci*, 1994,
16(3):22-33.

Segesten K: Patient advocacy—an important part of the daily work of
the expert nurse, *Scholarly Inquiry for Nursing Practice*, 1993,
7(2):129-135.

Weinert C, Burman ME: Rural health and health-seeking behaviors,
Annual Review of Nursing Research, 1994, 12.65-92.

Management of therapeutic regimen, community: ineffective—cont'd

Management of therapeutic regimen, families: ineffective

CLINICAL CONDITION/
MEDICAL DIAGNOSIS

Wife and mother with malnutrition and dehydration 2 months after a stroke, living with elderly husband and dependent daughter with chronic fatigue syndrome.

RELATED FACTORS

Sudden inception of caregiving role by husband and daughter; neglect of wife and mother

---

Patient goals
Expected outcomes
> Associated nursing/collaborative interventions *and scientific rationale*

Family will improve quality of care delivered to wife and mother as evidenced by the following:

Expresses desire to give required care to wife/mother
Expresses willingness to attend classes to master skills needed to manage caregiving tasks
Participates in development of plan of care
Prepares and provides nutritionally balanced meals
Supplements meals with high calorie drinks and up to 8 glasses of liquids a day
> Determine husband's and daughter's motivation to manage care of wife and mother in the home. *Sudden inception of caregiving role may have led to unrealistic expectations of their ability to provide care.*
> Monitor situation for signs of abuse and neglect; for example, administer Risk of Elder Abuse in the Home *(REAH) test. Abuse is often perpetrated by a dependent person.*
> Teach husband and daughter to include wife and mother with the problem-solving, especially how to frame problems so that reasonable solutions can be found. *Values, experience, and*

emotions are central to framing a problem; information alone is insufficient.

Visit family 2 or 3 times a week until plan of care is fully implemented and support services are in place. *Family members may have desire to care for ill member but lack skills and physical capability.*

Teach daughter to keep a written record of mother's food intake and to monitor body weight twice a week. *Food diary provides feedback to mother and daughter about adequacy of food intake.*

Family will accept assistance from outside medical and social resources as evidenced by the following:

Makes and keeps appointments with physicians and representatives of home health care agencies
Contacts volunteer services to locate individual willing to help with weekly shopping and housekeeping

Determine need for assistance in managing tasks of daily living; locate and access required services in the community. *There may not be sufficient energy and ability within the family to provide needed care.*

Refer daughter to physician to treat chronic fatigue syndrome.

Provide information about volunteer services in community that could assist with shopping and housekeeping. *Volunteers may provide sufficient supportive services to prevent excessive caregiver burden.*

Confer with wife's physician to request in-home services of physical therapist. *Physical therapists provide programs of daily exercises and activities that would increase her strength, and decrease caregiving burden.*

REFERENCES

Cartwright JC, Archbold PS, Stewart BJ, Limandri B: Enrichment processes in family caregiving to frail elders, *Adv Nurs Sci*, 1994, 17(1):31-43.

Given BA, Given CW: Family caregiving for the elderly, *Annual Review of Nursing Research*, 1991, 9:77-101.

Bowers BJ: Intergenerational caregiving: adult caregivers and their ageing parents, *Adv Nurs Sci*, 1987, 9(2):21-31.

Brandriet LM, Lyons M, Bentley J: Perceived needs of poststroke elders following termination of home health services, *Nursing Health Care*, 1994, 15(10):514-520.

Congdon JAG: Managing the incongruities: the hospital discharge experience for elderly patients, their families, and nurses, *Applied Nurs Res*, 1994, 7(3):125-131.

Davis LL, Grant JS: Constructing the reality of recovery: family home care management strategies. *Adv Nurs Sci*, 1994, 17(2):66-76.

Fulmer TT: Elder mistreatment, *Annual Review of Nursing Research*, 1994, 12:51-64.

Phillips LR, Rempusheski VF: Caring for the frail elderly at home: toward a theoretical explanation of the dynamics of poor quality caregiving, *Adv Nurs Sci*, 1986, 8(4):62-84.

Robinson KM: A social skills training program for adult caregivers, *Adv Nurs Sci*, 1988, 10(2):59-72.

Sims S, Boland D, O'Neill CA: Decision-making in home health care, *Western J Nurs Res*, 1992, 14(2):186-200.

Management of therapeutic regimen, individuals: effective

CLINICAL CONDITION/ MEDICAL DIAGNOSIS	RELATED FACTORS
Insulin-dependent older female with arthritis and obesity	Wishes to improve overall health status; expresses interest in seeking services of alternative health physician

Patient goals
Expected outcomes
> Associated nursing/collaborative interventions *and scientific rationale*

Negotiate collaboration between an internist and a physician who offers alternative health care as evidenced by the following:

Discusses plan to locate and access services of a physician who offers alternative health care
Makes and keeps appointment with both physicians
Continues to participate in diabetes education classes
Monitors own responses to new regimen
> Help patient to locate and access services of alternative health practitioner *to demonstrate confidence in patient's ability to improve health status.*
> Teach importance of continued monitoring of health status as advised by both physicians.
> Serve as advocate for patient in negotiation with health care providers.
> Acquaint patient with strategies to improve self-monitoring of sensations, symptoms, and power components of self-care. *Knowledge of theoretical underpinnings of self-care will increase patient's ability to become own advocate.*

Implement new health practices into activities of daily living as evidenced by the following:

Makes decision with family members to follow a vegetarian diet to bring down blood sugar and to decrease body weight

Joins local health club to engage in water exercises, swimming, and walking on treadmill.
Modifies recreational and volunteer activities to free time for health-related activities.

Provide information about risks associated with very low calorie diets (VLCD). *VLCDs should not be used for longer than 12 to 16 weeks; risks include nitrogen losses, increased tendency to develop gallstones, and cardiovascular problems.*

Provide information about metabolic changes associated with dieting, such as decrease in resting metabolic rate (RMR). *The decrease in RMR results from more efficient metabolism; that is, fewer calories are needed to support energy needs at rest. The decrease for women ranges from 10% to 30%.*

Discuss metabolic changes associated with dieting and exercise. *During periods of dieting, the energy requirement for a given activity decreases by 25%; therefore, weight loss is slower.*

Provide support to remain on dietary regimen to avoid yo-yo syndrome, that is, repeated dieting and refeeding with increases in body weight. *Repeated dieting and refeeding increase risks associated with dieting, and weight loss is more difficult to achieve.*

REFERENCES

Gast HL, Denyes MJ, Campbell JC, Hartweg DL, Schott-Baer D, Isenberg M: Self-care agency: conceptualizations and operationalization, *Adv Nurs Sci*, 1989, *12*(1):26-38.

Keeling A, Utz SW, Shuster III GF, Boyle A: Noncompliance revisited: a disciplinary perspective of a nursing diagnosis, *Nursing Diagnosis*, 1993, *4*(3):91-98.

Keller ML, Ward S, Baumann LJ: Processes of self-care: monitoring sensations and symptoms, *Adv Nurs Sci*, 1989, *12*(1):54-66.

Olson A: Women and weight control. In McElmurry BJ, Parker RS: *Annual review of women's health*, New York: 1993, National League for Nursing, pp. 199-242.

Weinert C, Burman ME: Rural health and health-seeking behaviors, *Annual Review of Nursing Research*, 1994, *12*:65-92.

Woods N: Conceptualizations of self-care: toward health-oriented models, *Adv Nurs Sci*, 1989, *12*(1):1-13.

GERTRUDE K. MCFARLAND, ELIZABETH KELCHNER GERETY, AND JOAN M. CALEY

Management of therapeutic regimen, individuals: ineffective

CLINICAL CONDITION/ MEDICAL DIAGNOSIS	RELATED FACTORS
Male police officer newly diagnosed with non–insulin-dependent diabetes	Powerlessness Perceived barriers versus perceived benefits

Patient goals
Expected outcomes
> Associated nursing/collaborative interventions *and scientific rationale*

Make effective choices in ADLs and achieve goals of treatment program as evidenced by the following:

Increases sense of control in making choices about treatment program

> Encourage patient to identify actual and/or potential barriers (e.g., food and family customs, ethnic health care practices, religious preferences, work schedule) that prevent him from engaging in treatment plan and feeling a sense of control over outcomes.

> Evaluate patient's attitudes, cultural beliefs, and values about current health state and treatment regimen. *Attitudes, beliefs, and values can serve as barriers or supports for further interventions in patient's management of therapeutic regimen.*

> Evaluate impact of diabetes regimen on current level of function, life-style, and employment.

> Explore with patient past experiences, strengths, problems in illness, threats to health, and other stressful situations in which patient has experienced powerlessness.

> Discuss patient's perspectives on his future health status, life-style, and career. *It is important to determine patient's perspectives of current health status and treatment regimen to collaborate with him in developing a practical plan for participating in treatment and in meeting treatment goals.*

311

Recognizes and accepts benefits of treatment

Discuss with patient consequences of not adhering to treatment regimen and possible negative outcomes. *Adequate understanding of illness, involvement in a treatment regimen and outcomes, serves as a basis for developing a plan for behavior change.*

Encourage patient to discuss perceived benefits of following prescribed regimen. *There is an increase in effective management of diabetes when patients perceive the benefits of following the treatment program.*

Provide feedback to patient on assessment of and choice of options *to facilitate making informed decisions and choices, thereby increasing feelings of control and adherence to treatment regimen.*

Collaborate with patient to develop plan that focuses on selected areas *to maximize patient's feelings of control. Capitalizing on strengths and starting with selected behavioral target areas for change are important beginning steps in developing a plan for patient to participate effectively in treatment program and to meet specific health goals.*

Meets goals of treatment program

Encourage patient to focus on single area and set small goals for a "trial period" *so that patient can obtain feedback on how to be successful in his plan.*

Collaborate with patient in setting mutual goals that are short- term, realistically manageable, and progressive *to reach ultimate, long-range goals.*

Support patient as he begins with plan, giving positive feedback and focusing on small achievements. *Small achievements and reaching short-term goals will decrease patient's sense of powerlessness and increase a sense of control over his health status and involvement in the treatment plan.*

Encourage patient to discuss and seek out additional resources that will help him obtain positive feedback on adherence to treatment regimen and enhance his feelings of satisfaction and achievement.

Monitor patient's progress at regular, scheduled intervals. Encourage patient to discuss setbacks as well as progress. *Management of chronic illness requires the nurse to keep in mind long-range planning with patient on more short-term, achievable goals that will contribute to the patient's ultimate long-term success.*

REFERENCES

Anderson RM, Fitzgerald JT, Oh MS: The relationship between diabetes-related attitudes and patients' self-reported adherence, *Diabetes Educator* 19(4):287, 1993.

Anderson RM and others: A comparison of the diabetes-related attitudes of health care professionals and patients, *Patient Education and Counseling* 21:41, 1993.

Burckhardt CS: Coping strategies of the chronically ill, *Nurs Clin North Am* 22(3):543, 1987.

Lubkin IM: *Chronic illness: impact and intervention*, ed 2, Boston, 1991, Jones & Bartlett.

Jensen L, Allen M: Wellness: the dialectic of illness, *Image: J Nurs Schol* 25(3):220, 1993.

Raymond NR, D'Eramo-Melkus G: Non–insulin-dependent diabetes and obesity in the Black and Hispanic population: culturally sensitive management, *Diabetes Educator* 19(4):313, 1993.

Seley JJ: Is noncompliance a dirty word? *Diabetes Educator* 19(5):386, 1993

Management of therapeutic regimen, individuals: ineffective—cont'd

Memory, impaired

CLINICAL CONDITION/ MEDICAL DIAGNOSIS	RELATED FACTORS
Elderly female admitted with recent diagnosis of mild head injury.	Temporary neurologic disturbance with inability to process new information.

Patient goals
Expected outcomes
    Associated nursing/collaborative interventions *and scientific rationale*

Recognize the need for cognitive rehabilitation as evidenced by the following:

Verbalizes awareness of memory deficit

Provide opportunity for patient to discuss concerns about impaired memory in supportive environment.

Assure patient that memory impairment is not unusual after neurologic trauma. *A therapeutic environment is created when staff acknowledge and respond to stated and unstated patient concerns.*

Maintain ability to attend to environmental routine as evidenced by the following:

Demonstrates ability to use an effective recording system (memory book)

Collaborate with family and significant others to identify previous organizational methods and styles. *Information is better learned and retained when it is related to previously learned skills and knowledge.*

Collaborate with other disciplines to determine appropriate therapeutic techniques and approaches.

Assist with selection of recording system that is meaningful to patient, such as daily calendar, note cards, memory book. *Adaptation and adjustment to disabilities are major areas of focus in course of recovery.*

Demonstrate method of recording meaningful
information in memory book.
Assist patient to record data in memory book.
Reinforce use of memory book for reference to
attend therapy sessions.
Monitor attendance at therapy sessions.
Provide feedback when therapy sessions are not
attended. *Decreased awareness results in an
inability to effectively use compensatory strategies.*
Provide feedback and validation as patient gains
independence in use of recorded information.
*Perceived ability to complete health practice
increases the likelihood of maintaining behavior.*

REFERENCES

Paulanka BJ, Griffin LS: Behavioral responses of memory impaired
clients to selected nursing interventions, *Physical Occupational
Therapy in Geriatrics*, 1993, 12(1), 65-78.

Rosenthal M: Mild traumatic brain injury syndrome, *Ann Emerg Med*,
1993, 22(6):1048-1051.

Roth EJ: The elderly stroke patient: principles and practices of
rehabilitation management, *Topics in Geriatric Rehabilitation*, 1988,
3(4):27-61.

Toglia JP: Generalization of treatment: a multicontext approach to
cognitive perceptual impairment in adults with brain injury, *Am J
Occupat Ther*, 1991, 45(6):505-516.

Uomoto JM: Neuropsychological assessment and cognitive
rehabilitation after brain injury, *Phys Med Rehab Clin*, 1992,
3(2):291-317.

Stuifbergen AK, Becker: Predictors of health-promoting lifestyles in
persons with disabilities. *Res Nurs Health*, 1994, 17:3-13.

Mobility, impaired physical

CLINICAL CONDITION/ MEDICAL DIAGNOSIS	RELATED FACTORS
Systematic lupus erythematosus (SLE)	Acute and chronic joint pain, fatigue

> **Patient goals**
> **Expected outcomes**
> Associated nursing/collaborative interventions *and scientific rationale*

Improve pain management as evidenced by the following:

Rates pain as a 3 or less on a scale of 0 to 10 over a 48-hour period (0, no pain; 10, worst pain)

Teach patient how to use a numerical pain scale.

Apply warm moist heat to affected joints.

Provide warm showers prn and at bedtime to promote comfort. Avoid excessively hot water *because this might increase fatigue*

Teach patient how to use progressive relaxation as an adjunct to analgesics prn and at bedtime. *Pain control is a major component in maintaining optimal muscle and joint mobility.*

Self-administers prescribed antiinflammatory and/or analgesic medications consistently and on schedule

Teach appropriate use of antiinflammatory medications and analgesics *which are most effective when administered on a consistent and fixed schedule to maintain adequate serum levels.*

Reports a minimum of 7 hours of uninterrupted sleep for 3 consecutive days

Provide egg-crate mattress or similar joint-cushioning material for patient's bed to increase comfort.

Suggest back massage at bedtime to promote sleep.

Counsel patient to limit naps to no more than two a day. *Excessive napping during the day can interfere with normal sleep patterns.*

Monitor patient's emotional response to disease

Mobility, impaired physical

process, *because emotional state may have an impact on patient's ability to manage pain.*

Protect currently affected (acute) joints while maintaining function of joints affected by chronic lupus symptoms as evidenced by the following:

Maintains full ROM in chronically affected joints
Coach patient through passive ROM before initiating active ROM twice daily to all but acutely affected joints *to ensure safety and efficiency.*

Rests and supports acutely affected joints
Provide rest and support to acutely affected joints *to stabilize and reduce stress on the joint and aid in muscle relaxation.*

Splint inflamed wrists and hands. *By immobilizing the joint, splinting can decrease pain and prevent contractures from forming in nonfunctional positions.*

Maintains daily exercise regimen as prescribed by physician and/or physical therapist
Balance rest therapy with active physical exercise program *to promote strength and function and to minimize fatigue related to activity level.*

Achieve optimal level of physical mobility as evidenced by the following:

Provides own daily self care within limits of any existing physical disabilities
Assist patient with task analysis of daily activities.
Teach patient how to use a walker and other assistive devices correctly.

Performs ADLs in a manner that promotes joint conservation and protection
Provide information about task simplification, assistive devices, and other energy-conserving techniques.
Identify resources within patient's social support systems and in wider community that may aid in meeting ADLs outside the bounds of

patient's current physical abilities (e.g. assistance with housework and transportation).

REFERENCES

Creason NS: Toward a model of clinical validation of nursing diagnoses: developing conceptual and operational definitions of impaired physical mobility. In Carroll-Johnson RM, ed: *Classification of nursing diagnoses: proceedings of the ninth conference*, Philadelphia, 1991, JB Lippincott.

Halverson PB, Holmes SB: Systemic lupus erythematosus: medical and nursing treatments, *Orthop Nurs* 11(6):17, 1992.

Krupp LS and others: A study of fatigue in SLE, *J Rheumatol* 17(11):1450, 1990.

Mehmert PA, Delaney CW: Validating impaired physical mobility, *Nurs Diagn* 2(4):143, 1991.

Quellet LL, Rush KL: A synthesis of selected literature on mobility: A basis for understanding impaired mobility, *Nurs Diagn* 3(2):72, 1992.

Mobility, impaired physical—cont'd

Noncompliance (therapeutic regimen)

CLINICAL CONDITION/ MEDICAL DIAGNOSIS	RELATED FACTORS
Degenerative joint disease (older adult)	Complexity of exercise regimen Side effects of medication

Patient goals
Expected outcomes
Associated nursing/collaborative interventions *and scientific rationale*

Integrate exercise prescription into ADLs as evidenced by the following:

Records in exercise log time and distance walked
Collaborate with patient/significant other to develop and implement a weekly exercise (activity/rest) plan.
Teach patient/significant other how to use exercise log.

Records joint pain on scale of 0 to 10 (0, no pain; 10, worst pain) before and after exercise and adjusts time and distance walked as appropriate

Modifies activities that consistently increase pain
Teach patient/significant other use of visual analog scale to record joint pain. *Logging exercise and rest may increase compliance with activity/rest prescription.*
Discuss pain log with patient/significant other and suggest ways to modify activity/rest plan.

Adhere to schedule for taking medications as evidenced by the following:

Takes nonsteroidal antiinflammatory drugs (NSAIDs) with food

Records medications taken and missed and any side effects
Collaborate with patient/significant other to implement plan for taking medications. *Active*

Noncompliance (therapeutic regimen)

319

participation in decision-making about therapeutic regimen may increase compliance.

Review side effects of medications (e.g., gastrointestinal irritation from NSAIDs).

Teach patient/significant other to record in pain log medication taken and missed.

Discourage patient from discontinuing medications without consulting physician.

Makes and keeps appointment to evaluate compliance with regimen

Make appointment to interview patient and conduct "pill count" to evaluate compliance with medication regimen. *Patient interview is the most accurate measure of compliance.*

REFERENCES

Conn VS, Taylor SG, Kelley S: Medication regimen complexity and adherence among older adults, *Image: J Nurs Scholar* 23(4):231-235, 1991.

Hegyvary ST: Patient care outcomes related to management of symptoms, *Ann Rev Nurs Res* 11:145-68, 1993.

Keeling A and others: Noncompliance revisited: a disciplinary perspective of a nursing diagnosis, *Nurs Diagn* 4(3):91-98, 1993.

Kison C: Health beliefs and compliance of cardiac patients, *Appl Nurs Res* 5(4):181-185, 1992.

Miller P and others: Regimen compliance two years after myocardial infarction, *Nurs Res* 39(6):333-336, 1990.

Miller P, Wikoff R, Hiatt A: Fishein's model of reasoned action and compliance behavior of hypertensive patients, *Nurs Res* 41(2):104-109, 1991.

Redeker NS: Health beliefs and adherence to chronic illness, *Image: J Nurs Scholar* 20(1):31-35, 1988.

Roberson MHB: The meaning of compliance: patient perspective, *Qual Health Res* 2(1):7-26, 1992.

Rogers A, Caruso CC, Aldrich MS: Reliability of sleep diaries for assessment of sleep/wake patterns, *Nurs Res* 42(6):368-372, 1993.

Wewers ME, Lowe NK: A critical review of visual analogue scales in the measurement of clinical phenomena *Res Nurs Health* 13:227,1990.

Noncompliance (therapeutic regimen)—cont'd

Nutrition, altered: less than body requirements

CLINICAL CONDITION/
MEDICAL DIAGNOSIS

RELATED FACTORS

Chronic obstructive
lung disease; oxygen
dependent

Inadequate intake of nutrients
Gastric distress

Patient goals
Expected outcomes
  Associated nursing/collaborative interventions *and*
    scientific rationale

Consume a well-balanced, high-calorie diet (2400 calories) as evidenced by:

Weight remains plus or minus three pounds from current and increases by one to two pounds per month

  Teach use of food diary *to facilitate self-monitoring.*
  Analyze with patient and wife the food diary
    weekly. *Documenting oral intake and patient's*
    progress facilitates early detection of inadequate
    intake and serves as a teaching tool.
  Help patient to identify food preferences including
    foods high in complex carbohydrates and
    protein. *Several small additions, such as adding*
    margarine or butter to hot cereal, will increase the
    caloric intake.
  Teach importance of oral hygiene before meals *to*
    enhance taste.
  Encourage a pattern of four to six small meals per
    day after rest periods. *Several small meals and*
    snacks are less fatiguing than three large meals.
  Schedule bronchodilators and steroids with
    food/milk products *to reduce the gastric irritation.*
  Establish a dietary prescription in collaboration
    with a dietician.

Establish a pattern of rest and activity as evidenced by:

Participates in activities of enjoyment and necessity

Teach pacing of ADLs.

Teach appropriate use of oxygen to increase ability to engage in exercise. *Independence in self-care will maximize the patient's self-esteem.*

Teach/monitor inspiratory muscle-training exercises as appropriate. *Increasing inspiratory muscle strength can help reduce shortness of breath.*

Teach patient self-care practices to prevent respiratory infection. If bronchitis develops, consult physician for antibiotic prescription as appropriate. *Infection increases the work of breathing.*

Facilitate patient's enrollment in an out-patient pulmonary rehabilitation program. *Group interactions provide reinforcement and support and an opportunity for socialization.*

Explain/review use of exercise log. *Exercise log reinforces positive behavior and promotes motivation.*

REFERENCES

Evans NJ: Feeding. In Bulecheck, GM and McCloskey JL, eds: *Nursing interventions—essential nursing treatment*, ed 2, Philadelphia, 1992, W.B. Saunders.

Rajcevich K and Wakefield B: Altered nutrition: less than body requirements. In Maas M, Buckwalter KC, Hardy M, eds: *Nursing diagnosis and interventions for the elderly*, Redwood City, Cal, 1991, Addison-Wesley.

Snyder M: *Independent nursing interventions*, Albany, NY, 1992, Delmar Publishers, Inc.

Weaver K: Reversible malnutrition in AIDS, *Am J Nurs* 91(9):25, 1991.

Nutrition, altered: less than body requirements—cont'd

Nutrition, altered: more than body requirements

CLINICAL CONDITION/
MEDICAL DIAGNOSIS

Obesity

RELATED FACTORS

Long-established overeating habits; no
regular pattern of exercise

Patient goals
Expected outcomes
   Associated nursing/collaborative interventions *and
   scientific rationale*

Verbalize need to lose weight

Demonstrates commitment to lose weight
   Assist patient to identify relationship between
      current health problems and excess weight.
   Explore motivation to lose weight.
   Reinforce commitment to lose weight. *Motivation
      occurs when the patient identifies a significant need.*
   Establish written contract with patient to use
      techniques to modify eating behaviors. *Provides
      patient and nurse with clear expectations about the
      agreed-upon goals and responsibilities each has in
      moving toward weight loss.*

Eat a well-balanced diet as evidenced by:

Chooses foods from the food pyramid groups
   Teach use of food diary in order *to facilitate self-
      monitoring*
   Analyze food diary with patient weekly. Include
      food eaten, time of day, surroundings,
      circumstances, and where eating occurs.
   Suggest techniques to change diet and eating
      behaviors.
   Identify low-calorie food preferences. *Identifying
      food preferences increases likelihood of compliance.*
   Encourage water consumption to eight glasses a
      day. *This provides adequate hydration necessary for
      body metabolism.*

Nutrition, altered: more than body requirements

Participate in activities to increase metabolic rate as evidenced by the following:

Increases use of energy utilization techniques
Explore current level of activity.

Discuss with patient methods to increase energy utilization techniques such as parking the car well away from an entrance, using stairs instead of elevators, and walking to work or shopping instead of driving. *Initially, increasing energy utilization techniques is easier to accomplish than a formal exercise program and provides positive reinforcement.*

Encourage patient to commit to using at least one energy utilization technique. *Commitment increases likelihood of follow-through.*

Praise patient accomplishments. *This provides positive reinforcement.*

Engages in regular exercise for 20 minutes at least three times a week
Explain relationship between exercise, weight loss, and hypertension. *Knowledge increases likelihood of compliance.*

Offer pamphlets/samples of exercise.

Encourage patient to decide on exercise regime. *Patient involvement increases adherence to exercise program.*

Review use of exercise log. *Exercise log reinforces positive behavior and promotes motivation.*

Review health precautions to take when exercising; e.g., check pulse; stop exercising if experiencing muscle or chest pain, etc.

Achieve gradual weight loss to 20% to 30% over ideal weight as evidenced by:

Loses 1 to 2 pounds per week
Monitor weight weekly or twice weekly in order *to provide feedback/reinforcement.*

REFERENCES

Crist JK: Weight management. In Bulechek G, McCloskey J eds: *Nursing interventions—essential nursing treatment*, ed 2, Philadelphia, 1992, W.B. Saunders

Nutrition, altered: more than body requirements—cont'd

Mahan LK, Arlin MT. *Krause's food, nutrition and diet therapy*, ed 8, Philadelphia, 1992, W.B. Saunders

Resnick BM: Geriatric motivation—clinically helping the elderly to comply, *J Gerontol Nurs*, 17(5):17, 1991.

Snyder M: *Independent nursing interventions*, Albany, NY, 1992, Delmar Publishers.

Stechel SB: *Patient contracting*, Norwalk, Conn, 1982, Appleton-Century-Crofts.

Vickers MJ: Understanding obesity in Women, *J Obstet Gynecol Neonat Nurs* 22(1), 17, 1993.

Nutrition, altered: more than body requirements—cont'd

Nutrition, altered: risk for more than body requirements

CLINICAL CONDITION/ MEDICAL DIAGNOSIS	RISK FACTORS
Obesity	Disruption of significant relationship
	Dysfunctional pattern of intake

Patient goals
Expected outcomes
 Associated nursing/collaborative interventions *and*
  scientific rationale

Alter pattern of intake as evidenced by the following:

Holds present weight for 1 week followed by loss of 1 to 2 lb per week until desired weight is achieved
 Develop a method for patient to keep a daily record of intake and cues associated with intake.

Verbalizes the relationship between experience of loss and pattern of intake
 Analyze weekly log to determine relationship of patient's feelings to pattern of intake.
 Have patient identify desired weight.
 Contract with patient for desired weekly weight loss.
 Develop with patient a diet prescription.
 Evaluate intake patterns for balance in major food groups.

Limits alcohol intake to one drink, containing no more than 1 oz of alcohol, per week
 Alert patient to dangers of using alcohol as a coping strategy.
 Have patient log alcohol intake along with food intake.

Increase energy expenditure as evidenced by the following:

Translates awareness of need for increased physical activity into common energy expending activities, e.g., uses stairs, walks to grocery store

Participates in energy-expending diversional activities for 30 minutes daily

Help patient to identify, select, and participate in one or more energy-expending activities on a daily basis. Record activity, type, and length.

Monitor involvement in selected activities.

Patients need help incorporating exercise into their daily lives. Planning to exercise three times a week is more difficult to implement than exercising daily, i.e. making a life-style change.

Engage in relationships that facilitate positive coping as evidenced by the following:

Seeks support and assistance from selected relationships

Assist patient in identifying pattern of social relationships using social network tool.

Help patient to verbalize his/her responses to efforts to increase or strengthen social network.

Maintain an atmosphere of genuineness, empathy, and unconditional positive regard.

Monitor influence of social interaction on food intake.

REFERENCES

Allan JD: Exercise program. In Bulechek GM, McClosky JC, eds: *Nursing interventions—essential nursing treatments*, ed 2, Philadelphia, 1992, WB Saunders.

Anderson GH, Hrboticky N: Approaches to assessing the dietary component of the diet-behavior connection, *Nutr Rev Suppl* 42 50, May 1986.

Bodkin WL, Hansen BC: Nutritional studies in nursing, *Ann Rev Nurs Res* 9:203, 1991.

Brewerton TD, Hefferman MM, Rosenthal NE: Psychiatric aspects of the relationship between eating and mood, *Nutr Rev Suppl* 78, May 1986.

Crist JK: Weight management. In Bulechek GM, McCloskey JC, eds: *Nursing interventions—essential nursing treatments*, ed 2, Philadelphia, 1992, WB Saunders.

Lean GR, Chamberlain K: Comparison of daily eating habits and maintaining a weight loss, *J Consult Clin Psychol* 61:108, 1973.

Miller, KD: Compulsive overeating, *Nurs Clin North Am* 26(3), 677-97, 1991.

Riley, EA: Codependency and the eating disorder client, *Nurs Clin North Am* 26(3):765, 1991.

Underwood BA: Evaluating the nutritional status of individuals: a critique of approaches, *Nutr Rev Suppl* 213, May 1986.

Nutrition, altered: risk for more than body requirements—cont'd

Oral mucous membrane, altered

CLINICAL CONDITION/ MEDICAL DIAGNOSIS	RELATED FACTORS
Cancer	Trauma associated with chemotherapy

> **Patient goals**
> **Expected outcomes**
> > Associated nursing/collaborative interventions *and scientific rationale*

Maintain a comfortable and functional oral cavity

Demonstrates knowledge of a routine oral hygiene regimen

Provide verbal and written information on how to prevent, recognize and treat stomatitis. *Patients who received education materials have a lower incidence of severe stomatitis.*

Demonstrates absence from oral inflammation and infection

Examine oral cavity daily for inflammation, infection, or ulceration. *White or yellow patches may indicate Candida albicans.*

Establish a mouth care regimen before and after meals and at bedtime *to prevent infection.*

Increase mouth care to every 2 hours and twice at night for severe stomatitis. *Omission of oral hygiene for periods of 2 to 6 hours nullifies past benefits.*

Remove dentures. Brush, soak, and cleanse thoroughly. In case of severe stomatitis instruct patient to remove dentures for at least 8 hours daily. *Dentures will irritate inflamed mucosa and cause necrotic ulceration, bleeding, pain when eating or talking.*

Select a small soft toothbrush for removal of dental debris. To soften toothbrush, soak in hot water before brushing, and rinse in hot water during brushing. Rinse well after use and store in a cool dry place. *Toothbrushes may be contraindicated in severe stomatitis, thrombocytopenia, and neutropenia.* Use a finger wrapped in gauze to help remove dental debris.

Use toothpaste designed for fragile, sensitive mucosa.

Use toothettes or disposable foam swabs *to stimulate gums and clean oral cavity.* Avoid use of lemon-glycerine swabs, *which irritate the oral mucosa and contribute to tooth decalcification.*

Encourage flossing between teeth twice a day with unwaxed dental floss if platelet levels are above 50,000/mm. *Unwaxed fiber strands separate when pressed against the flat tooth surface, permitting cleansing of a larger surface area.* Alternatives to unwaxed floss include waxed dental tape or a double strand of waxed floss.

Encourage frequent rinsing of mouth with mouthwashes and gargles *to cleanse the mouth, reduce microscopic flora, and soothe and relieve local discomfort.*

Chlorhexidine gluconate is an antimicrobial mouthwash that can be used prophylactically *to reduce the incidence and severity of mucositis. Solutions stronger than 0.5% may cause mucosal burning and browning of teeth.*

Sodium bicarbonate helps remove thick mucus. Mix 1 quart of lukewarm water, $1/2$ tsp baking soda, and $1/2$ tsp salt. Change solution daily.

Warm saline is a nonirritating and efficient way to apply heat and cleanse inflamed mucus membranes. *It is economical, readily available, isotonic, and it facilitates the granulation process.* Saline may not be effective in removing hardened crusts or debris.

Avoid the use of hydrogen peroxide solutions. *Peroxide may promote bacterial growth and destroy newly granulating cells.*

Administer oral antibacterial or antifungal agents as prescribed. *Candida albicans* can be treated with a nystatin mouth rinse or troche. Nonspecific stomatitis can be treated with a mixture of 60 ml tetracycline 125 mg, 120 ml of diphenhydramine 25 mg/10 ml and 60 ml of kaolin-pectin.

Oral mucous membrane, altered—cont'd

Maintains symptomatic relief of mucosal dryness with moistening agents and/or agents that increase the flow of saliva

Instruct patient to avoid tobacco, alcohol, and commercial mouthwashes, *which dry the oral mucosa*. Avoid hot, coarse, spicy foods and citrus juices, *which irritate the mouth*.

Encourage patient to take frequent sips of fluids. Have a fluid available throughout the night.

Encourage the use of synthetic saliva products when mouth feels dry.

Provide hard, sour, sugarless gum or candy *to stimulate saliva production. Caution patient that the chronic use of oral lozenges and candy can lead to oral mucosal damage caused by pressure and changes in oral osmolarity*.

Provide adequate room humidification.

Apply vitamin A & D ointment in a lanolin-petrolatum based lip balm *to keep lips moist and to promote healing of cracked lips*.

Administer sialogogues (products that increase the flow of saliva) as prescribed.

Reports oral comfort in swallowing and talking

Modify diet to include soft or pureed foods. *Foods with high water content or those served in cream sauces or gravy are easy to swallow even without normal amounts of saliva.*

Apply topical analgesics such as viscous lidocaine or administer systemic analgesics as prescribed.

REFERENCES

Graham KM and others: Reducing the incidence of stomatitis using a quality assessment and improvement approach, *Cancer Nurs* 16:2, 1993.

Hill C and others: Oral care, *Oncol Nurs Forum* 19:6, 1992.

Holmes S: The oral complications of specific anticancer therapy, *Int J Nurs Stud* 28:4, 1991.

Kenny SA: Effect of two oral care protocols on the incidence of stomatitis in hematology patients, *Cancer Nurs* 13:6, 1990.

Miaskowski C, Rostad M: Implementing the ANA/ONS Standards of Oncology Nursing Practice, *J Nurs Qual Assur* 4:3, 1990.

Weimart TA: Common ENT emergencies: the acute nose and throat, Part 2, *Emerg Med* 30:24:6, 1992.

Zerba MG and others: Relationships between oral mucositis and treatment variables in bone marrow transplant patients, *Cancer Nurs* 15:3, 1992.

Oral mucous membrane, altered—cont'd

Pain (acute)

CLINICAL CONDITION/ MEDICAL DIAGNOSIS	RELATED FACTORS
Inoperable cancer (2 days postoperative)	Inadequate pain relief from prn analgesic Reluctance to take pain medication

Patient goals
Expected outcomes
  Associated nursing/collaborative interventions *and scientific rationale*

Obtain pain relief in hospital and at home as evidenced by the following:

Verbalizes comfort and pain relief after taking analgesic
Reports 3 to 4 hours of uninterrupted sleep at night
  Collaborate with physician to establish a regular schedule for administration of parenteral and/or oral narcotics.

  Collaborate with physician to provide upward adjustment of dose when substituting oral for parenteral narcotic

  Use a flow sheet to monitor pain in terms of quality, intensity, duration, and effects of narcotics and comfort measures *to determine adequacy of pain medication.*

  Teach patient/significant other to continue scheduled narcotic use at home to maximize pain relief.

  Provide patient/significant other with verbal and/or written, accurate information about narcotic analgesics.

  Assist patient/significant other with downward adjustment of narcotic (if indicated) after completion of chemotherapy. *Collaboration with physician and patient/significant other provides opportunity for joint evaluation of analgesic regimen.*

Pain (acute)

Augment narcotic-induced pain relief as evidenced by the following:

Uses music tapes, TV, and radio for diversion
Learns/uses progressive muscle relaxation
Collaborates with nurse to test/evaluate selected cognitive and physical measures to augment comfort and pain control

> Teach patient use of selected strategies to augment pain relief (relaxation, guided imagery, diversion). *Diversion through use of auditory stimulation (music) may augment pain relief by release of endorphins.*
>
> Evaluate use of physical measures, massage, heat, etc, to increase patient comfort.
>
> Teach patient/significant other to use daily log of pain and activities to determine what precipitates/relieves pain.
>
> Teach family members to use back massage and other comfort-inducing measures. *Use of comfort measures, e.g., back rub, massage, clean sheets, may facilitate restful night's sleep and increase ability to cope with pain.*

REFERENCES

Acute Pain Management Guideline Panel: *Acute pain management: operative or medical procedures and trauma. Clinical practice guidelines*, AHCPR Pub. No. 92-0032. Rockville, Md: 1992, Agency for Health Care Policy and Research, Public Health Service, U.S. Department of Health and Human Services.

Davis GC: The meaning of pain management: a concept analysis, *Adv Nurs Sci* 15(1):77-86, 1992.

Greipp ME: Undermedication for pain: an ethical model, *Adv Nurs Sci* 15(1):44-53, 1992.

Herr KA, Mobily PR: Comparison of selected pain assessment tools for use with the elderly, *Appl Nurs Res* 6(1):39-46, 1993.

Hegyvary ST: Patient care outcomes related to management of symptoms, *Ann Rev Nurs Res* 11:145-168, 1993.

Kolcaba KY. Holistic comfort: operationalizing the construct as a nurse-sensitive outcome, *Adv Nurs Sci* 15(1):1-10, 1992.

McDonald DH: Gender and ethnic stereotyping and narcotic analgesic administration, *Res Nurs Health* 17:45-49, 1994.

Mersky H: Development of a universal language of pain syndromes. In Bonica JJ and others, eds: *Advances in pain research and therapy*, vol 5, New York, 1978, Raven Press.

Scandrett-Hibdon S, Uecker S: Relaxation training. In Bulechek GM, McCloskey JC, eds: *Nursing interventions—essential nursing treatments*, ed 2, Philadelphia, 1992, WB Saunders.

Pain (acute)—cont'd

Stewart M: Measurement of clinical pain. In Jacox A, ed: *Pain: a source book for nurses and other health professionals*, Boston, 1977, Little, Brown.

Taylor G: Pain, *Ann Rev Nurs Res* 5:23, 1987.

Twycross RG: Narcotic analgesics in clinical practice. In Bonica JJ and others, eds: *Advances in pain research and therapy*, vol 5, New York, 1983, Raven Press.

Pain, chronic

CLINICAL CONDITION/ MEDICAL DIAGNOSIS	RELATED FACTORS
Laminectomy	Inadequate knowledge of chronic pain management

> **Patient goals**
> **Expected outcomes**
>> Associated nursing/collaborative interventions *and scientific rationale*

Take an active role in pain management as evidenced by the following:

Identifies measures that have helped relieve pain in the past
Verbalizes desire to gain control over pain
> Elicit patient's ideas about measures to control pain.
> Pay attention to language used to describe pain and its severity.
> Teach early intervention in the pain experience.
> Elicit patient's knowledge of analgesics and nonsteroidal antiinflammatory drugs (NSAIDs) used to control pain.

Records pain episodes, measures used to control pain, and pain relief
> Teach and monitor use of pain log to record type of pain, measures used to control pain, and pain relief obtained. *Recording pain experiences and measures used to relieve pain increases patient's perception of control.*
> Teach and monitor use of pain log to record all medications patient is taking. *Combinations of prescription and over-the-counter drugs place individuals at risk for adverse drug reactions.*

Implement a mutually established pain management program as evidenced by the following:

**Collaborates with physician and pharmacist in
selection of cost-effective analgesic/NSAID**
**Expresses willingness to try new strategies to
augment pain relief**
**Practices and records relaxation with music sessions
in pain log**
Uses heat and rest to augment pain relief

Discuss importance of trying a pain-control
technique more than one time. *Pain relief
obtained from a pain control measure may differ
from day to day; measure may not be effective the
first time used.*

Coach and monitor relaxation practice sessions.

Instruct in safe use of heating pad; use moist heat;
e.g., Thermophore. *Moist heat helps to relieve pain
and promotes relaxation/rest.*

REFERENCES

Pain Management Guideline Panel: *Acute pain management: Operative
or medical procedures and trauma. Clinical practice guidelines.* AHCPR
Pub. No. 92 0032, Rockville, MD: 1992, Agency for Health Care
Policy and Research, Public Health Service, U.S. Department of
Health and Human Services.
Davis GC: Measuring the clinical outcomes of the patient with
chronic pain. In Waltz CF, Strickland OL, eds: *Measurement of
nursing outcomes,* vol 1. *Measuring client outcomes,* New York 1988,
Springer, pp. 160-184.
Geach B: Pain and coping, *Image: J Nurs Scholar* 19(1):12, 1987.
Hegyvary ST: Patient care outcomes related to management and
symptoms, *Ann Rev Nurs Res* 11:145-168, 1993.
Kolcaba KY. Holistic comfort. operationalizing the construct as a
nurse-sensitive outcome, *Adv Nurs Sci* 15(1):1 10, 1992.
McCaffery M: *Nursing management of the patient with pain,* ed 2,
Philadelphia 1979, JB Lippincott.
McDonald DH: Gender and ethnic stereotyping and narcotic
analgesic administration, *Res Nurs Health* 17(1):45-49, 1994.
Moran KJ: The effects of self-guided imagery and other-guided
imagery on chronic low back pain. In Funk SG and others, eds: *Key
aspects of comfort,* New York 1989, Springer, pp. 160-165.
Pollow RL and others. Drug combinations and potential for risk of
adverse drug reaction among community-dwelling elderly *Nurs Res*
43(1):44-49, 1994.
Schorr JA: Music and pattern change in chronic pain, *Adv Nurs Sci*
15(4):27-36, 1993.
Whipple B: Methods of pain control: review of research and literature,
Image: J Nurs Scholar 19(3):142, 1987.
Wild LR: Caveat emptor: a critical analysis of the costs of drugs used
for pain management, *Adv Nurs Sci* 16(1):52-61, 1993.
Wilkie DJ and others: Use of the McGill Pain Questionnaire to
measure pain; a metaanalysis *Nurs Res* 39(1):36, 1990.

Pain, chronic—cont'd

Parent-Infant-Child attachment, altered: risk for

CLINICAL CONDITION/ MEDICAL DIAGNOSIS	RISK FACTORS
Prematurity	Separation

> **Patient goals**
> **Expected outcomes**
> Associated nursing/collaborative interventions *and scientific rationale*

Share feelings about altered parental role as evidenced by:

Verbalize experience of pregnancy and delivery

Provide an opportunity for parents to discuss their feelings about their high-risk pregnancy and premature delivery. *Parents are often unprepared for the premature birth and have unresolved pregnancy and childbirth issues in the immediate postpartum period.*

Help parents examine reasons for their infant's premature birth. *Feeling guilty is a common response after a premature birth. Self-blame may offer some parents a sense of control over the future.*

Express feelings about having a hospitalized premature infant.

Create a caring environment so that parents will feel comfortable sharing their feelings.

Validate the emotional reactions of parents by informing them about the common responses about premature infants. *Parents of premature infants express feelings of disappointment, helplessness, isolation, uncertainty about the infant's survival and prognosis, and loss of the role as primary caregiver for their infant.*

Monitor parents' response to having a preterm infant, accepting individual and gender differences in coping styles. *There is variability in parents' adaptation to the premature birth. There are*

> *no prescribed stages of parental adjustment to a premature birth.*

Accept parents' need to ask questions about other infants in the unit. *Parents cope by comparing their infant's condition to that of other infants in the unit.*

Refer parents to parent support groups or other parents of premature infants.

Refer parents to appropriate religious support. *Seeking religious explanations for the premature birth is a coping strategy for some parents.*

Utilize support systems

Assist parents to share information with family, friends, and other parents. *Assisting parents to provide information may enhance the support they receive from others.*

Refer to social services as needed.

Parents will acquire adequate information as evidenced by the following:

Become familiar with the hospital unit environment

Acquaint parents with the environment of the hospital unit. *The sights and sounds of the hospital unit are stressors for parents.*

Introduce parents to the personnel of the unit and explain each staff member's role and any rotating patterns of staffing.

Use written and audiovisual materials to educate and reinforce parent teaching.

Learn about the infant's condition

Provide parents with complete and honest information, and arrange periodic patient care conferences with the parents. *Information should be provided in a respectful, unbiased, and caring manner that allows parents to communicate their feelings, ideas, and questions.*

Provide consistent information between health care members, avoiding any criticism of each other's care.

Acquaint parents with the infant's physical appearance and behaviors by performing a physical examination of the infant in the presence of the parents. *The infant's physical appearance and behaviors are stressors for parents.*

Emphasize the individual behavioral responses of the infant, including those infant cues that signal appropriate stimulation. *Parents usually elicit positive behaviors in their infants, such as smiling, which promote parent-infant attachment. However, some parents may not be able to elicit positive behaviors due to a lack of knowledge about appropriate infant stimulation and therefore, need education.*

Participate in the care of their infant as evidenced by the following:

Express desired level of participation in the care of their infant

Ask parents how often they wish to call and visit.

Identify any circumstances that may affect the parents' ability to call or visit. *Other life stressors or inadequate child care for other children may make it difficult for parents to visit their infant frequently.*

Monitor parents' desired level of participation in care and decision making, including when the parents want to be notified of changes in the condition or treatment of their infant. *Parents desire different levels of involvement in the care of their hospitalized infant.*

Participate in setting visitation rights and limits to their infant

Support parents' need for unrestricted visitation.

Arrange unit activities, such as patient care rounds or unit meetings, so that parents do not have to leave their infant's bedside during the activity.

Ask parents to identify those other individuals who have the parents' permission to visit their infant. *Parents, not unit personnel, should identify appropriate visitors for the infant.*

Have adequate resources for visiting and caring for their infant

Assess any financial concerns. *Parents may lack the financial resources to travel to the hospital or care for their infant after discharge.*

Refer to appropriate resources.

Demonstrate attachment behaviors to the infant

Allow the parents to visit the infant soon after the infant's admission to the unit and to hold the infant when the infant is stabilized. *Attachment behaviors include maintaining close proximity to the infant.*

Remove mechanical barriers such as non—life-sustaining equipment and phototherapy lights.

Provide photographs of the infant.

Visit the mother in her hospital room if she is unable to visit her infant, and transport the infant to her room when the infant's condition permits.

Call the parents if they are unable to call or visit their infant.

Encourage parents to name their infant, and refer to the infant by his or her first name.

Participate in infant caregiving from the beginning of the infant's hospitalization

Encourage parents to participate in caregiving to the infant. *Caregiving is one component of the parental role, and an alteration in the parental role is a stressor for parents of premature infants.*

Offer parents the opportunity to participate in infant caregiving during the acute and convalescent stages of hospitalization. *Mastery of the new parental role cannot be achieved without direct participation in caregiving.*

Schedule appointments for parents to learn or participate in infant caregiving.

Plan infant caregiving, such as bathing and feeding, at the time of the parents' visits.

Encourage parents to participate in caregiving that is exclusively within the domain of the parents, such as skin-to-skin contact and breastfeeding. *Mothers of premature infants have commented that breastfeeding is the one activity that only they can do for their infant.*

Reinforce parents' success in infant caregiving. *Positive feedback enhances self-esteem and competence, and increased competence facilitates attachment.*

Document parent caretaking so that the parents' ability to provide care to their infant is consistently supported by the hospital staff. *Parents should have adequate opportunity to master those infant caregiving activities that will be required after discharge.*

Parents view themselves as the primary nurturer and caregiver for the infant as evidenced by the following:

View the nurse as a professional rather than as a substitute parent for their infant

Establish "milestone" caregiving activities for which the parents want to be a participant, such as the first tub bath. *Parents mourn the loss of the anticipated role as primary caregiver, and have blurred boundaries between themselves and the nurse.*

Request parents' permission before photographing their infant for special holidays, such as Christmas.

Provide only those clothes and toys that parents have purchased or approved for the infant.

Maintain a professional relationship with the infant and family.

REFERENCES

Affleck G, Tennen H: The effect of newborn intensive care on parents' psychological well-being, *Children's Health Care*, 1991, 20(1):6.

Affonso DD, Hurst I, Mayberry LJ, Haller L, Yost K, Lynch ME: Stressors reported by mothers of hospitalized premature infants, *Neonatal Network*, 1992, 11(6):63.

Affonso D, Bosque E, Wahlberg V, Brady JP: Reconciliation and healing for mothers through skin-to-skin contact provided in an American tertiary level intensive care nursery, *Neonatal Network*, 1993, 12(3):25.

Griffin T: Nurse barriers to parenting in the special care nursery, *J Perinatal Neonatal Nurs*, 1990, 4(2):56.

Harrison H: The principles of family-centered neonatal care, *Pediatrics*, 1993, 92(5):643.

Hayes N, Stainton MC, McNeil D: Caring for a chronically ill infant: a paradigm case of maternal rehearsal in the neonatal intensive care unit, *J Pediat Nurs*, 1993, 8(6):355.

McNeil D: Uncertainty, waiting, and possibilities: Experiences of becoming a mother with an infant in the NICU, *Neonatal Network*, 1992, 11(7):78.

Mercer RT, Ferketich SL: Predictors of parental attachment during early parenthood, *J Adv Nurs*, 1990, 15:268.

Miles MS, Funk SG, Kasper MA: The stress response of mothers and fathers of preterm infants, *Res Nurs Health*, 1992, 15:261.

Miller DB, Holditch-Davis D: Interactions of parents and nurses with high-risk preterm infants, *Res Nurs Health*, 1992, 15:187.

Sharp MC, Strauss RP, Lorch SC: Communicating medical bad news: parents' experiences and preferences, *J Pediatr*, 1992, 121:539.

Parental role conflict

CLINICAL CONDITION/ MEDICAL DIAGNOSIS	RELATED FACTORS
Childhood Chronic Illness	Home care of a child with special technologic needs

Patient goals
Expected outcomes
> Associated nursing/collaborative interventions *and scientific rationale*

Participate in technology-related care as evidenced by the following:

Maintains desired levels of participation with health professionals
Participates in routine and complex caretaking activities
Makes independent, safe decisions related to acute episodes of the illness, equipment malfunction, or need for professional assistance
Adapts information for the development of a personal style of performing skills

> Monitor parents' desired level of participation in care and decision making.
> Provide consistent contact with health professionals for information gathering and follow-up.
> Determine style of parental relationship with health professionals: e.g., limited contact, recipients of care, monitors of care, and managers of care, *because they differ according to the level of trust in professionals, information gathering style, and decision- making patterns.*
> Monitor knowledge base and competency related to equipment and required technical care.
> Assess level of anxiety related to skill performance.
> Teach equipment operation, maintenance, safety, and necessary back- up.
> Teach CPR as necessary.

Parental role conflict

Provide opportunities to master required home health-care skills when the child is hospitalized.

Teach factors that increase frequency of complications, such as exposure to infections and immobility.

Review management of acute episodes.

Evaluate parents' understanding of special care and provide clarification as needed. *Learning is a complex process that requires time for integration into the family's current lifestyle. Continual assessment of barriers to learning, anxiety and competency enhance the process.*

Develop plans for ordering supplies and contacting vendors.

Express feelings and concerns about parental role demands as evidenced by the following:

Verbalizes feelings and perceptions of self, role change, fears, and level of stress

Maintains roles of primary caretaker, educator, protector, and disciplinarian

Has adequate financial resources

Has minimal health problems related to stress

Maintains desired level of contact with significant others for emotional and caretaking support

Monitor parents' perception of current situation as they compare with previous parenting patterns.

Help parents to verbalize any fears, expectations for the future, and feelings of isolation and overwhelming responsibility.

Determine extended family and friends' positive and negative reactions to child's situation.

Assist the parents to involve the child in age-appropriate self care and home responsibilities

Discuss ways to maintain appropriate parent child relationship without overprotectiveness, guilt, or anger.

Assess financial status and concerns and refer to appropriate resources.

Counsel parents to develop strategies for the future to facilitate expression of feelings and concerns.

Parental role conflict—cont'd

Refer to support groups and parents in similar situations as available and desired by the parents.

Assess involvement in community religious groups.

Teach parents about specific strategies used by families in difficult situations, such as acquiring social support, reframing, seeking social support, mobilizing of family to acquire and accept support and passive appraisal. *Families of technology-assisted children often lack financial resources, feel isolated, receive unwanted advice from others, and expend tremendous energy mobilizing community assistance and support.*

Incorporate technology in family life as evidenced by the following:

Evaluates family boundaries, goals, patterns of interaction, and values in relation to the health of the child

Develops adjustment strategies and problem-solving and adaptive coping skills

Integrates new patterns of behavior and responsibility into individual, family, and school routines

Assist family to identify stressors and strains related to incorporation of the technology, specific strengths related to the stage of development/career, and resources. *Long term effects of pediatric home care vary over time and warrant continual reevaluation.*

Assist family to determine their accord about competencies as a family, such as quality of marital communication, shared orientation to childrearing and illness management, and satisfaction with quality of life. *Adaptability is the ability of the family to reorganize its power structure, roles, and rules. Emotional bonding, boundaries, supports, and time for recreation influence family cohesion.*

Help parents incorporate necessary lifestyle changes.

Provide anticipatory guidance regarding schooling
and/or child care.

Help family to plan and implement necessary
social and environmental adaptations at home
and school.

Assist parents to involve siblings in the care of the
child and home responsibilities.

Assist parents to involve the child in age-
appropriate self-care and home responsibilities.
*A family management style develops when a family
incorporates the care of a chronically ill child.*

REFERENCES

Knafl KA, Cavallari KA, Dixon DM: *Pediatric hospitalization: family and
nurse perspectives,* Glenview, Ill, 1988, Foresman.

Knafl KA, Deatrick JA: Family management style: concept analysis
and development, *J Ped Nurs* 5:4-14, 1990.

Leonard BJ, Johnson AL, Brust JD: Caregivers of children with
disabilities: a comparison of those managing "OK" and those
needing more help, *Child Health Care* 22(2):93-105, 1993.

Olson, D and others: *Families: what makes them work,* Beverly Hills,
Cal, 1983, Sage.

Perkins MT: Parent nurse collaboration: using the caregiver identity
emergence phases to assist parents of hospitalized children with
disabilities, *J Ped Nurs* 8(1):2-9, 1993.

Ray LD, Ritchie JA: Caring for chronically ill children at home: factors
that influence parents' coping, *J Ped Nurs* 8(4):217-225, 1993.

Redman BK: *The process of patient education,* ed 7, St. Louis, 1993,
Mosby.

Teague BR and others: "High-tech" home care for children with
chronic health conditions: a pilot study, *J Ped Nurs* 8(4):226-232,
1993.

Thomas VM and others: Caring for the person receiving ventilatory
support at home: care giver's needs and involvement, *Heart Lung*
21(2):180-186, 1992.

Turner-Henson A, Holaday B, Swan JH: When parenting becomes
caregiving: caring for the chronically ill child, *Fam Comm Health*
15(2):19-30, 1992.

Parental role conflict—cont'd

Parenting, altered

CLINICAL CONDITION/ MEDICAL DIAGNOSIS	RELATED FACTORS
Mother experiencing major depression	Inadequate role identity; unrealistic expectations

Patient goals
Expected outcomes
    Associated nursing/collaborative interventions *and scientific rationale*

Provide safe environment for child as evidenced by the following:

Remains physically and psychologically safe

Provide physically and psychologically safe environment for the child, which is the basic function of a parent.

Assess degree of risk to child's physical and psychological safety.

Contact other family members or appropriate authorities if child's safety seems jeopardized. *Deficiencies in this area may range from routinely ignoring a child's diet or personal hygiene to homes with multiple safety hazards to severe physical abuse.*

Provide interventions that are designed to focus the parent's awareness of the child's needs. In situations where the parent(s) cannot provide for the minimum safety and physiologic needs of the child, mechanisms designed by the community must be engaged to remove the child to a safer environment.

Achieve role identity as parent as evidenced by the following

Identifies socially expected parenting behaviors

Identify major components and priorities within role identity (i.e., child of one's parents, spouse, career identity)

Parenting, altered

Identify source of verbalized "ideal" parenting behavior.

Identify perception of specific parenting behaviors.

Encourage patient to verbalize presence or absence of effective role models.

Encourage patient to verbalize incongruence between "ideal" parenting behaviors and actual behaviors.

Incorporates concept of "parent" as integral part of role identity

Observe parent-child interactions for congruence between verbalized "ideal" of parent behavior and actual behavior.

Provide opportunity for parent to explore role identity through individual counseling or group interaction.

Provide learning opportunities for additional parenting behavior.

Provide opportunity for parent to observe or experience effective parenting behaviors.

Provide opportunity for parent to implement alternative parenting behaviors.

Give positive reinforcement for additional parenting behavior that will support incorporation of concept of "parent" into role identity. *Parenting is a learned behavior. In many communities the opportunity for observing parenting behavior is limited, and persons rely on their perception of how they were parented. Interventions that provide information about alternative parenting behaviors and opportunity to discuss the changes in life-style required as a parent broaden the perspective of the parent and aid in internalizing the parenting role.*

Acquire realistic expectations of self, spouse, and infant or child within family as evidenced by the following:

Develops realistic expectations of self, spouse and infant or child

Assist patient to identify present expectations of self, spouse and infant or child.

Assist patient to identify areas of failure to meet expectations of self.

Assist patient to identify areas where others fail to meet expectations.

Provide opportunity for patient to express feelings about unmet expectations.

Encourage patient to speculate on reasons for expectations being unmet.

Encourage patient to acknowledge own responsibility for attempting to meet expectations as well as realistic limits of self and others.

Help patient to develop realistic expectations as result of increased knowledge of normal development and basic needs.

Develops strategies that increase the possibility that expectations will be met

Help patient to develop alternative strategies to increase possibility of having expectations met (e.g., discussing expectations with spouse, identifying steps that must occur in order to meet expectations). *Many parents have unrealistic expectation of their role and abilities as a parent, of their spouse's role and abilities, and the role and ability of the child in the relationship. This may lead to increased frustration and anxiety as the expected behaviors are not manifested. Since anxiety is frequently transformed into anger or depression, the potential for disruption of parenting function is great. Helping the parent to identify the source of the anger and develop more realistic expectations diffuses the anxiety and offers opportunity to develop alternative behaviors.*

REFERENCES

Bigner JJ: *Parent-child relations: an introduction to parenting*, New York, 1989, Macmillan Publishing Co.

Denehy JA: Interventions related to parent-infant attachment, *Nurs Clin North Am* 27(2):4225, 1992

Gross D: At risk: children of the mentally ill, *J Psychosoc Nurs* 28(8):14, 1989

Hall LA, Gurley DN, Sachs B, Kryscio RJ: Psychosocial predictors of maternal depressive symptoms, parenting attitudes, and child behavior in single-parent families, *Nurs Res* 40(4):214, 1991

Parenting, altered—cont'd

Karl D: The consequences of maternal depression for early mother-
infant interaction: a nursing issue, *J Ped Nurs* 6(6):384, 1991

Knafl KA and Deatrick JA: Family management style: concept analysis
and development, *J Ped Nurs* 5:4, 1990.

Martel LK: Postpartum depression as a family problem. *MCN* 15(2):90,
1990

Norris DM, Hoyer PJ: Dynamism in practice: parenting within King's
framework, *Nurs Sci Quart* 6(2):79, 1993

Olshansky, EF: Parenting, Altered. In McFarland, GK and Thomas,
MD: *Psychiatric mental health nursing: application of the nursing
process*, New York, 1991, JB Lippincott.

Senner A: Munchausen syndrome by proxy, *Comp Ped Nurs* 12(5):345,
1989

Parenting, altered, risk for

CLINICAL CONDITION/ MEDICAL DIAGNOSIS	RISK FACTORS
Growing preterm infant (6 months of age)	Inadequate knowledge

> **Patient goals**
> **Expected outcomes**
>> Associated nursing/collaborative interventions *and scientific rationale*

Acquire adequate knowledge base for effective parenting as evidenced by the following:

Verbalizes desired knowledge about specific aspects of parenting

Assist parent(s) to identify knowledge deficits related to caring for a growing preterm infant.

Identify learning readiness and learning capability of parent(s).

Provide information related to normal growth and development as well as specific information for growing preterm infant.

Teach parent(s) skills and behaviors related to caring for a growing preterm infant.

Demonstrates more effective parenting behavior, such as providing for child's physical, psychological, emotional, and social needs

Provide opportunity for parent(s) to test out new information.

Encourage age-appropriate play activities between parent(s) and child.

Encourage age-appropriate caretaking activities by parent(s). *Lack of information, lack of role models, lack of external resources, and ineffective coping skills may all be decreased through appropriate patient-education methods.*

Experience emotional, social and physical support as evidenced by the following:

Recognizes realistic limitations of self and support systems

Assist parent(s) to identify specific areas of needed emotional, social, or physical support.

Assist parent(s) to identify specific strengths of parent(s) and support systems.

Encourage parent(s) to express feelings about areas of need.

Activates additional support systems as needed

Provide information about additional resources available to meet areas of need.

Assist parent(s) to select appropriate resources to supplement self and support system.

Act as liaison or advocate as needed in obtaining help from appropriate resources. *Many of the defining characteristics of Altered Parenting are the result of insufficient emotional, social, or physical support. Persons whose own basic needs for safety, nutrition, or love have not been met will be unable to meet the needs of another. Once specific areas of deficiencies have been identified, the nurse may offer information about services available to provide the support needed.*

REFERENCES

Denehy JA: Interventions related to parent-infant attachment, *Nurs Clin North Am* 27(2):4225, 1992

Griffin T: Nurse barriers to parenting in the special care nursery, *J Peri Neo Nurs*, 4(2).56, 1990

Hardy JB, Streett R: Family support and parenting education in the home: an effective extension of clinic-based preventive health care services for poor children, *J Pediatr* 115:927-931, 1989

McCain GC: Parenting growing preterm infants, *Ped Nurs* 16(5):467, 1990

Younger JB: A model of parenting stress, *Res Nurs Health*, 14(3);197, 1991

Zahr LK: The relationship between maternal confidence and mother-infant behaviors in premature infant, *Res Nurs Health*, 14(4):279, 1991

Parenting, altered, risk for—cont'd

Peripheral neurovascular dysfunction, risk for

CLINICAL CONDITION/ MEDICAL DIAGNOSIS	RISK FACTORS
Bone fractures of upper or lower extremity	Mechanical compression, (e.g., tourniquet, cast)

Patient goals
Expected outcomes
    Associated nursing/collaborative interventions *and scientific rationale*

Maintain neurovascular integrity to the extremity as evidenced by the following:

Experiences absence of pain, pallor or cyanosis, pulselessness, paresthesia, and paralysis ("five P's")

Perform neurovascular assessment every hour for first 24 hours; then every 2 hours for 8 hours; then every 4 hours. Continue as long as mechanical compression is present (extremity cast, check involved distal extremity; spica or body cast, check all 4 extremities; halo cast, check cranial nerves).

Observe capillary filling after compression of arteries of extremity. *Failure of circulatory return to extremity when pressure is released indicates arterial injury.*

Feel and compare temperature of both extremities.

Observe color of skin.

Observe for presence and amount of edema; e.g., insert fingers under cast or measure circumference of extremities. *As swelling within muscle compartment increases, neurovascular compromise occurs.*

Palpate pulses at least every 2 hours. Report absent or diminished pulses (1 or less on 4+ scale).

Monitor oxygen saturation by pulse oximetry. *Oxygen saturation may be compromised even in presence of palpable peripheral pulses.*

Monitor for evidence of paresthesia, and decreased or absent sensation including 2-point discrimination. *Two-point discrimination is best check of sensitivity.*

Assess mobility of involved extremity (flexion, extension, abduction, and adduction) of fingers and toes. Bring tips of thumb and fingers together to form circle. *Impossible to perform circle maneuver if radial, ulnar, and median nerves are not intact to intrinsic muscles.*

Assess for pain out of proportion to injury. *The primary concern of neurovascular dysfunction is impairment of nerves or blood vessels distal to the area of the cast, splint, or traction. Early detection of neurovascular compromise can avoid irreversible and permanent damage.*

Progresses through cast, splint, or brace therapy without experiencing complications

Document and report immediately and persistently, if necessary, any evidence of neurovascular compromise. *Permanent and irreversible damage resulting in paresis, paralysis, or amputation can occur rapidly, within 4-12 hours.*

Elevate extremity to level of heart until edema is controlled. Avoid elevating above person's central venous pressure (normal CVP = 6-13 cm H_2O pressure; 2.5 cm = 1 inch). *Elevating extremity aids venous return to decrease edema. Elevating above person's CVP impedes arterial flow and increases rather than decreases edema.*

Apply icebags to lateral surfaces of cast or traction for 24-48 hours —avoid placing over arterial areas. *Cold decreases edema; applying over artery could impede arterial flow.*

Avoid pressure over peroneal nerve.

Observe for paresthesia at anterior surface of affected leg, dorsum of foot, and great toe and inability to dorsiflex foot or extend toes. *Pressure on peroneal nerve can result in permanent foot drop.*

Split cast down one or both sides and rewrap splint cast with elastic bandage if necessary;

remove traction or splint and reapply more loosely. *Irreversible and permanent damage can result in 6 hours if pressure is not relieved.*

Notifies nurse or physician of signs and symptoms of peripheral neurovascular compromise while in the hospital and after discharge

Instruct client and significant other about signs and symptoms of peripheral neurovascular compromise.

Emphasize importance of notifying nurse or physician immediately of numbness or tingling, increasing pain, increased swelling, or change in color. *Complications from cast, splint, or traction therapy can occur at any time. Changes in body weight, edema loss, and softening of the cast can create changes in neurovascular status.*

Prevent compartment syndrome and Volkmann's ischemic fracture resulting from compression or severance of an artery as evidenced by the following:

Normal compartment pressure (< 10 mm Hg), adequate tissue perfusion as noted by brisk (< 3 sec) capillary refill, and normal ROM in all extremities

Assess for increasing and progressive pain on passive motion every 1-2 hours. *Pain on passive motion is earliest and most significant sign of compartment syndrome.*

Assess for evidence of pallor or cyanosis. *Tissue damage results when oxygen is reduced because of lack of blood supply; hypoxia resulting from entrapment of vessels or nerves can result in ischemic contracture or ischemic myositis.*

Immobilize traumatized extremity. *Movement of arm or leg can result in further injury to nerves and blood vessels.*

Perform and document tissue pressure readings. *Normal tissue pressure is 0 to 10 mm Hg. Increase in pressure recordings denotes impending compartment syndrome.*

Report immediately tissue pressure readings of 30

mm Hg or above. *Pressures of 30 mm Hg or above can result in irreversible damage if not relieved within 6 hours; 30 mm Hg is criterion used for surgical decompression. If pressure in compartment equals diastolic blood pressure, microcirculation ceases.*

REFERENCES

David HG: Pulse oximetry in closed limb fractures, *Ann Royal Coll Surg of Eng*, 73:283-284, 1991.

Harris IE: Supracondylar fractures of the humerus in children, *Orthopedics*, 15, 811-817, 1992.

Hawkins BJ, Bays PN: Catastrophic complication of simple cast treatment—Case report, *J Trauma*, 34:760-762, 1993.

Myerson M, Manoli A: Compartment syndromes of the foot after calcaneal fractures, *Clin Orthop Related Res*, 290:142-150, 1993.

Negri L, Weber W, Haus J, Krugerfranke M: Use of pulse oximetry in compartment syndrome, *Anaesthetist*, 40:680-681, 1991.

Peck SA: Crush syndrome: pathophysiology and management, *Orthop Nurs*, 9(3):33-40, 1990.

Ross D: Acute compartment syndrome, *Orthop Nurs*, 10(2):33-38, 1991.

Woll TS, Duwelius PJ: The segmental tibial fracture, *Clin Orthop Related Res*, 281:204-207, 1992.

Peripheral neurovascular dysfunction, risk for—cont'd

Personal identity disturbance

CLINICAL CONDITION/ MEDICAL DIAGNOSIS	RELATED FACTORS
Borderline personality disorder (BPD)	History of severe, traumatic interpersonal experiences

Patient goals
Expected outcomes
> Associated nursing/collaborative interventions *and scientific rationale*

Maintain a positive concept of personal identity over time as evidenced by the following:

Distinguishes between self and non-self and responds to others as separate from self

> Develop a trusting, accepting relationship with patient.

> Support the patient's independence and autonomous ventures *to reinforce establishment of separate, differentiated relationships with others in the environment and support existing ego strengths.*

> Maintain personal boundaries and clarify expectations about the nurse-patient relationship *to decrease ambivalence and anxiety.*

> Encourage independent decision making, providing nonjudgemental feedback.

Integrates thoughts, emotions, and behaviors into an organized cohesive, continuing self

> Show empathy and awareness of the patient's vulnerability to feelings of abandonment and aloneness. *These internal states may trigger anger, anxiety, and acting-out by the patient.*

> Modify environment stressors *to decrease a sense of threat, disorganization, and overstimulation for the patient.*

> Teach patient stress management strategies.

> Teach patient to record thoughts and feelings *to reinforce a continuous sense of self and decrease fragmentation.*

> Assess patient's ability to differentiate between

Personal identity disturbance

356

internal and external stimuli *to evaluate reality-testing.*

Monitor mental status *to identify presence of organic causes of symptoms and reality-testing difficulties.*

Demonstrates positive acceptance and identification of self

Encourage patient to discuss personal values, beliefs, and goals for the future.

Encourage patient to discuss relationships and experiences that have influenced self-concept in order *to assess impact of events on development of self.*

Support positive self-designations and self-affirmation statements *to reinforce positive self-image and competencies.*

REFERENCES

Buck MH: The personal self. In Roy SC, Andres A, eds: *The Roy adaptation model*, Norwalk, Conn, 1991, Appleton & Lange.

Kerr NJ: Ego competency: a framework for formulating nursing care, *Perspect Psychiatr Care* 26(4):30, 1990.

Hauser ST and others: Paths of adolescent ego development: links with family life and individual adjustment, *Psychiatr Clin N Amer* 13(3):489, 1990.

Lego S: The fear of moving beyond one's parents, *Perspect Psychiatr Care* 26(1):28, 1990.

LeMone P: Analysis of a human phenomenon: self-concept, *Nurs Diagnosis* 2(3):126, 1991.

Masterson J: *Psychotherapy of the borderline adult*, New York, 1976, Brunner/Mazel.

Perry JC and others: Psychotherapy and psychological trauma in borderline personality disorder, *Psychiatr Ann* 20(1):33, 1990.

Ricci MS: Aloneness in tenuous self-states, *Perspect Psychiatr Care* 27(2):7, 1991.

Sayre J: Psychodynamics revisited: an object-relations framework for psychiatric nursing, *Perspect Psychiatr Care* 26(1):7, 1990.

Sebastian L: Promoting object constancy-writing as a nursing intervention, *J Psychosoc Nurs* 29(1):21, 1991.

Personal identity disturbance—cont'd

Poisoning, risk for

CLINICAL CONDITION/ MEDICAL DIAGNOSIS	RISK FACTORS
Elderly woman with reduced vision and hearing	Large stock of medications stored in an inappropriate place; poor lighting

> **Patient goals**
> Expected outcomes
> > Associated nursing/collaborative interventions *and scientific rationale*

Adapt home environment to reduce risk of accidental poisoning as evidenced by the following:

Selects an appropriate storage area for medications
Permanently removes all cleaning supplies from bathroom
Discards outdated prescription and over-the-counter drugs

Collaborate with patient to establish a separate storage area for medications.

Evaluate with patient contents of medicine cabinet and discard outdated medications.

Replaces 25- and 60-watt bulbs with 100-watt bulbs where appropriate
Keeps hall and bathroom lights on during evening and night
Keeps a flashlight at bedside, in kitchen, and next to favorite chair in living room

Teach patient to keep environment well lighted.

Assist patient with selection of places to keep flashlights in case of power failure.

Place list of emergency telephone numbers near telephone.

Provide patient with information about life-line service available from local hospital.

Establish a safe method for taking medications as evidenced by the following:

**Uses magnifying glass to check contents of each
bottle of medication.**
**Sets up medications for 24-hour period in well-lighted
area.**
**Demonstrates agreed-on method to set up
medications.**
**Counts with nurse amount of medication remaining
in containers**

Help patient to develop a way to identify
medications accurately.

Discuss and demonstrate way to set up medications
for 24 hours. *Setting up medication for 24-hour
period decreases risk of missing a dose or taking an
extra dose.*

Monitor medication taking.

Seek medical evaluation of reduced vision as evidenced by the following:

Schedules an appointment for visit from social worker
**Makes and keeps appointment to see
ophthalmologist**
**Family members agree to assist with transportation to
keep appointments**

Provide patient with list of medical and financial
resources in community.

Help patient to make appointments.

Develop plan with patient and family for medical
evaluation.

REFERENCES

Janken JK, Cullinan CL: Auditory sensory/perceptual alteration:
suggested revision of defining characteristics. *Nurs Diagnosis*, 1990,
1(4):147-154.

Neill KM: The need for safety. In Yura H, Walsh MB, eds: *Human needs
and the nursing process.* Norwalk, CT, 1983, Appleton-Century-
Crofts

Nelson MA: Economic impoverishment as a health risk:
methodologic and conceptual issues. *Advanc Nurs Sci*, 1994,
16(3):1-12.

Williams MA: The physical environment and patient care. *Ann Rev
Nurs Res*, 1988, 6:61-84

Post trauma response

CLINICAL CONDITION/
MEDICAL DIAGNOSIS | RELATED FACTORS

Multiple injuries | Overwhelming guilt about auto accident: temporary loss of mobility

Patient goals
Expected outcomes
  Associated nursing/collaborative interventions *and scientific rationale*

Use new coping strategies to deal with excessive feelings of guilt as evidenced by the following:

Decreases excessive verbalization of details of accident.
Schedules regular visits with minister or psychologist.
Develops an objective appraisal of the event
  Explore guilt feelings with patient. Pace intervention to readiness for assistance. *Free expression of feelings is more productive after initial period of denial.*
  Support the use of appropriate defense mechanisms.
  Provide consultation or referral to deal with excessive feelings of guilt.
Maintains relationship with significant other
  Contact family of significant other to obtain information about injury of significant other.
  Arrange for telephone and personal visits with significant other.
  Allow for privacy during interactions with significant other. *This will enable patient to deal with feelings of guilt.*

Maintain relationship with family and friends as evidenced by the following:

Accepts assistance of parents and siblings to deal with outside obligations.
Asks parents to manage insurance and legal aspects of accident.

Initiates telephone visits with friends and personal visits with close friends

Provide family members with information about patient's physical status.

Instruct family members about importance of frequent, short visits from family members and close friends.

Request family members to bring meaningful personal items for patient's use.

Discuss with family an interim-interaction approach; answer patient's questions about accident but avoid excessive details, including pictures. *The preceding actions help patient, family, and significant other to express and accept feelings and reactions to the traumatic event.*

Maintain structural and physiological integrity of body systems as evidenced by the following:

Retains muscle strength in unaffected limbs
Retains full ROM in affected limbs
Skin remains intact with no redness, abrasions
Circulation and sensory and motor functions remain intact in affected limbs

Instruct and assist with active ROM in unaffected limbs.

Assist with passive ROM in affected limbs (within limits imposed by injuries).

Make small changes in body position every 2 hours.

Monitor and massage pressure-prone areas of skin.

Monitor warmth, sensation, and movement of fingers and toes in casted extremities. *Providing ROM and proper position assists in maintaining structural integrity of body systems.*

Maintains pretrauma pattern of urine and bowel elimination

Monitor adequate fluid and fiber intake to prevent bladder and bowel elimination problems.

Provide for adequate intake of fluids and foods high in fiber.

Use assistive devices to enhance self-care ability as evidenced by the following:

Transfers from bed to wheelchair with assistance of one person
Attends physical therapy sessions twice a day to gain muscle strength and learn crutch walking
Practices crutch walking with nursing assistance
Resumes responsibility for ADLs gradually within limits of injuries

Guide patient in learning transfer techniques.

Arrange for physical therapy.

Praise patient for small gains in ADLs.

Monitor for side effects of increased activity, e.g., increased discomfort or pain in affected limbs.

Focus on taking more responsibility for ADLs helps patient to control intrusive thoughts about accident.

REFERENCES

Beyea SC: Concept analysis of feeling: a human response pattern. *Nurs Diagn*, 1990, 1 (3):97-101.

Komnenich P, Feller C: Disaster nursing. *Ann Rev Nurs Res*, 1991, 9:123-134.

McCloskey JC, Bulechek GM: Coping enhancement. In *Nursing interventions classification (NIC)*, St. Louis, 1992, Mosby, pp. 183-184.

Murphy SA: Human responses to catastrophe. *Ann Rev Nurs Res*, 1991, 9:57-76.

Oberst MT: Response to Coping amid uncertainty: an illness trajectory perspective. *Scholary Inquiry for Nursing Practice*, 1993, 7(1):33-35.

Thompson JM, McFarLand GK, Hirsch JE, Tucker SM: Posttrauma response. In *Mosby's clinical nursing* ed 3, St. Louis, 1993, Mosby, pp. 1629-1631.

Wiener CL, Dodd MJ: Coping amid uncertainty: an illness trajectory perspective. *Scholary Inquiry for Nursing Practice*, 1993, 7(1):17-31.

Post trauma response—cont'd

Powerlessness

CLINICAL CONDITION/ MEDICAL DIAGNOSIS	RELATED FACTORS
Cancer requiring frequent hospitalizations; undifferentiated schizophrenia	Controlling or authoritative health care environment; life-style of helplessness

Patient goals
Expected outcomes
    Associated nursing/collaborative interventions *and scientific rationale*

Experience an increased sense of control over life situation and own activities along with a decrease in a life-style of helplessness as evidenced by the following:

Verbalizes positive feelings about own ability to achieve mastery in role performance

Assist patient to identify preferences, needs, values, and attitudes that may affect role performance.

Mutually explore with the patient readiness to initiate and sustain health-promoting behaviors.

Discuss with the patient desirable health behaviors.

Identify with the patient undesirable health behaviors and assist patient to formulate specific plans to avoid such behaviors.

Identify with the patient situations in which powerlessness is experienced.

Explore reality perceptions and clarify if necessary by providing information or correcting misinformation. *Verbalizing, exploring feelings increases understanding of individual coping styles and defense mechanisms.*

Provide consistent caregivers.

Modify the environment if needed to facilitate the patient's active involvement in self-care.

Encourage a sense of partnership with the health care team and reinforce the patient's right to ask questions

Powerlessness

363

Provide procedural and sensory information related to specific treatment interventions for cancer; consider utilizing peer models who demonstrate successful mastery *because such actions promote mastery and reduce anxiety.*

Engages in problem-solving behaviors

Help the patient develop awareness of care aspects that are patient-controlled.

Eliminate unpredictability of events by informing and involving patient in scheduling.

Provide for patient's privacy needs.

Limit the use of medical jargon.

Alleviate physical discomfort that diminishes energy reserve.

Provide positive reinforcement for increasing involvement in self-care.

Provide relevant learning material about clinical conditions, i.e., cancer and schizophrenia.

Assist the patient to maintain realistic expectations through strategies such as proximal goal setting.

Involve the patient in role play in order to strengthen ability to express concerns.

Teach coping skills; e.g., relaxations, distraction, visual imagery, comforting and positive self-talk, self monitoring. *Focused coping strategies enhance potential for mastery over specific aspects of care.*

Integrates therapeutic regimen into lifestyle

Provide opportunity for the expression of positive emotions (e.g., hope, faith, sense of purpose).

Help the patient identify strength and improvements in condition and mastery of self-care and coping resources.

Involve the family or significant others in reinforcing and supporting health enhancing behaviors.

Facilitate continuity of significant roles that the patient fills in everyday life or help the patient find alternative roles, interests and use of talents.

Assist the patient in planning tasks that may deplete energy so that support systems are available.

Support involvement in self-help groups or self-help education when indicated. *Social support systems provide ongoing reinforcement of health-desirable behaviors and enhance compliance.*

REFERENCES

Braden CJ: A test of the self-help model: learned response to chronic illness experience, *Nurs Res* 39(1):42, 1990.

Burckhardt CS: Coping strategies of the chronically ill, *Nurs Clin North Am* 22(3):543, 1987.

Fleury JD: Empowering potential: a theory of wellness motivation, *Nurs Res* 40(5):286, 1991.

Lambert C, Lambert V: Psychosocial impacts created by chronic illness, *Nurs Clin North Am* 22(3):527, 1987.

LaMontagne LL: Bolstering personal control in child patients through coping interventions, *Pediatric Nursing* 19(3):235, 1993.

McFarland GK, McFarlane EA: *Nursing diagnosis and intervention,* ed 2, St. Louis, 1993, Mosby.

Miller JF: *Coping with chronic illness: overcoming powerlessness,* ed 1, Philadelphia, 1992, F.A. Davis.

Swearingen PL: *Manual of medical surgical nursing care: nursing interventions and collaborative management,* ed 3, St. Louis, 1994, Mosby.

Thompson J, McFarland G, Hirsch J, Tucker JM: *Mosby's clinical nursing,* ed 3, St. Louis, 1993, Mosby.

Powerlessness—cont'd

Protection, altered

CLINICAL CONDITION/ MEDICAL DIAGNOSIS	RELATED FACTORS
Hematologic cancer	Altered immune and hematopoietic function

Patient goals
Expected outcomes
  Associated nursing/collaborative interventions *and scientific rationale*

Maintain protective defenses as evidenced by the following:

Establishes a pattern of personal hygiene consistent with other demands of daily living
  Teach strategies to promote personal and environmental cleanliness.
  Assist with daily shower and oral hygiene. *Skin and mucous membranes are the frontline of defense and cleanliness decreases exposure to microbes.*
  Monitor vital signs. *Early report of abnormal vital signs (e.g., fever) can reduce complications.*

Incorporates safety measures, prevent infection, bleeding
  Teach and demonstrate safety precautions to patient and family.
  Re-orient and assist patient during periods of confusion. *Injury from falls and trauma have a high risk of complications due to deficient protective mechanisms.*

Restore protective defenses as evidenced by the following:

Maintains normal body weight and fluid balance
  Establish diet plan in collaboration with patient and dietitian.
  Weigh patient daily.
  Offer small frequent meals.
  Prescribe dietary supplement as needed.
  Encourage fluid intake.

Monitor intake and output. *Nausea, vomiting, anorexia, diarrhea, and stomatitis are associated with therapy and impact nutritional status and fluid balance.*

Incorporates period of rest before or after activities

Teach measures to conserve energy (e.g., pacing of ADLs).

Symptoms resolve in response to therapy.

Provide comfort for symptoms (e.g., chills, fever, myalgias). *Flu-like symptoms cause distress and may lead to stress and decreased quality of life.*

Promote protective defenses as evidenced by the following:

Reports increased sense of well-being

Initiate stress management.

Teach relaxation exercises.

Teach alternate coping strategies.

Assist with communication between patient and family.

Provide supportive nurse interactions.
Psychoneuroimmunology provides rationale for mind body interaction, stress and immunodepression, and justifies interventions of touching, listening, and caring attitudes of the nurse.

REFERENCES

American Nurses Association, Oncology Nursing Society: *Standards of oncology nursing practice,* Kansas City, 1987, American Nurses Association.

Brophy LR, Sharp EJ: Physical symptoms of combination bitherapy; a quality of life issue. *Oncol Nurs Forum* 18(1):25-30, 1991.

Groer M: Psychoneuroimmunology, *Am J Nurs* 91(8)33, 1991.

Sheppard KC: Altered protection: A nursing diagnosis. In R Carroll-Johnson, ed: *Classification of nursing diagnoses: proceedings of the ninth conference,* Philadelphia, 1991, J.B. Lippincott.

Volker Di Neoplasia In PG Beare, JL Myers: *Principles and practice of adult health nursing,* ed 2, St Louis, 1994, Mosby.

Protection, altered—cont'd

Rape-trauma syndrome (acute)

CLINICAL CONDITION/ MEDICAL DIAGNOSIS	RELATED FACTORS
Raped by acquaintance	Fear of reprisal; anxiety about AIDS

Patient goals
Expected outcomes
> Associated nursing/collaborative interventions *and scientific rationale*

Obtain relief from emotional responses to rape experience as evidenced by the following:

Accepts immediate and ongoing counseling from rape-crisis center staff
> Acknowledge appropriateness and support of patient responses to victimization.
> Provide empathetic support during physician and police interviews.
> Provide for continuity of support throughout entire emergency room experience.

Identifies individuals in family and peer group who would provide support

Verbalizes decrease in fears, anxieties, and concerns
> Help patient identify, select, and contact individual with whom rape experience could be discussed. *Women who receive crisis support recover more quickly than those who do not.*
> Assist with identifying and avoiding individuals who are upsetting.
> Assist significant other to focus on subjective experience of rape rather than on whether rape occurred. *A nonjudgmental attitude helps to alleviate feelings of guilt and self blame.*

Assume decision-making role as evidenced by the following:

Asks questions that enable her to make decisions about health care

Offer information about medical and legal options
to facilitate making choices.

Identify decisions that can be postponed

- *Rape challenges an individual's sense of power,*
  autonomy, and control; making own decisions can
  maintain power, sense of control, and feeling of
  responsibility.

Verbalizes concern of exposure to HIV or AIDS
infection

Makes appointment to discuss HIV testing and
accepts written information about ethical issues
surrounding HIV testing

Help patient identify fears related to rape,
pregnancy, HIV transmission. *Patient's*
verbalization of concern of AIDS will enable her to
seek and accept help toward recovery.

Discuss benefit of periodic HIV testing, 5-year
window of infection, and right to know
assailant's HIV status versus right to privacy and
informed consent.

Provide written information about ethical issues
related to HIV testing and potential loss of
employment and access to health insurance if
seropositive.

- *Individual has the right to know benefits and risks*
  of HIV testing and status of debate about ethical
  and legal issues.

Cope with concern for personal safety as evidenced
by the following:

Asks family member/peer to stay with her for a few
days.

Set goal of returning to usual activities by a specified
date.

Collaborate with patient to identify safety
measures to decrease vulnerability.

Provide a list of immediate and long-term
responses to rape experience, e.g., nightmares,
flashbacks; emphasize reactions are not
unusual.

REFERENCES

Blair T, Warner CG: Sexual assault. *Topics in Emergency Medicine,* 1992, 14(4):58.

Burgess AW, Baker T: AIDS and victims of sexual assault. *Hospital and Community Psychiatry,* 1992, 43 (5):447.

Burgess AW and others: HIV testing of sexual assault populations: ethical and legal issues. *J Emerg Nurs,* 1990, 16 (5):331.

Larson E, Ropka ME: An update on nursing research and HIV infection. *Image: J Nurs Scholar,* 1991, 23:4-12.

Ledray LE: Counseling rape victims: the nursing challenge. *Perspective on Psychiatric Care,* 1990, 26 (2)21.

McArthur MJ: Reality therapy with rape victim. *Arch Psychiatr Nurs,* 1990, 6:360.

Turner JG: Acquired immunodeficiency syndrome. *Ann Nurs Res,* 1990, 8:195-210.

Turner JG: AIDS-related knowledge, attitudes, and risk for HIV infection among nurses. *Ann Rev Nurs Res ,* 1993, 11:205-224.

Visser E: AIDS as a result of incest. *AIDS Patient Care,* 1992, 6(3):113.

PAMELA KOHLBRY, AUDREY M. MCLANE

Rape-trauma syndrome: compound reaction

CLINICAL CONDITION/ MEDICAL DIAGNOSIS	RELATED FACTORS
Did not seek medical/ psychological help to deal with trauma	Inadequate support system; inability to resolve rape-trauma experience

---

Patient goals
Expected outcomes
  Associated nursing/collaborative interventions *and scientific rationale*

Develop significant other or family support as evidenced by the following:

Verbalizes that significant other has begun to express warmth and concern
  Assist significant other or family to focus on the subjective experience of rape.
  Help patient identify individuals with whom the rape experience could be discussed.

Accepts and keeps appointment with counselor at rape crisis center
  Refer patient and significant other to rape counseling center.
  Assist patient and significant other with seeking individual and group counseling. *Group counseling assists members with changing negative attitudes and behaviors.*
  Determine need for family members to seek counseling. *Failure of significant other or family to provide support leads to feelings of guilt and self-blame; feelings require resolution before current physical and emotional problems can be successfully treated.*

Make realistic decisions about actual or potential health problems as evidenced by the following:

Keeps follow-up medical appointments

Takes medication in keeping with prescribed regimen
Makes appointment to discuss HIV testing and accepts written information about ethical and legal issues surrounding HIV testing

Teach importance of medication regimen.

Monitor adherence to medical regimen.

Discuss benefit of periodic HIV testing, 5-year window of infection, and right to know assailant's HIV status vs right of privacy and informed consent.

Provide written information about ethical issues related to HIV testing and potential loss of employment and access to health insurance if seropositive. *Individual has the right to know benefits and risks of HIV testing and status of the debate about ethical and legal issues.*

Cope with cognitive and emotional responses to rape and other stressor as evidenced by the following:

Verbalizes anger and resolves self-blame.
Keeps and discusses feelings recorded in separate journal

Teach and monitor use of journal to express anger and related feelings. *Discussing anger and related feelings enables couple to support one another.*

Provide and discuss written list of long-term responses to rape experience; emphasize that reactions are not unusual.

Monitor resolution of symptoms with Rape-Trauma Symptom Rating Scale.

Practices relaxation and cognitive coping strategies
Participates in rape support group

Teach relaxation strategies.

Teach use of cognitive coping strategies such as thought stopping, desensitization, guided imagery, and refuting irrational ideas.

Resume a satisfying life-style as evidenced by the following:

Reestablishes intimate relationship with significant other
Reports feeling more secure
Maintains contact with legal system

Collaborate with patient in pacing social activities.
Select strategies to protect from future assaults.
Monitor and support patient's experiences with
legal system.

REFERENCES

Blair T, Warner CG: Sexual assault. *Topics in Emergency Medicine*, 1992, 14(4):58.

Burgess AW, Baker T: AIDS and victims of sexual assault. *Hospital and Community Psychiatry*, 1992, 43(5):447.

Burgess AW and others: HIV testing of sexual assault population: ethical and legal issues. *J Emerg Nurs* , 1990, 16(5):331.

Larson E, Ropka ME: An update on nursing research and HIV infection. *Image: J Nurs Scholar*, 1991, 23:4-12.

Ledray LE: Counseling rape victims: the nursing challenge. *Perspective on Psychiatric Care*, 1990, 26(2):21.

Ledray LE: A nursing developed model for the treatment of rape victims. In American Academy of Nursing From accommodation to self-determination: nursing's role in the development of health care policy, Kansas City, MO, 1982, American Academy of Nursing.

McArthur MJ: Reality therapy with rape victims. *Arch Psychiatr Nurs*, 1990, 6:360.

Turner JC: Acquired immunodeficiency syndrome. *Ann ReviewNurs Res*, 1990, 8:195-210.

Turner JC: AIDS-related knowledge, attitudes, and risk for HIV infection among nurses. *Ann Rev Nurs Res*, 1993, 11:205-224.

Visser E: AIDS as a result of incest. *AIDS Patient Care*, 1992, 6(3):113.

Rape-trauma syndrome: compound reaction—cont'd

Rape-trauma syndrome: silent reaction

CLINICAL CONDITION/ MEDICAL DIAGNOSIS	RELATED FACTORS
Concern for personal safety	Anxiety, denial

Patient goals
Expected outcomes
    Associated nursing/collaborative interventions *and scientific rationale*

Cope with personal safety concern as evidenced by the following:

Verbalizes feeling of insecurity
    Establish a trusting relationship with patient.
    Actively listen to patient's perceptions of increased vulnerability.
    Collaborate with patient to identify safety measure to decrease vulnerability.

Makes some progress in relating anxiety about safety to the rape event
    Assist patient to identify source of anxiety about personal safety.
    Provide opportunity to discuss safety concerns with a female police officer. *Establishing a trusting relationship and providing direct assistance with safety measures may reduce anxiety enough to enable patient to deal with the unidentified problem of rape.*

Decrease reliance on denial to maintain sense of well-being as evidenced by the following:

Begins to verbalize feelings of anger and shame related to rape.
Verbalizes fear of male friends and relatives since rape
    During routine interview, ask patient if anyone has ever attempted to assault her or hurt her in any way.

Avoid direct questioning; allow patient to continue
at own pace to reveal details of the rape event.
Determine readiness for referral to rape counselor.
*Avoiding direct confrontation of denial may enable
patient to begin to deal with fears and anxieties
associated with the rape.*

Reveals some details of rape experience
Help patient identify specific concerns related to
rape experience, e.g., concern about pregnancy,
sexually transmitted diseases (STDs).

**Assume decision-making about health-care needs as
evidenced by the following:**

Asks questions about health care resources
Offer information about medical and legal options
to facilitate making choices.
Identify decisions that should be made soon and
those that can be postponed.
Verbalizes fear of HIV and AIDS
**Does not return to full denial during discussion of HIV
testing**
Offer information about HIV testing. Discuss
benefit of periodic HIV testing, 5-year window
of infection, and right to know assailant's HIV
status vs right of privacy and informed consent.
Provide written information about ethical issues
related to HIV testing and potential loss of
employment and access to health insurance if
seropositive. *Individual has the right to know
benefits and risks of HIV testing and status of
debate about ethical and legal issues.*

**Cope with cognitive and emotional responses to
rape experience as evidenced by the following:**

Verbalizes anger and resolves self-blame
Practices cognitive coping strategies
Participates in rape support group
Teach use of cognitive coping strategies such as
thought stopping, desensitization, guided
imagery, refuting irrational ideas.

Provide information about support group opportunities and benefits.

Teach and monitor use of journal to express anger and related feelings. *Discussion of fear, anger, and related feelings enables individual to obtain support from group.*

REFERENCES

Blair T, Warner CG: Sexual assault. *Topics in Emergency Medicine,* 1992, 14(4):58.

Burgess AW, Baker T: AIDS and victims of sexual assault. *Hospital and Community Psychiatry,* 1992, 43(5):447.

Burgess AW and others: HIV testing of sexual assault populations: ethical and legal issues. *J Emerg Nurs,* 1990, 16(5):331.

Larson E, Ropka ME: An update on nursing research and HIV infection. *Image: J Nurs Scholar,* 1991, 23:4-12.

Ledray LE: Counseling rape victims: the nursing challenge. *Perspective on Psychiatric Care,* 1990, 26(2):21.

McArthur MJ: Reality therapy with rape victims. *Arch Psychiatr Nurs,* 1990, 6:360.

Turner JG: Acquired immunodeficiency syndrome. *Ann Review Nurs Res,* 1990, 8:195-210.

Turner JG: AIDS-related knowledge, attitudes, and risk for HIV infection among nurses. *Ann Rev Nurs Res,* 1993, 11:205-224.

Visser E: AIDS as a result of incest. *AIDS Patient Care,* 1992, 6(3):113.

KAREN B. INABA, GERTRUDE K. MCFARLAND

Relocation stress syndrome

CLINICAL CONDITION/ MEDICAL DIAGNOSIS	RELATED FACTORS
Pelvic fracture (Indochinese refugee)	Sudden environmental change within context of recent migration

Patient goals
Expected outcomes
    Associated nursing/collaborative interventions *and scientific rationale*

Adapt to sudden change associated with hospitalization and migration as evidenced by the following:

Demonstrates reduced levels of fear and anxiety

Establish a supportive relationship with patients *to build trust and a sense of security.*

Orient patient to new surroundings and routines *to decrease unfamiliarity, uncertainty, and a sense of disruption.*

Assess patient's current level of stressors (e.g., resettlement and acculturation stress, developmental crises, family roles, impact of changed health status) *to determine patient's appraisal of relocation events and level of loss and vulnerability.*

Provide structure and consistent caregivers whenever possible *to minimize further changes for the patient and establish predictable relationships.*

Communicates about changes and losses associated with relocation (e.g., loss of culture, status, roles, social network) and describes impact on coping with changed health status

Provide opportunities for patient to verbalize feelings about perceived or actual changes and losses associated with relocation *to acknowledge distress, facilitate grieving, and promote problem-solving.*

Use consultants when appropriate (e.g., language translators, volunteers from culture-specific community programs) *to maximize communication between the patient and care providers.*

Acknowledge patient's positive statements about new environment and acceptance of changed surroundings.

Assess for dysfunctional grieving responses (e.g., explore somatic complaints) and make psychiatric referrals if indicated.

Maintains a sense of self-worth and positive personal identity during transition to new setting

Acknowledge patient's cultural preferences whenever possible (e.g., diet, family involvement, communication patterns) and incorporate into care.

Protect patient's privacy and encourage participation in decision making about care *to decrease powerlessness, uncertainty, and feelings of marginality.*

Assess sources of support for patient (e.g., family, friends, ethnic community, religious organizations) and facilitate contact.

Accepts support from appropriate resources during adjustment period to hospitalization as evidenced by the following:

Verbalizes acceptance of referrals to community agencies and health care providers prior to discharge

Initiate early discharge planning for culturally relevant follow-up in the community.

Initiate early patient predischarge teaching, working with language translators and others in the patient's support system.

Refer patient to relevant self-help support groups (e.g., resettlement classes, ethnic clinics, church groups) *to rebuild disrupted social network, promote feelings of universality, decrease isolation, and increase support during the adjustment period and convalescence.*

REFERENCES

Aroian KJ: A model of psychological adaptation to migration and resettlement, *Nurs Res* 39(1)5, 1990.

Aroian KJ: Mental health risks and problems encountered by illegal immigrants, *Issues Ment Health Nurs* 14:379, 1993.

Cravener P: Establishing therapeutic alliance across cultural barriers, *J Psychosoc Nurs* 30(12):10, 1992.

Gass KA, Gaustad G, Oberst MT, Hughes S: Relocation appraisal, functional independence, morale, and health of nursing home residents, *Issues in Ment Health Nurs* 13:239, 1992.

Kinzie JD: Therapeutic approaches to traumatized Cambodian refugees, *J Traum Stress* 2(1):75, 1989.

Kinzie JD and others: The prevalence of posttraumatic stress disorder and its clinical significance among southeast Asian refugees, *Am J Psychiatry* 147(7):913, 1990.

Lee E: Cultural factors in working with southeast Asian refugee adolescents, *J Adolesc* 11(2):167, 1988.

Leininger M: Becoming aware of types of health practitioners and cultural imposition, *J Transcult Nurs* 2(1): 32, 1991.

Ramey L, Cloud J: Relocation success: a model for mental health counselors, *J Ment Health Couns* 9(3): 150, 1987.

Starker JE: Psychosocial aspects of geographic relocation: the development of a new social network, *Am J Health Promot* 5(1): 52, 1990.

Role performance, altered

CLINICAL CONDITION/ MEDICAL DIAGNOSIS	RELATED FACTORS
Chronic obstructive pulmonary disease	Inadequate role performance; decline in strength and endurance

Patient goals
Expected outcomes
> Associated nursing/collaborative interventions *and scientific rationale*

Engage in functional role performance within limitations of health status changes as evidenced by the following:

Describes realistic expectations for self and behaviors necessary for fulfilling modified role expectations
> Encourage patient to express concerns and feelings about chronic illness, physical limitations, and other losses.

Determines nature of role performance disturbance (e.g., role failure, role loss, interpersonal role conflict, or role insufficiency) to assess limitations and plan strategies to cope with role changes
> Assess scope and nature of situational transition experienced by patient *to determine degree of crisis created by changes.*
> Determine role of the patient within family and social contexts *to identify responsibilities and expectations held by patient and others.*
> Determine cultural factors influencing role expectations and performance.
> Encourage patient to clarify role expectations with family or partner and discuss potential impact of changed role performance.

Uses constructive strategies to cope with situational transition related to changes in health status
> Assist patient in identifying strengths and resources, including positive role models *to increase and reinforce functional role performance.*
> Teach patient specific strategies to cope with physical disability (e.g., problem-focused

strategies of positioning and breathing techniques; emotion-focused strategies of relaxation exercises).

Discuss impact of role changes with family or partner *to assess degree of support available to patient and to increase collaborative problem-solving.*

Use role playing *to teach new behaviors, provide opportunities for role rehearsal, and reinforce desired changes.*

Assist patient and family or partner in identifying previous coping strategies and resources to apply to current situation.

Provide patient with positive feedback for initiating and practicing new behaviors *to reinforce changes and build self-esteem related to role transition.*

Seeks assistance from appropriate resources within the health care system and community

Initiate early discharge planning and collaborate with patient and family or partner in planning rehabilitation care *to maximize a sense of control and decrease anxiety.*

Provide patient with referrals to relevant self-help support groups in the community *to facilitate reference group interaction, information-sharing, and advocacy.*

REFERENCES

Andrews HA: Overview of the role function mode. In Roy SR, Andrews A, eds: *The Roy adaptation model*, Norwalk, Conn, 1991, Appleton & Lange.

Doyle DL, Stern PA: Negotiating self-care in rehabilitation nursing, *Rehabil Nurs*, 1992, 17(6):319.

Gift AG, Austin DJ: The effects of a program of systematic movement on copd patients, *Rehabil Nurs*, 1992, 17(1):6.

Gillis DA: Role supplementation to overcome intrafamilial role insufficiency following physical disability, *Rehabil Nurs*, 1988, 13(1):19.

Johnson JL, Morse JM: Regaining control: the process of adjustment following myocardial infarction, *Heart Lung*, 1990, 19(2):126.

Kersten L: Changes in self-concept during pulmonary rehabilitation, Part I, *Heart Lung*, 1990, 19(5):456.

Kersten L: Changes in self-concept during pulmonary rehabilitation, Part II, *Heart Lung*, 1990, 19(5):463.

Musolf JM: Easing the impact of the family caregiver's role, *Rehabil Nurs*, 1991, 16(2):82.

Sexton DL, Munro BH: Living with a chronic illness-the experience of women with chronic obstructive pulmonary disease (COPD), *West J Nurs Res*, 1988, 10(1):26

Role performance, altered—cont'd

Self-care deficit (Bathing/Hygiene/Dressing/ Grooming/Feeding/Toileting)

CLINICAL CONDITION/
MEDICAL DIAGNOSIS

Post-cerebrovascular
accident (CVA)

RELATED FACTORS

Disability requiring modified life-style

> **Patient goals**
> Expected outcomes
>> Associated nursing/collaborative interventions *and scientific rationale*

Modify life-style to maximize self-care ability and increase independence within limitations.

Recognizes that self-care practices are necessary for managing activity within limitations

Provide opportunity for expression of feelings related to CVA and physical limitations (e.g., denial, anxiety, or depression).

Encourage patient to identify motivations to engage in self-care behaviors.

Assist patient to identify factors that support or hinder self-care activity.

Provide factual or technical information relevant to meet self-care requisites. *Adequate information will allow the patient to be as independent as possible, to make intelligent decisions about his or her care, and to decrease anxiety.*

Discuss with patient a means of negotiating and instilling a sense of responsibility or commitment to self-care (i.e., contract learning). *A sense of responsibility gives a patient some form of control during a time of uncertainty and powerlessness.*

Consistently convey value of patient's knowledge and competence necessary to engage in health promoting self-care activities.

Demonstrates self-care activities as much as possible within limitations

Assist patient to set short-term, realistic, and attainable goals.

Assist patient to make free choices of self-care activity and methods of assistance. *A chance of free choice will give patient a sense of control and self-esteem.*

Allow patient to make own schedule for ADLs.

Provide sufficient time and personal care supplies necessary for self-care.

Provide patient and family support and knowledge to empower them to manage self-care limits more effectively. *Education and support reinforce positive psychological and social outcomes, and reduce fear and anxiety related to physical limitations.*

Avoid emphasis on self-care limitations that could heighten self- criticism and lower physical self-concept.

Assist patient to select self-care practices that enhance adjustment to disability (e.g., maintaining balanced exercise and rest regimen).

Encourage patient to engage in ADLs for herself or himself as much as possible.

Explore the use of self-help devices or assistive devices to help patient become more self-sufficient.

Provide assistance, supervision, and teaching as necessary to improve self care practices.

Provide opportunity for building self-care confidence by frequent reinforcement of positive feedback. *Positive reinforcement emphasizes the need for continuing self-care behaviors*

Allow patient to explore feelings associate with positive changes.

Uses strengths and weaknesses to engage in self-care activities within limitations

Assist patient to identify and utilize own strengths, intact roles, and resources to maximize sense of ability for regaining control.

Assist patient to identify past self-care abilities and present limitations. *Self-care abilities and perceived self-efficacy have an effect on self-care behavior.*

Facilitate discussion by patient and family of topics that are not related to disability (e.g., current events, hobbies, recreational interests, family activities).

Encourage patient to maintain previously learned self-care activities.

Assist patient to identify previous coping behaviors and support system for problem solving to generate a sense of hope and self- control. *Patients using problem-focused coping strategies appear to have less psychosocial difficulty with post-CVA adjustment.*

Reassess goals periodically and set new goals as possible.

Reinforce patient's progress, no matter how small, with positive feedback.

Utilizes available support system and community resources

Assess the family's willingness to support patient's self-care limitations, changed life-style, and patient's ability to increase independence.

Actively include family and significant others in entire stroke rehabilitation process. *The perceived beliefs of significant others are important for patient's adherence to medical regimen.*

Teach the family the role of supervision rather than the role of activity maintenance. *The pessimistic attitude of a family member impedes the patient from doing what she or he is capable of doing and leads to regression and low self-esteem.*

Assist patient and family to utilize available resources such as Medicare, Social Security, and disability insurance.

Encourage patient and family to utilize community resources such as stroke support group, interest group, senior citizen center, or adult day care for diversional activity.

Keep patient's significant others who can influence patient, informed of patient's progress, so they can give patient positive feedback. *Family could provide validation of worth to the patient in the family within the patient's ability to function.*

REFERENCES

Barron M: Life after stroke, *Nurs Times*, 1992, 88(10):32.

Borgman MF, Passarella P: Nursing care of the stroke patient using Bobath principles: an approach to altered movement, *Nurs Clin North Am*, 1991, 26(4):1019.

Bronstein KS: Psychosocial components in stroke: implication for adaption, *Nurs Clin North Am*, 1991, 26(4):1007.

Farzan DT: Reintegration for stroke survivors: home and community consideration, *Nurs Clin North Am*, 1991, 26(4):1019.

Sutton P: Positive progress, *Nurs Times*, 1992, 88(5):38.

Walkins M: Can you tread this emotional high wire? *Prof Nurse,* 1993, 8(9):604.

Self-esteem disturbance

CLINICAL CONDITION/ MEDICAL DIAGNOSIS	RELATED FACTORS
Rheumatoid arthritis (elderly patient)	Reduced self-care ability; limited coping mechanisms

Patient goals
Expected outcomes
    Associated nursing/collaborative interventions *and scientific rationale*

Experience and maintain self-esteem as evidenced by the following:

Identifies strategies for coping with negative feelings about self

Help patient to describe effects of illness on self-appraisal, daily activities, family, and friends. *Rheumatoid arthritis accompanied by functional incapacities may be associated with decreased levels of self-esteem.*

Convey respect and acceptance of the patient as a unique individual. *Creating an atmosphere of acceptance and interest is important so that the patient can begin to explore presenting problems and the significance of current experiences.*

Encourage discussion of illness *to facilitate acceptance of reality of illness. Patients who accept the reality of a disease and integrate this reality into their own self-concept experience higher levels of self-esteem.*

Discourage the use of palliative coping responses (e.g., wishful thinking, ruminating on past problems and failures) *because these coping behaviors are associated with ongoing lowered self-esteem.*

Inspire hope by describing situations in which other patients have managed similar difficulties.

Help patient set initial goals that can be achieved within a short period.

Encourage decision-making in planning and directing own care *to promote patient autonomy and to decrease avoidance of constructive problem-solving.*

Teach meditation and relaxation skills *to provide the patient with the ability to successfully cope with stressors and to improve his/her self-esteem and life satisfactions.*

Facilitate participation in treatment modalities that emphasize support, acceptance, and belonging.

Encourage development of a health-promoting activity such as an exercise program, to extent possible. *Participation in a regular exercise program increases self-esteem.*

Achieves goals within family and social environment that reflect awareness of personal talents and limitations

Encourage identification and description of existing strengths and potentials.

Acknowledge recognition of patient's expertise or knowledge *to reinforce patient's recognition of existing strengths and competencies.*

Encourage patient to initiate realistic activities in which success can be anticipated *because failure and negative feedback from others can influence patient's self-confidence.*

Help patient strengthen desired coping skills and become involved in actions to meet goals within the patient's functional capacity. *Strengthening a positive coping response lessens the patient's tendency to avoid problems or stressors.*

Monitor extent to which patient's family influences patient's perception of self.

Teach family members to recognize the influence of their interactive style on patient's perceptions of self.

Encourage participation in volunteer programs (e.g., programs sponsored by church affiliation or a community-based programs) *to reinforce perception to self and others of ability to make positive contributions to others.*

Teach patient to create and maintain relationships that provide successful social interaction.

Maintains self-care skills necessary for functioning in society as evidenced by the following:

Engages in daily activities to meet personal needs (e.g., personal hygiene practices, good grooming,

meal preparation, home maintenance, planning leisure time) to extent possible

Monitor ongoing pain levels as well as patient's expectations of pain control. *Acute and chronic arthritic pain affects an individual's ability to maintain routine self-care skills.*

Monitor patient's ability to identify and accurately report symptoms.

Compare subjective descriptions with objective measurements *to determine possible discrepancies between the patient's ability and willingness to participate in self-care skills.*

Encourage participation in treatment modalities such as an ADL group that focus on learning or relearning how to live independently in a community and achieving highest level of functional capacity.

Emphasize the importance of participating in activities that maximize the patient's ability to maintain optimal health, personal hygiene, and independent living (e.g., meal planning and preparation, money management and leisure time). *Maintaining optimal level of health and functioning aids in maintaining self esteem, as well as optimal social functioning.*

REFERENCES

Bednar RL, Wells MG, Peterson SR: *Self-esteem: paradoxes and innovations in clinical theory and practice,* Washington, DC, 1989, American Psychological Association.

Bonheur B, Young SW: Exercise as a health-promoting lifestyle choice, *Applied Nurs Res* 4(1):2, 1991.

Cornwell CJ, Schmitt MH: Perceived health status, self-esteem and body image in women with rheumatoid arthritis or systemic lupus erythematosus, *Res Nurs Health* 13:99,1990.

Greenblatt F: Maintaining self-esteem, *J Long Term Care Admin* 20(4):7, 1992.

McFarland GK, Wasli EL, Gerety EK: *Nursing diagnoses and process in psychiatric mental health nursing,* ed 2, Philadelphia, 1992, JB Lippincott.

Norris J: Nursing intervention for self-esteem disturbances, *Nurs Diagnosis* 3(2):48, 1992.

O'Brien M: Multiple sclerosis: the relationship among self-esteem, social support, and coping behavior, *Applied Nurs Res* 6(2):54, 1993.

Pigg JS, Schroeder PM: Frequently occurring problems of patients with rheumatic diseases: the ANA outcome standards for rheumatology nursing practice, *Nurs Clin North Am* 19(4):697, 1984.

Walsh A, Walsh PA: Love, self-esteem, and multiple sclerosis, *Soc Sci Med* 29(7):793, 1989.

White NE, Richter JM, Fry C: Coping, social support, and adaptation to chronic illness, *Western J Nurs Res* 14(2):211, 1992.

Self-esteem, chronic low

CLINICAL CONDITION/ MEDICAL DIAGNOSIS	RELATED FACTORS
Eczematous dermatitis (young female adult)	Repeated negative and stressful interpersonal relationships

---

Patient goals
Expected outcomes
  Associated nursing/collaborative interventions *and
    scientific rationale*

Develop more positive self-evaluations as evidenced by the following:

Increase in positive statements about self and own capabilities

  Explore with patient nature of feelings about self
    and extent of existence and change over time *to
    help the patient begin to understand the associations
    between repeated negative interpersonal statements
    and current state of low self-esteem.*

  Demonstrate empathy.

  Help patient describe experiences that make her
    feel worthwhile and good about herself.

  Convey genuine interest in and concern for patient
    to reinforce sense of self-worth.

  Teach patient to recognize negative and distorted
    thoughts about self *so that she can begin to learn
    techniques for interrupting or stopping self-defeating
    thoughts.*

  Support patient's endeavors to practice techniques
    to stop and replace negative and self-defeating
    thoughts about self.

  Encourage identification and description of
    realistic and positive self assessments.

Engage in constructive interpersonal relationships as evidenced by the following:

Develops positive interpersonal relationships

Teach patient to observe pattern of interactions with mother, significant other, employer, and friends.

Help patient to identify and describe problems in relating to these people.

Suggest that patient keep journal *to assist in problem solving and obtaining feedback.*

Teach patient strategies for building self-confidence (e.g., improving communications skills, making constructive use of defenses, developing hobbies and interests, and developing personal opinions about issues).

Evaluates self as able to deal with interpersonal relationships

Acknowledge to patient that she does have choices in life.

Discourage rumination about past failures.

Assist patient in setting realistic goals for improving interpersonal relationships.

Role play a variety of ordinary interpersonal encounters *to help patient become aware of strengths and difficulties in interactions with mother, significant other, employer, and friends.*

Evaluate need for referral to specific additional treatment modalities (e.g., brief psychotherapy, social skills training, women's issues group therapy, or women's support group). *These modalities can serve as additional resources for helping the patient learn new skills in establishing and maintaining constructive interpersonal relationships.*

Develop more healthful physical life-style as evidenced by the following:

Participates in planning to make life-style changes to enhance physical health and well-being

Assess patient's current physical health status.

Teach patient to recognize relationship between physical health and positive feelings about self.

Assist patient in identifying ways to promote health and well-being.

Reinforce health-promoting practices such as
exercise, relaxation, and diversional activity.

REFERENCES

Antonucci TC, Peggs JF, Marquez JT: The relationship between self-esteem and physical health in a family practice population, *Family Pract Res J* 9(1):65, 1989.

Bonheur B, Yong SW: Exercise as a health-promoting lifestyle choice, *Appl Nurs Res* 4(1):2, 1991.

Crouch MA, Straub V: Enhancement of self-esteem in adults, *Fam Community Health* 6(2):65, 1983.

Decarlo JJ, Mann WC: The effectiveness of verbal versus activity groups in improving self-perceptions of interpersonal communication skills, *Am J Occup Ther* 39(1):20, 1985.

Kinney CK, Mannetter R, Carpenter MA: Support groups. In Bulechek GM, McCloskey JC: *Nursing interventions: essential nursing treatments*, ed 2, Philadelphia, 1992, WB Saunders.

Norris J: Nursing intervention for self-esteem disturbances, *Nursing Diagnosis*, 3(2):48, 1992.

Prehn RA, Thomas P: Does it make a difference? The effect of a women's issues group on female psychiatric inpatients. *J Psychosoc Nurs Ment Health Serv*, 28(11):34, 1990.

Stanwyck DJ: Self-esteem through the life span, *Fam Community Health* 6(2):11, 1983.

Self-esteem, situational low

CLINICAL CONDITION/ MEDICAL DIAGNOSIS	RELATED FACTORS
Adjustment disorder with work inhibition (Female administrator in complex health care organization that is undergoing restructuring)	Organizational instability; impending job loss

---

Patient goals
Expected outcomes
    Associated nursing/collaborative interventions *and scientific rationale*

Regain former realistic positive self-esteem as evidenced by the following:

Increases confidence in handling job situation

Encourage identification and description of changes in feelings about self.

Assist patient in clearly describing previous state of positive self-evaluation.

Assess patient's perception of the current situation, availability of supportive resources, and current coping strategies *to obtain information about patient's educations, counseling, support, and referral needs.*

Explore with patient current employment environment in organization (e.g., degree of organizational instability, level of interpersonal conflict, extent of personal involvement, impending threat to current job).

Help patient to assess realistic options for self within current organization and other potential employment opportunities, short-term and long-term, *to assist patient in identifying and mobilizing own resources and strengths.*

Engage patient in problem solving (e.g., assess realities of situation, examine personal assets and strengths, identify incremental goals, develop action plan to meet goals). *These actions promote awareness of positive relationship between self-esteem and effective problem solving.*

Increases ability to problem solve, set goals, and take action

Help patient to explore community groups and resources that could help with problem solving and decision making about transitions.

Offer patient reading materials that might assist in problem solving.

Teach conflict-resolution skills.

Teach patient constructive defenses against attacks from others *to help patient regain sense of competency and control.*

Assist patient to identify available resources for exploring job opportunities.

Increases understanding of situational factors and self-behaviors that have an impact on current situation

Assist patient in describing current level of on-the-job performance; perceptions of feeling valued, needed, or important in relation to the overall organization; and impact of current situation on other aspects of daily living.

Help patient identify previous problem-solving strategies and strengths, limitations, and potentials.

Offer hope that situation can be handled, by describing others who have overcome similar job instabilities.

Suggest that patient keep journal *to assist in problem solving and obtaining feedback.*

Support patient's decision-making efforts. *These actions create a supportive reality-based environment for effective problem solving and feedback.*

Maintain physical health as evidenced by the following:

Improves balance between physical and mental health states

Assess patient's current physical health status.

Teach patient awareness of potential harmful effects of negative self-talk.

Teach patient about relationship between physical health and positive feelings about self *to promote awareness of positive relationship between self-esteem and physical health.*

Assist patient in identifying ways to promote health and well-being.

Reinforce health-promoting practices, such as exercise program, use of relaxation techniques, and diversional activity. *These types of activities serve to reduce anxiety, and they facilitate exploration of constructive problem solving.*

REFERENCES

Antonucci TC, Peggs JF, Marquez JT: The relationship between self-esteem and physical health in a family practice population, *Family Pract Res J* 9(1):65, 1989.

Bonheur B, Young SW: Exercise as a health-promoting lifestyle choice, *Appl Nurs Res* 4(1):2, 1991.

Crouch MA, Straub V: Enhancement of self-esteem in adults, *Fam Community Health* 6(2):65, 1983.

DeCarlo JJ, Mann WC: The effectiveness of verbal versus activity groups in improving self-perceptions of interpersonal communication skills, *Am J Occup Ther* 39(1):20, 1985.

Gilberts R: The evaluation of self-esteem, *Fam Community Health* 6(2):29, 1983.

Hagerty BM and others: Sense of belonging: a vital mental health concept, *Arch Psychiatric Nurs* 6(3):172, 1992.

LeMone P: Analysis of a human phenomenon: self-concept, *Nurs Diagnosis* 2(3):126, 1991.

Norris, J: Nursing intervention for self-esteem disturbances, *Nurs Diagnosis* 3(2):48, 1992.

Self-esteem, situational low—cont'd

Self-mutilation, risk for

CLINICAL CONDITION/ MEDICAL DIAGNOSIS	RELATED FACTORS
Borderline personality	Psychosis; history of physical, emotional, or sexual abuse

> **Patient goals**
> Expected outcomes
>   Associated nursing/collaborative interventions *and scientific rationale*

Experience fewer episodes of self-mutilation as evidenced by the following:

Identifies and manages anxiety
Develop trusting relationship with patient.

Assist patient in recognition of anxiety and situations in which he/she becomes anxious. *This step is necessary before plans for reducing anxiety can be developed.*

Explore with patient approaches to reduce anxiety (e.g., music, physical activity).

Constructively uses resources to deal with stressors
Create nonthreatening environment *because an increase in stressors can lead to self-mutilation.*

Assist patient to identify perceived stressors.

Explore with patient past successes in reducing stress *to capitalize use of patient's strengths.*

Collaborate with patient to develop a plan to cope with stressors.

Have patient demonstrate use of stress-reduction techniques.

Demonstrate self-differentiation
Engage patient in values clarification, self-appraisal, and identification of ideal self *to develop clearer sense of self-identity.*

Provide opportunities in which patient can maximize use of his/her strengths *to enhance self-esteem.*

Offer unconditional positive regard when interacting with patient *to enhance feelings of self-esteem.*

Displays positive family interactions.

Determine to what extent the patient's self-perception is affected by his/her dysfunctional family.

Discuss alternative strategies with patient to enhance family interaction (e.g., family therapy) *so as to decrease any stress or threat to self.*

REFERENCES

Favazza A: Why patients mutilate themselves, *Hosp Community Psychiatry* 40(20):137, 1989.

Feldman M: The challenge of self-mutilation: a review, *Compr Psychiatry* 29(2):252, 1988.

Kernberg O: The borderline self-mutilant: a psychodynamic approach, *J Pers Dis* 1:344, 1987.

Rosen PM, Walsh BW, Rode SA: Interpersonal loss and self-mutilation, *Suicide Life Threat Behav* 20:177, 1990.

Rosen S, Collins KJ: Six case studies depicting the deliberate self-harm syndrome, *Curationis* (South Africa) 16(1):50, 1993.

Sebree R, Popkess-Vawter S: Self-injury concept formation: nursing diagnosis development, *Persp Psych Care* 27(2):27, 1991.

Valente S: Deliberate self-injury: management in a psychiatric setting, *J Psychosoc Nsg* 29(12):19, 1991.

Self-mutilation, risk for—cont'd

Sensory/perceptual alteration (auditory)

CLINICAL CONDITION/ MEDICAL DIAGNOSIS	RELATED FACTORS
Schizophrenia disorder, undifferentiated type	Traumatic emotional event; poor symptom management skills

---

Patient goals
Expected outcomes
    Associated nursing/collaborative interventions *and scientific rationale*

Experience reduction in hallucinations and/or distress they cause as evidenced by the following:

Recognizes auditory hallucinations as part of disease of schizophrenia, and that they can be managed

Use empathy and listening in the relationship with patient. *Schizophrenic patients are sensitive to the clinical relationship, which can produce feelings of safety and understanding, or helplessness and being controlled.*

Assist in developing a frame of reference for understanding the voices and the role of increased stress.

Discuss type of relationships that are particular sources of stress.

Identifies actions to be taken which are specific and meaningful to self

Monitor use of denial as way to deal with anxiety. *Frequently daily life events are overestimated or negatively perceived, increasing helplessness and contributing to relapse.*

Teach to recognize early signs of relapse in self, i.e., rejecting or alienating others, forgetting to take medicine, not keeping appointments.

Develop cognitive and behavioral coping strategies to deal with traumatic emotional event as evidenced by the following:

Reports fewer hallucinations and/or feelings of distress as he/she goes about daily routines

Teach strategies to deal with traumatic emotional event, such as appraising correctly daily life events or one's coping abilities.

Teach strategies to deal with social contexts in which hallucinations are experienced.

Demonstrates ways to handle hallucinations and to share with others

Teach use of diversional activities, e.g., self-talk, tapes, enjoyable events.

Provide opportunity to exchange experiences with others.

REFERENCES

Corrigan PW, Storzbach DM: Behavioral interventions for alleviating psychotic symptoms, *Hosp Community Psychiat* 44(8):341, 1993.

Eckman TA, Wirshing WC, Marder SR: Technique for training schizophrenic patients in illness self management: a controlled trial, *Am J Psychiatry* 149(11):1549, 1992.

Harmon RB, Tractnack SA: Teaching hospitalized patients with serious, persistent mental illness, *J Psychosoc Nurs Ment Health Serv* 30(7):33, 1992.

Kavanagh DJ: Schizophrenia. In Wilson PH, ed: *Principles and practice of relapse prevention*, New York, 1992, Guilford Press.

Liberman RP, ed: *Handbook of psychiatric rehabilitation*, New York, 1992, Macmillan.

Liberman RP, Corrigan PW: Designing new psychosocial treatments for schizophrenia, *Psychiatry* 56(3):238, 1993.

Mills PD, Hansen JC: Short-term group interventions for mentally ill young adults living in a community residence and their families, *Hosp Community Psychiat* 42(11):1144, 1991.

Mueser KT: Schizophrenia. In Bellack AS, Hersen M, eds: *Handbook of behavior therapy in psychiatric settings* New York, 1993, Plenum Press.

UCLA Social and Independent Living Skills Series 1990. Available from Dissemination Coordinator, Camarillo UCLA Research Center, P.O. Box 6022, Camarillo CA, 93011-6022.

Wasylinki DA: Psychotherapy of schizophrenia revisited, *Hosp Community Psychiat* 43(2):123, 1992.

Sensory/perceptual alteration (auditory)—cont'd

Sexual dysfunction

CLINICAL CONDITION/ MEDICAL DIAGNOSIS	RELATED FACTORS
Generalized anxiety disorder	Misinformation or inadequate knowledge
	Conflicting values

> **Patient goals**
> Expected outcomes
>   Associated nursing/collaborative interventions *and scientific rationale*

Verbalize increased knowledge about sexual concerns as evidenced by the following:

Identifies personal sexual concerns

Assist patient in identifying possible factors that may contribute to sexual dysfunction. *Medications, alcohol or drug abuse, or clinical conditions can effect sexual functioning.*

Encourage patient to describe current sexual interactions and behavior patterns (e.g., compatibility with sexual partner; comfort with sexual interactions or frequency of sexual interactions). *Patients need reassurance from authoritative source that it is permissible to think, read, talk, and fantasize about sex.*

Provide privacy when discussing sexual matters. Provide climate in which patient can openly discuss concerns. Use nonjudgmental attitude. *Comfort factors show respect to client and promote expression of feeling.*

Acknowledge patient's feelings of anxiety about discussing sexual concerns *to establish rapport and create an internal state of trust for patient*

Verbalizes knowledge about human sexuality

Explore patient's knowledge deficit about sexuality (e.g., how did patient learn about sexuality? What is patient's understanding about normal sexual functions?)

Dispel any myths or misinformation patient may have about sexual activities (e.g., that masturbating will make you crazy). *Patients need to have myths dispelled and be provided with accurate information about sexual functioning.*)

Use terminology that patient understands (e.g., does patient know what the words coitus and sexual intercourse mean?)

Clarify with patient any uncertainties about terminology being used (slang or street terminology can have a variety of meanings). *Because the same words may have different meaning for different people, the nurse must be constantly prepared to define or clarify the meaning of a word or phrase.*

Identify and discuss personal sexual beliefs and values as evidenced by the following:

Selects socially acceptable behaviors consistent with personal beliefs and values

Explore with patient beliefs and values regarding sexuality, without placing your own personal beliefs or values on the patient (e.g., how do factors, such as patient's early childhood beliefs, religious beliefs, and perceptions of parental attitudes toward sex affect present beliefs and values?)

Offer suggestions to patient about alternative sexual behaviors or outlets within own scope of knowledge and level of comfort.

Allow patient the opportunity to discuss suggestions. *Make facts available whenever patient needs or asks for them; this builds trust, orients, enables decision making, and decreases anxiety, frustration, or other distressing feelings that hinder realistic action, thereby helping the patient focus on deeper concerns.*

Listen to what the patient has to say without jumping to conclusions or interpreting behavior prematurely. Provide specific facts that address expressed needs. *Careful listening conveys respect and promotes self-esteem and a sense of security and safety.*

Attend closely to verbal and nonverbal signals suggesting anxiety or indications that a problem is more extensive than originally presented. *Nonverbal behavior often conveys more directly the feelings and is often the key to the message.*

Assist the patient in describing behavior rather than labeling (e.g., "I have difficulty becoming sexually aroused" instead of "I am frigid"). Help the patient determine whether behavior is helpful or useful in reaching goals, instead of labeling behavior as good or bad. *Patients need help in arriving at their own answers and determining what is right or wrong; do not judge for the patient what is right or wrong, normal or abnormal. Patients must decide what is normal for themselves.*

Teach patient assertive communication skills so that patient can say "no" or not do something. *Assertiveness training provides the patient with the behavioral repertoire needed to interact successfully with others.*

Encourage communications between partners. Recommend a self-help program or refer to individual or group counseling, as appropriate.

REFERENCES

Annon JS: The PLISSIT model: a proposed conceptual scheme for the behavioral treatment of sexual problems, *Journal of Sex Education Therapy* 2(1):1, 1976.

Dickman GL, Livingston CA: Sex Therapy. In McFarland GK, Thomas MD: *Psychiatric Mental Health Nursing, Application of Nursing Process*, Philadelphia, 1991, J.B. Lippincott.

Driscoll CE, Arnold J, Jones JG, Phillips DM: Common sexual problems in family practice, *Medical Aspects of Human Sexuality* February:51, 1991.

Gender AR: An overview of the nurse's role in dealing with sexuality, *Sexuality and Disability* 10(2):71, 1992.

Matocha LR, Waterhouse JK: Current practice related to sexuality, *Res Nursing Health* 16.371, 1993.

Otman US: Psychosocial and sexual implications of genitourinary cancers, *Seminars in Oncology Nursing* 9(4):286, 1993.

Ridley PJ: Kautman's theory of shame and identity in treating childhood sexual abuse, *J Psychosocial Nurs* 31(6):13, 1993.

Tepper MS: Sexual Education in spinal cord injury rehabilitation: current trends and recommendations, *Sexuality and Disability* 10(1):15, 1992.

Sexual dysfunction—cont'd

Sexuality patterns, altered

CLINICAL CONDITION/ MEDICAL DIAGNOSIS	RELATED FACTORS
Myocardial infarction (MI)	Knowledge deficit

Patient goals
Expected outcomes
  Associated nursing/collaborative interventions *and scientific rationale*

Attain satisfying level of sexual activity compatible with functional capacity as evidenced by the following:

Verbalizes knowledge related to the resumption of sexual activity

Provide specific information to patient and partner about limitations; correct myths and misinformation; address issues with sensitivity to customs and cultural issues. *Patients who receive education and counseling report improved sexual satisfaction and performance because of decreased anxiety.*

Use information about premorbid sexual activity obtained through sexual history as basis for teaching and counseling; assess for long-standing sexual dysfunction, which can be caused by a psychogenic problem. *Assessment of patterns of sexual activity provides basis for individualized counseling and can help identify previous patterns that caused physiologic and psychologic stress.*

Examine concerns about sexuality and adequacy of sexual function. *Issues that may influence resumption of sexual activity are: fear of sudden death or precipitation of symptoms such as angina, dyspnea, and palpitations; perceived change in body image; depression, which can affect ability to invest*

Sexuality patterns, altered

emotionally and be a factor in sexual dysfunction; forced dependency; changes in feelings of self-worth; and attractiveness to sexual partner.

Assess level of comfort in discussing topic alone or with partner; provide opportunity for both. *Individual counseling allows discussion of issues that may cause discomfort if discussed with partner present (e.g., concerns about extramarital sexual relationships or concerns about coital death).*

Address stress, fears, and sexual concerns of partner and examine relationship with sexual partner. *Partner should be included in the counseling process; if not he/she may become overprotective and seek to limit those activities that are seen as potentially harmful to patient.*

Teach patient about possible side effects of drugs such as digitalis, hypnotics, tranquilizers, and diuretics. *Commonly prescribed medications may affect libido and cause inorgasmia and/or erectile problems.*

Assess physical status that indicates when sexual activity can be resumed: patient's general health, tolerance for physical activity before MI, extent of myocardial damage, frequency and severity of angina or arrhythmias, and patient's ability to tolerate progression of activity. *Base advice to patient on consultation with physician. Depending on individual case, patient may resume sexual intercourse 3 to 6 weeks after MI.*

Evaluate physical status with low-level treadmill test, portable ECG recording made during moderate exercise, or by two flight stair-climbing test followed by resting ECG recording before discharge. *The O_2 demand of intercourse is in the 4 to 5 MET (metabolic equivalent) range. The ability to exercise at 5 or 6 METs and attain a heart rate of 115 to 120 beats per minute without such symptoms as ischemic changes or significant arrhythmias signifies that resumption of sexual activity will be safe.*

Sexuality patterns, altered—cont'd

Resumes sexual activity at or near premorbid level

Assist patient in developing individualized plan of progressive physical and sexual activity based on physiologic limitations. *Sexual activity should be resumed gradually. Similar to any physical activity, sexual intercourse places increased demands on the cardiovascular system.*

Instruct about potential for angina during sexual intercourse and how to respond (if angina is experienced, stop intercourse and take nitroglycerine; may resume after relief is obtained). *If couple is advised that angina may occur and they know what to do, they may be better able to cope if they do encounter this problem. Additional medication may be needed to prevent angina.*

Advise patient to avoid sexual activity for 2 or more hours after eating. *Angina may occur because of increased blood flow to GI organs and increase demands caused by sexual activity. This results in decreased blood flow to myocardium.*

Advise patient to avoid sexual activity after excessive alcohol intake. *Alcohol causes decreased cardiac output, which may decrease the amount of exercise that can be performed without provoking angina.*

Teach patient warning signs that must be reported to physician: rapid pulse or respiratory rate that persists 4 to 5 minutes after orgasm, feeling of extreme fatigue after sexual activity, anginal symptoms during or after sexual activity. *Potentially significant dysrhythmias and arrhythmias can be precipitated by sexual activity. Cardiovascular symptoms that occur during sexual activity may require further evaluation, use of medication, and physical conditioning, which would allow the patient to exercise in greater comfort.*

REFERENCES

Fridlund B, Hogstedt B, Lidell E, and Larsson PA: Recovery after myocardial infarction: effects of a caring rehabilitation programme, *Scandinavian Journal of Caring Sciences* 5(1), 1991.

Sexuality patterns, altered—cont'd

Glick DF: Home care of patients with cardiac disease. In Kinney MR, Pack DR, Andreoli KG, Zipes DP: *Comprehensive cardiac care*, St. Louis, 1991, Mosby.

Hamilton GA: The importance of systematic inquiry in nursing research: an example; women and recovery from acute myocardial infarction, *Vard I Norden—Nursing Science and Research in the Nordic Countries* 11(2), 1991.

Hamilton GA, Seidman RN: A comparison of the recovery period for women and men after an acute myocardial infarction, *Heart and Lung* 22(4): 1993.

Jones C: Sexual activity after myocardial infarction, *Nursing Standard* 6(48): 1992.

Low KG: Recovery from myocardial infarction and coronary artery bypass surgery in women: psychosocial factors, *Journal of Women's Health* 2(2), 1993.

Miller NH: Cardiac rehabilitation. In Kinney MR, Pack DR, Andreoli KG, and Zipes DP: *Comprehensive cardiac care*, St. Louis, 1991, Mosby.

Piper KM: When can I do "it" again nurse? Sexual counseling after a heart attack, *Professional Nurse* 8(3), 1992.

Seidl A, Bullough B, Haughey B, Scherer Y, Rhodes M, and Brown G: Understanding the effects of a myocardial infarction on sexual functioning: a basis for sexual counseling, *Rehabilitation Nursing* 16(5), 1991.

Skin integrity, impaired

CLINICAL CONDITION/ MEDICAL DIAGNOSIS	RELATED FACTORS
Pressure ulcer	Physical immobilization
	Altered circulation

Patient goals
Expected outcomes
    Associated nursing/collaborative interventions *and scientific rationale*

Manifest intact skin in area of disruption as evidenced by the following:

Skin lesion clean and healing

Perform assessment of wound (Stage 1-4) and surrounding skin as a baseline and document daily or when dressing is changed.

Provide wound treatment based on stage and drainage, using gauze, polyurethane film, hydrocolloid, foam, absorptive dressing, hydrogel.

Debride and clean wound as ordered.

Ambulate patient if possible.

When patient is in bed, turn every 1-2 hours; use all four sides (lateral, prone, dorsal) unless contraindicated.

Position patient off pressure ulcer.

Use a pressure-relieving therapy bed.

Keep pressure off skeletal prominences by positioning patient with pillow and/or foam devices.

Do not position directly on trochanter *because higher interface pressures and lower transcutaneous O_2 tension occurs.*

Use lifting devices and/or sheets to position patients.

Do not drag patient *because dragging causes shear.*

Use static devices (filled with foam or water, air, or gel) as necessary.

Do not massage skin; *rubbing may cause additional trauma.*

Prevent head of bed elevation of more than 30 degrees for long periods *because shearing forces are generated on sacrum, causing mechanical stress.*

Use underpads or briefs that absorb moisture and leave a quick-drying surface toward the skin if skin is continuously moist (incontinence, perspiration, drainage). *Excessive moisture reduces the resistance of skin to ulceration and increases risk of pressure sore formation fivefold.*

Avoid use of doughnuts and rubber rings *because these increase pressure and damage tissue.*

Have patient do active ROM or do passive ROM for patient every 2 hours *to promote circulation to skin and to alter weight-bearing.*

Elevate legs to prevent edema. *Edema slows oxygen diffusion and metabolic transport from capillary to cell.*

Teach patient to change position if possible.

Provide the following:
- Increased calories and protein *because tissues are more vulnerable to necrosis with smaller amounts of pressure if the diet is deficient in these.*
- Increased fluid intake to prevent dehydration (2600 ml/day if possible).
- Supplement iron and vitamin C as needed. *Vitamin C is important for wound healing, fosters collagen synthesis and capillary function; iron improves oxygen carrying capacity of blood.*

Monitor laboratory values that have an impact on skin and report abnormalities: HCT/Hbg *because low levels compromise oxygen delivery to tissues;* BUN *because elevated levels may indicate renal disease, which may affect albumin;* albumin *because low amounts cause interstitial edema, which impedes exchange of nutrients and waste products;* bilirubin *because levels may indicate liver disease, which may affect albumin;* arterial blood gases *because it indicates oxygen available for tissues.*

Patient/significant other demonstrates proper skin care

Teach patient/significant other above
   interventions.
Teach to call physician regarding signs and
   symptoms of infection or worsening of ulcer.

REFERENCES

Barnes S: Patient/family education for the patient with pressure
   necrosis, *Nurs Clin North Am*, 22(2):463, 1987.
Robel L: Nutritional implications in the patient with pressure sores,
   Nurs Clin North Am, 22(2):379, 1987.
Gosnell D: Assessment and evaluation of pressure sores, *Nurs Clin
   North Am,* 22(2):399, 1987.
How to predict and prevent pressure ulcers, *AJN*, 92(7):52, 1992.
Maklebust J: Pressure ulcer update, *RN*, 54(12):56, 1991.
Quick Reference Guide for Clinicians Agency for health Care Policy &
   Research: Pressure ulcers in adults: prediction and prevention,
   Decubitus, 5(3):26, 1992.
Yen PK: Eat right to avoid pressure ulcers, *Geriatric Nursing*, 11(5):255,
   1990.

Skin integrity, impaired, risk for

CLINICAL CONDITION/ MEDICAL DIAGNOSIS	RISK FACTORS
Acute CVA	Prolonged bedrest

Patient goals
Expected outcomes
Associated nursing/collaborative interventions *and scientific rationale*

Maintain intact skin tissue as evidenced by the following:

No reddened areas, no broken skin

Assess patient for the following risk factors or use a risk assessment scale: incontinence, immobility, inactivity, poor nutrition, edema, diminished sensation, decreased mental status.

Inspect skin for redness, cyanosis, blistering, temperature, and pulses daily.

Keep skin clean and dry after washing.

Prevent extremes in environmental temperature and humidity.

Lubricate dry skin *because dry skin results in reduced pliability, fissuring, and cracking.*

Keep pressure off skeletal prominences by positioning patient with pillows or foam devices.

Ambulate patient if possible.

Use all four sides (lateral, prone, dorsal) unless contraindicated. When patient is in bed, turn every 1-2 hours.

Do not position directly on trochanter *because higher interface pressures and lower transcutaneous O_2 tension occurs.*

Do not drag patient; *dragging causes shear.* Use lifting devices/sheets to position patient.

Teach patient to change position if possible.

Use static devices (filled with foam or water, air or gel) as necessary.

Do not massage skin; *rubbing may cause additional trauma.*

Prevent head of bed elevation of more than 30 degrees for long periods. *Shearing forces are generated on sacrum, causing mechanical stress.*

Use underpads or briefs that absorb moisture and leave a quick-drying surface toward the skin if skin is continuously moist (incontinence, perspiration, drainage). *Excessive moisture reduces the resistance of skin to ulceration and increases risk of pressure sore formation fivefold.*

Avoid use of doughnuts and rubber rings *because these increase pressure and damage tissue.*

Provide adequate nutrition, including the following: sufficient calories and protein because *tissues are more vulnerable to necrosis with small amounts of pressure if the diet is deficient in calories and protein;* fluid intake adequate to prevent dehydration (2600 ml/day if possible).

Have patient do active ROM or do passive ROM for patient every 2 hours in order *to promote circulation to skin and to alter weight-bearing.*

Elevate legs to prevent edema. *Edema slows oxygen diffusion and metabolic transport from capillary to cell.*

Monitor blood chemistry levels that have an impact on skin and report abnormalities when present: Hct/Hbg *because low levels compromise oxygen delivery to the tissue;* BUN *because elevated levels may indicate renal disease, which may affect albumin;* albumin *because low amounts cause interstitial edema, which impedes exchange of nutrients and waste products;* bilirubin *because elevated levels may indicate liver disease, which may affect albumin;* arterial blood gases *because of indication of oxygen available for tissues.*

Returns demonstration of proper skin care.

Teach patient/significant other above interventions.

Teach to call physician if symptoms worsen.

Skin integrity, impaired, risk for—cont'd

REFERENCES

Barnes S: Patient/family education for the patient with pressure necrosis, *Nurs Clin North Am*, 22(2):463, 1987.

Bergstrom N, et al: The Braden scale for predicting pressure sore risk, *Nurs Res*, 36(4):205, 1987.

Bobel L: Nutritional implications in the patient with pressure sores, *Nurs Clin North Am*, 22(2):379, 1987.

How to predict and prevent pressure ulcers, *AJN*, 92(7):52, 1992.

Maklebust J: Pressure ulcers: etiology and prevention, *Nurs Clin North Am*, 22(2):359, 1987.

Pressure ulcers in adults: prediction and prevention, *Decubitus*, 5(3):26, 1992.

Yen PK: Eat right to avoid pressure ulcers, *Geriatric Nurs*, 11(5):255, 1990.

Skin integrity, impaired, risk for—cont'd

Sleep pattern disturbance

CLINICAL CONDITION/ MEDICAL DIAGNOSIS	RELATED FACTORS
Major medical illness	Disruptions in life-style or usual sleep habits

---

Patient goals
Expected outcomes
Associated nursing/collaborative interventions *and scientific rationale*

Understand factors contributing to sleep pattern disturbances as evidenced by the following:

Participates in determining potential or actual causes for inadequate sleep

Compare patient's current sleep pattern with usual sleep habits before hospitalization or current episode of sleep disturbance.

Monitor and discuss possible causes for disturbed sleep (e.g., patient's worries, concerns, pain).

Encourage expression of concerns if and when patient is unable to sleep.

Confer with family or significant others about potential causes of sleep disturbance.

Evaluate effects of patient's medications (e.g., steroids, diuretics) that may interfere with sleep. *Emotional problems may occur when corticosteroids are used, including mood swings, insomnia, etc.*

Observe and monitor patient's daytime habits and activities.

Verbalizes understanding of specific plan to manage or correct causes of inadequate sleep

Plan daytime activities to assure adequate physical and mental activity.

Discourage daytime napping only if daytime naps negatively affect nighttime sleep. *Unsynchronized circadian sleep-wake cycles result from short naps dispersed over a 24-hour period.*

Monitor patient to avoid excessive time in bed (if medically appropriate).

Sleep pattern disturbance

Sleep through the night or at least for increased lengths of uninterrupted periods as evidenced by the following:

Falls asleep within 30 minutes of going to bed

Determine patient's usual nighttime habits and provide for routine as closely as possible (e.g., provide warm milk if allowed on medical regimen and if no nighttime voiding problem exists). Explain reasons for any necessary modifications in usual routine. *Changing a person's usual pattern of food intake in the evening has been found to impair subsequent sleep.*

Decrease fluid intake before bedtime (if wakening for frequent voiding occurs).

Have patient empty bladder at bedtime.

Avoid caffeine for 4 hours before sleep (if fluids are needed, substitute decaffeinated drinks).

Promote relaxation at bedtime: select interventions approved by the patient (e.g., provide soft music, back massage, security objects; suggest guided imagery techniques; teach muscle-relaxation techniques).

Provide patient with comfortable environment to promote sleep or rest (e.g., turn off lights; provide adequate room ventilation; provide warmth or coolness as needed; avoid noise disturbances). *Cortical inhibition on reticular formation is eliminated during sleep, enhancing autonomic responses; thus, cardiovascular responses to noise are greater during sleep.*

Avoid strenuous physical or mental activity just before bedtime.

Minimal number of essential interruptions occur

Sleeps during longer intervals between nursing care functions

Verbalizes feeling of being rested or refreshed after nighttime sleeping

Schedule assessments or interventions to allow for longer sleep periods (e.g., check vital signs and turn patient at same time). *Sleep deprivation occurs with frequent interruption of sleep and may*

Sleep pattern disturbance—cont'd

413

impair recovery because of psychologic and physiologic disturbances. Patient's own circadian rhythm is disturbed by interruptions.

Explain to patient the need for essential interruptions.

Help patient to maintain a normal day/night pattern to facilitate night sleeping.

Provide sedation as prescribed, if necessary, temporarily.

Determine effectiveness of sedative prescribed (i.e., optimal dosage, no rebound effects).

Monitor level of daytime alertness and daytime functioning.

REFERENCES

Becker PM, Jamieson AO: Common sleep disorders in the elderly: diagnosis and treatment, *Geriatrics* 47(3):41-48, 1992.

Edwards GB, Schuring LM: Pilot study: validating nurses' observations of sleep and wake states among critically ill patients, using polysomnography, *Am J Crit Care* 2(2):125-131, 1993.

Jensen DP, Herr KA: Sleeplessness, *Advances in Clinical Nursing Research* 28(2):385-403, 1993.

Johnson JE: A comparative study of the bedtime routines and sleep of older adults, *J Community Health Nurs* 8(3):129-136, 1991.

Johnson JE: Progressive relaxation and the sleep of older women, *Appl Nurs Res* 4(4):165-170, 1991.

Spenceley SM: Sleeping inquiry: A look with fresh eyes, *Image* 25(3):249-256, 1993.

Topf M: Effects of personal control over hospital noise on sleep, *Res Nurs Health* 15:19-28, 1992.

Sleep pattern disturbance—cont'd

Social interaction, impaired

CLINICAL CONDITION/ MEDICAL DIAGNOSIS	RELATED FACTORS
Chronic undifferentiated schizophrenia	Knowledge/skill deficit about enhancing mutuality
	Absence of available significant other

Patient goals
Expected outcomes
    Associated nursing/collaborative interventions *and*
      scientific rationale

Improve social competence in interpersonal interactions and enhance social network as evidenced by the following:

Identifies strengths and limitations in current patterns of social interaction

    Assess with the patient the strengths and limitations of current social interaction style.

    Observe and assist the patient to identify nonverbal behaviors of which he/she may not be aware.

    Review the patient patterns of relating with family/peers.

    Encourage the patient to express feelings and perceptions of social skills. *Self-perceptions can be altered to promote adaptive changes and growth.*

    Explore with the patient feelings that cause discomfort in social situations.

    Help patient to identify situations in which others are alienated because of patient's behavior.

Utilizes enhanced social skills in both familiar and new interpersonal situations in order to enhance mutuality

    Provide opportunities for meaningful task performance within the milieu.

    Facilitate conversation between patient and peers or significant others to enhance mutuality.

    Help patient to identify others with whom he/she feels comfortable and encourage interactions and activities with them.

Social interaction, impaired

Provide feedback about observed interactions; consider use of videotaping to review learning.

Structure milieu to provide opportunities for socialization (small areas for reading, games, refreshments).

Use social skill training to assist patient to identify strategies and role play more effective behavior, obtain social reinforcement, and practice the behavior in a real situation.

Modeling, structuring and providing feedback promote learning and awareness of positive actions and problem areas.

Increase interactions with others as evidenced by the following:

Resumes or adds to socialization, activities with expressed satisfaction in interpersonal relationships

Encourage visits and involvement of family or significant others.

Use creative activities to provide opportunities for self-expression and demonstration of talent, as well as group interaction.

Help patient identify opportunities for increased social interaction.

Encourage attendance at activities, resumption of hobbies or involvement in affiliative groups or volunteer work to expand social networks.

Provide positive reinforcement for demonstration of more effective social skills.

These actions provide increased opportunity for positive social reinforcement and repetition of successful social behaviors.

REFERENCES

Liberman RP, DeRisi WJ, Mueser KT: *Social skills training for psychiatric patients*, New York, 1989, Pergamon Press.

Manderino M, Bzdek V: Social skill building with chronic patients, *J. Psychosoc Nurs Ment Health Serv* 25(9):18, 1987.

McFarland GK, McFarlane EA: *Nursing diagnosis and intervention*, ed. 2, St. Louis, 1993, Mosby.

Mertzanakis C: Improving social skills, *Nursing Times* 86(44):44, 1990.

Reed PG: Self-transcendence and mental health in oldest-old adults, *Nurs Res* 40(1):5, 1991.

Topf M, Dambacher B: Teaching interpersonal skills: a model for facilitating optimal interpersonal relations, *J. Psychosoc Nurs* 19:29, 1981.

Watkins AJ, Kligman EW: Attendance patterns of older adults in a health promotion program, *Public Health Reports*, 108(1):86, 1993.

Social isolation

CLINICAL CONDITION/ MEDICAL DIAGNOSIS	RELATED FACTORS
Third degree burns Facial disfigurement	Loss of significant relationship and of work role Inability to engage in or sustain satisfying relationships

> **Patient goals**
> Expected outcomes
> > Associated nursing/collaborative interventions *and scientific rationale*

Develop a trusting relationship as evidenced by the following:

Expresses feelings of aloneness, absence of supportive significant others, and feelings of rejection

Facilitate and explore expressions of feelings.

Explore dynamics of past relationships: process and outcome.

Engage in active listening.

Alert patient to negative self-talk and discuss inaccuracies of perception.

Assess social skills through varied behavioral observation. Incorporate findings into personalized strategies for successful socialization.

Assess situational and chronic low self-esteem. Assess need for referral.

Help patient to recognize bodily reactions to cognitions. *Awareness is a first step in gaining control over thoughts, feelings, and behaviors.*

Reduce degree of social isolation as evidenced by the following:

Regularly participates in a pertinent, therapeutic group meeting

Invites at least one person to visit home at regular intervals

Selects and participates in at least one leisure group activity every 2 weeks

Structure with patient a self-modification program using self-selected strategies.

Provide information about available pertinent groups (e.g., social skills training, cognitive reappraisal, social support).

Provide positive reinforcement for even the slightest movement toward involvement with others.

Develop one or two meaningful relationships as evidenced by the following:

Identifies one or two individuals who are important and why they are important

Interacts with these individuals regularly, e.g., one phone call per week.

Identify barriers to forming meaningful relationships.

Discuss relationship of personal responsiblity and social isolation.

Discuss and analyze at each visit positive and negative aspects of interpersonal interactions that occurred in previous week.

Discuss reality and risks and benefits of opening oneself to others.

Develop interest in volunteering to assist someone or an organization as evidenced by the following:

Makes at least one phone call per week for 3 weeks, inquiring about volunteer service

Discuss satisfaction that can be experienced through helping others.

Provide patient with information about volunteer possibilities in immediate vicinity. *Engaging in volunteer activities provides recognition and allows patient to experience satisfying personal relationships.*

Contract with patient for at least one phone call to a volunteer service per week. Elicit feelings about the phone call at next session.

Expand and engage in new interest as evidenced by the following:

Engages in one satisfying leisure activity appropriate to developmental stage with another individual(s) on a regularly planned basis.

Negotiate with patient to complete a leisure assessment.

Discuss findings of leisure assessment; elicit feelings regarding assessment and finding.

Explore with patient obstacles to involvement in one leisure activity identified as interesting.

Help patient to engage in strategies to overcome obstacles.

REFERENCES

Elsen J, Blegen M: Social isolation. In Maas M, Buckwalter KC, Hardy M, eds: *Nursing diagnoses and interventions for the elderly*, Philadelphia, 1991, WB Saunders.

Kinney CK, Mannettu R, Carpenter MA: Support groups. In Bulechek GM, McCloskey JC, eds: *Nursing interventions: essential nursing treatments*, ed 2, Philadelphia, 1992, WB Saunders.

Lien-Greschen: Validation of social isolation related to maturational age: elderly, *Nursing Diagnosis*, 4(1)37, 1993.

Norris J: Nursing intervention for self-esteem disturbances, *Nursing Diagnosis* 3(2)48, 1993.

Pender NJ: Self-modification. In Bulechek GM, McCloskey J, eds: *Nursing interventions: treatment for nursing diagnoses*, Philadelphia, 1985, WB Saunders.

Russel D: The measurement of loneliness. In Peplau LA, Perlman D, eds: *Loneliness*, New York, 1982, John Wiley & Sons.

Scandrett-Hibdon S: Cognitive reappraisal. In Bulecheck GM, McCloskey JC, eds: *Nursing interventions: essential nursing treatments*, ed 2, Philadelphia, 1992, WB Saunders.

Stevens SR: Post-trauma response. In Thompson JM, McFarland GK, Hirsch JE, and Tucker SM: *Mosby's clinical nursing*, ed 3, St. Louis, 1993, Mosby.

Whalen, P. Tu, solou (you, alone): alienation and resocialization of the elderly. *J Gerontol Nurs* , 6,348, 1980.

Spiritual distress (distress of the human spirit)

CLINICAL CONDITION/ MEDICAL DIAGNOSIS	RELATED FACTORS
HIV/AIDS	Fear, hopelessness, guilt, and sense of alienation

Patient goals
Expected outcomes
   Associated nursing/collaborative interventions *and scientific rationale*

Improve personal harmony and serenity as evidenced by the following:

Makes positive statements about self and life
Achieves high Existential Well-being score (40-60) on the Spiritual Well-being Index
Expresses a sense of hope, forgiveness, and loss of guilt
Expresses a sense of meaning in illness and purpose in life

   Encourage expression of feeling through presence, active listening, and being nonjudgmental. *Presence and active listening will help to build trust and positive regard.*

   Encourage storytelling by encouraging patient to review life story; share stories of others who have found meaning in diversity. *Storytelling will help the nurse to develop a better understanding of the patient and help the patient find meaning in life.*

   Monitor hope and existential well-being with the Spiritual Well-Being Index and the Hopelessness Scale. *there is a positive relationship between spiritual well-being and hope in persons with AIDS.*

   Inspire hope by referring to AIDS as a chronic illness; inform patient that newer treatments can prolong life for many years.

Improve personal harmony and connections with friends, family, members of personal faith and culture, and other support systems as evidenced by the following:

Initiates and maintains ongoing relationship with other individual
Explores, discusses, and maintains ongoing relationships with family, culture, and faith system
Participates in AIDS support group and systems

Encourage patient to continue relationships with significant others; realize that many of patient's significant others may be ill or have died from AIDS. *Helping patients cope with and express grief over losses will help them cope with own personal loss of future.*

Encourage patient to contact and communicate with family members and members of faith system. *Support system and spiritual heritage are important for persons coping with chronic illness; they help prevent alienation and are often helpful for finding meaning and purpose in life.*

Help the patient deal with the hurtful and destructive elements from family and spiritual heritage; be compassionate and open to nontraditional (blood and surrogate) families that seek reentry to faith system.

Provide information of AIDS support systems in community; collaborate with social worker in seeking out and encouraging participation in the support systems.

Familiarize self with African-American and Hispanic-American family systems. *African-American and Hispanic-American cultures have strong family systems and beliefs, and are statistically in a high-risk group for AIDS/HIV.*

Improve harmony with God, Supreme Being, or Power beyond self as evidenced by the following:

Scores high on the Spiritual Well-Being Scale; acknowledges that there is a loving and forgiving God

Expresses sense of being loved by friends or family.

Provide, encourage, and help with prayer or meditation; use uplifting stories or music in accordance with patient's preference.

Refer and collaborate with spiritual counselor to help affirm the individual and resolve feelings of anger, isolation, guilt, and past life hurts.

Help individual to realize that there is a forgiving and all-loving God. *Many persons with AIDS feel a sense of alienation with their formal source of faith or religion and have a picture of God as punishing and unforgiving. Faith system can be a primary source of being connected with a power beyond oneself and feeling a sense of love and oneness with others.*

REFERENCES

Bufford RK, Paloutzian RF, Ellison CW: Norms for the spiritual well-being scale, *J Psychology and Theology*, 1991, 19(1):56-70.

Carson V, Soeken KL, Shanty J, Terry L: Hope and spiritual well-being: essentials for living with AIDS, *Perspectives in Psychiatric Care*, 1990, 26(2): 2834.

Carson V, Soeken KL, Grimm PM: Hope and its relationship to spiritual well-being. *J Psychology and Theology*, 1988, 16(2): 159-167.

Fryback PB: Health for people with a terminal diagnosis, *Nursing Science Quarterly*, 1993, 6(3): 147-159.

Heliker D: Reevaluation of a nursing diagnosis: spiritual distress. *Nursing Forum*, 1992, 27(4): 15-20.

Landau-Stanton J, Clements CD, Tartaglia AE: Spiritual, cultural and community systems. In Landau-Stanton JB, Clements C: *AIDS Health and Mental Health*, New York, 1993, Brunner/Mazel Publishers, pp 267-299.

Reed PG: An emerging paradigm for the investigation of spirituality in nursing, *Res Nurs Health*, 1992, 15: 349-357.

Spiritual distress (distress of the human spirit)—cont'd

Spiritual well-being, potential for enhanced

CLINICAL CONDITION/ MEDICAL DIAGNOSIS	RELATED FACTORS
A 47-year-old business executive receiving daily radiation after mastectomy	Expresses renewed appreciation of life; wishes to reestablish relationships with estranged family members

Patient goals
Expected outcomes
> Associated nursing/collaborative interventions *and scientific rationale*

Find greater self-awareness and acceptance as evidenced by the following:

Discusses the meaning of health in her life
Formulates new goals
Expresses hope for the future

> Use "kything" to bring about a spiritual connection. The process of kything includes: choosing to be a healing force in an individual's life; becoming quiet and centered; holding individual in awareness; and joining self with other in spirit.

> Ask individual to tell her story and describe what is most meaningful in her life. *Meanings change as life unfolds.*

> Seek to understand the situation as it is being experienced by the individual; remain focused on what individual is relating.

> Assess the individual's inner strengths and ability to seek meaning and fulfillment in life, e.g., use Assessing the Spiriting Process tool.

> Help individual uncover the meaning of health in her life through the reassessment of priorities. *Priorities change when individuals face their own mortality.*

> Help individual find things to hope for. *Hope enables individuals to continue to enjoy their lives.*

Renew relationships with family members as evidenced by the following:

Writes a personal letter to each family member expressing desire to spend time with them and recalls enjoyment of past experiences

Follows letter with personal telephone contact to arrange a family meeting at their convenience

Modifies daily activities to provide more time to build family relationships

Help individual to use inner strength to make first move toward reconnecting with family. *Facing own mortality increases significance of family, friendships, and love.*

Identify caring behaviors in nurse-patient relationship and use as basis for teaching new caring behaviors. *Caring and being cared for promotes an individual's survival.*

Seek opportunity to help family members recognize individual's need for renewed relationships.

REFERENCES

Burkhardt MA, Nagai-Jacobson MG: Reawakening spirit in clinical practice, *J Holistic Nurs*, 12(1):9-21, 1994.

Dossey B, Frisch NC, Guzzetta CE, Burkhardt MA: American Holistic Nurses Association. In Carroll-Johnson RM, Paquette M: *Classification of nursing diagnoses: proceedings of the tenth conference*, Philadelphia, 1994, J.B. Lippincott Co, pp 160-167.

Fryback PB: Health for people with a terminal diagnosis, *Nursing Science Quarterly*, 6(3):147-159, 1993.

Mansen TJ: The spiritual dimension of individuals: conceptual development. *Nursing Diagnosis*, 4(4):140-147, 1993.

Newman MA: Theory for nursing practice, *Nursing Science Quarterly*, 7(4):153-157, 1994.

Ray V: *Green spirituality: reflections on belonging to a world beyond myself*, New York, 1992, Harper-Collins.

Spiritual well-being, potential for enhanced—cont'd

Suffocation, risk for

CLINICAL CONDITION/ MEDICAL DIAGNOSIS	RELATED FACTORS
Alcohol abuse	Smokes in bed; frequent emesis

Patient goals
Expected outcomes
    Associated nursing/collaborative interventions *and
      scientific rationale*

Recognize increased risk of suffocation as evidenced by the following:

Permanently removes all smoking materials from bedside

Establishes a separate area in home for smoking; outside when weather is mild

    Teach patient/spouse dangers of smoking in bed.
    Teach patient/spouse dangers of second-hand smoke.
    Refer patient to smoking cessation clinic.

Verbalizes understanding of risks associated with drinking behaviors

Spouse demonstrates side-lying position and use of supports to keep patient on side following bouts of drinking.

    Use anatomic drawings to teach patient/spouse danger of inhaling expelled gastric contents.
    Teach spouse to position patient on side to avoid inhaling own vomit. *Knowledge of safety measures will help spouse to reduce risk of suffocation.*

Participate in alcohol rehabilitation program as evidenced by the following:

Acknowledges problem with alcohol abuse

Verbalizes knowledge of adverse effects of excessive drinking

    Offer patient and spouse opportunity to discuss their perceptions of patient's drinking behavior.
    Assist patient in examining consequences of drinking behavior.

Suffocation, risk for

Joins Al-Anon (spouse)
Enters alcohol treatment program (patient)
Provide patient and spouse with list of alcohol
treatment programs in the community.
Negotiate weekly telephone follow-up with
patient/spouse.

REFERENCES

Estes NM, Smith-DiJulio K, Heineman ME: *Nursing diagnosis of the alcoholic person*, St. Louis, 1980, Mosby.

Hall JM: How lesbians recognize and respond to alcohol problems: a theoretical model of problematization. *Adv Nurs Sci*, 1994, 16(3): 46-63.

Hawks JH, Lindeman J, Bartek JK: A validation study, altered family processes: alcoholism. Abstract. In Carroll-Johnson RM, Paquette M, eds: *Classification of nursing diagnoses: proceedings of the tenth conference*, Philadelphia, 1994, J.B. Lippincott, pp 316-317.

Hughes TL: Research on alcohol and drug use among women: A review and update. In McElmurry BJ, Parker RS, eds: *Annual Review of Women's Health*, New York, 1993, National League for Nursing Press, pp. 245-285.

Huckstadt A: Locus of control among alcoholics, recovering alcoholics, and non-alcoholics. *Res Nurs Health*, 1987, 10:23-28.

O'Connell KA: Smoking cessation: research on relapse crises. *Annual Review of Nursing Research*, 1990, 8:83-100.

Rosenfeld SN and Stevenson JS: Perception of daily stress and oral coping behaviors in normal, overweight, and recovering alcoholic women. *Res Nurs Health*, 1988, 11:166-174.

Sullivan EJ and Handley SM: Alcohol and drug abuse in nurses. *Annual Review of Nursing Research*, 1992, 10:113-125.

Sullivan EJ and Handley SM: Alcohol and drug abuse. *Annual Review of Nursing Research*, 1993, 11:281-297.

Swallowing, impaired

CLINICAL CONDITION/ MEDICAL DIAGNOSIS	RELATED FACTORS
Right cerebrovascular accident (CVA) with paralysis of left side of face and mouth.	Decreased gag reflex and oral sensations; delayed swallow mechanism.

Patient goals
Expected outcomes
> Associated nursing/collaborative interventions *and scientific rationale*

Swallow food and liquids safely as evidenced by the following:

Swallows without aspirating

> Feed patient only when alert. *Lethargy hinders safe swallowing.*

> Supervise during feeding *to promote safe swallowing.*

> Check affected side of mouth for pocketing during and after meals. *Pocketing of food may occur on the affected side of mouth because of paralysis or weakness leading to high risk for aspiration.*

> Place emergency equipment at patient's bedside and meal site *in case of choking.*

> Minimize distractions in the environment *to keep patient focused on safe swallowing technique.*

> Feed patient one small bolus of food at a time, starting with $1/4$ to $1/2$ teaspoon and never exceeding 1 teaspoonful. *Small boluses are easier to swallow and manipulate for patients with impaired oral control.*

> Avoid mixing food textures, e.g., beef barley soup. *Varied food textures are more difficult for dysphagic patients to manage and may increase risk for aspiration.*

> Place foods on unaffected side of mouth *to promote optimal oral control.*

> Use verbal cueing, naming each bite of food, where placed, and when to swallow. *Cueing provides sequencing for patient.*

Follow recommendations of speech therapist for compensatory strategies *to reduce risk of aspiration and improve swallowing efficiency.*

Position patient upright with head flexed slightly forward in chin tuck position at mealtimes. *Chin tuck position reduces the likelihood of aspiration during swallowing by narrowing the pharyngeal space, facilitating laryngeal excursion, and decreasing the speed of bolus transit.*

Keep patient in upright position for at least $1/2$ hour after meals. *This position reduces the risk of aspiration.*

Encourage patient to rotate head toward the affected side. *This position causes bolus to lateralize away from direction of rotation when swallowing, thus directing bolus to functional side.*

Provide rest periods before and during feeding *to ensure optimal participation in eating.*

Praise small gains in ability to swallow. *Positive reinforcement enhances confidence in swallowing ability.*

Monitor for signs of aspiration (elevated temperature, upper airway congestion, wet voice quality). *Aspiration is a common complication for dysphagic patients, requiring continual monitoring.*

Collaborate with dietician and speech therapist to develop a plan for introduction and progression of fluids. Introduce thick liquids first. Progressively add thin liquids, beginning with juices with the most taste (citrus) and most sensation (carbonated beverages). Add thin liquids without much taste last (water and tea). *Thick liquids provide more sensation in the dysphagic patient's mouth and throat and are therefore easier to control and swallow.*

Collaborate with dietician and speech therapist to develop a plan for introduction and progression of foods. Introduce foods with pureed consistency first. Progressively add soft (ground) foods, then solid foods beginning with those that require the least chewing. *Foods that are cohesive and soft are easiest to control in the mouth and swallow safely.*

Maintain adequate nutrition and hydration as evidenced by the following:

Maintains stable weight

Encourage intake of 2000 calories every 24 hours. *Adequate intake prevents weight loss and decreases risk of muscular wasting.*

Provide mouth care before and after meals. *Mouth care stimulates salivation.*

Schedule tube feedings in such a manner as *to avoid interference with oral feeding and to facilitate stimulation of appetite.*

Determine patient's food preferences from patient and family members *to increase the probability of sufficient nutritional intake.*

Provide high calorie nutritional supplement 2 hours after meals and at bedtime. *Providing nutritional supplements enhances the likelihood of attaining and maintaining desired nutritional status.*

Provide small frequent meals. *Small meals enhance the likelihood of maximal caloric intake.*

Weigh patient at least twice a week.

Monitor caloric intake. *Monitoring decreases the risk of weight loss.*

Maintains minimum fluid intake of 1500 ml every 24 hours

Monitor intake and output. *Monitoring decreases the risk of dehydration.*

Determine patient's liquid preferences from patient and family members *to increase the likelihood of required fluid intake.*

Evaluate need for supplemental tube feeding *to maintain adequate nutrition and hydration.*

Learn safe swallowing techniques and participate in care management as evidenced by the following:

Family members assist patient with feeding with less supervision over time

Reassure family members about actual or potential improvements in swallowing. *Progress may be slow, so indications reflecting improvement need to be highlighted for family.*

Reinforce with patient and family that swallowing problems may be temporary. *Accurate, hopeful information may help the patient and family cope with the present impairment.*

Collaborate with speech therapist to teach and reinforce knowledge and understanding of compensatory swallowing techniques.

Family members describe and demonstrate pertinent safety techniques
Family members provide encouragement and support during meals

Advise family about proper food selection for home use. *Assistance may be required to translate hospital techniques to home environment.*

Teach Heimlich maneuver to family members *to prepare for possible emergency.*

Collaborate with speech therapist and family to ensure that family members participate in patient's swallowing therapy sessions. *Observation and practice with patient's swallowing therapy will decrease anxiety.*

REFERENCES

Bronstein K, Popovich J, Stewart-Amidel C: *Promoting stroke recovery*, St. Louis, 1991, Mosby.

Carr E, Mitchell J: A comparison of the mealtime care given to patients by nurses using two different meal delivery systems, *Internat J Nurs Studies*, 1991, 28(1):19.

Emich-Herring B, Wood P: A team approach to neurologically based swallowing disorders, *Rehabilitation Nursing*, 1990, 15(3):126.

Horner J, Massey EW: Managing dysphagia—special problems in patients with neurologic disease, *Postgraduate Medicine*, 1991, 89(5):203.

Price M, Dilorio M: Swallowing—a practice guide, *Am J Nurs*, 1990, 90(7):42.

Rubin-Terrado M, Linkenheld D: Don't choke on this—a swallowing assessment, *Geriatric Nurs*, 1991, 12(6):288.

Saltzman LS, Rosenberg CH, Wolf RH: Brainstem infarct with pharyngeal dysmotility and paralyzed vocal cord—management with a multidisciplinary approach, *Archives of Physical Medicine and Rehabilitation*, 1993, 74(2):214.

Welch MV, Logemann JA, Rademaker AW, Kahrilas PJ: Changes in pharyngeal dimensions effected by chin tuck, *Archives of Physical Medicine and Rehabilitation*, 1993 74(2):178.

Williams MJ, Walker GT. Managing swallowing problems in the home, *Caring Magazine*, 1992, 11(12):59.

Yen PK: When swallowing is a problem, *Geriatric Nurs*, 1991, 12(6):313.

Thermoregulation, ineffective

CLINICAL CONDITION/ MEDICAL DIAGNOSIS	RELATED FACTORS
Premature infant	Immature thermoregulatory system

Patient goals
Expected outcomes
  Associated nursing/collaborative interventions *and*
    scientific rationale

Establish normothermia as evidenced by the following:

Maintains temperature within normal range

Adjust environmental temperature to infant's needs by using an incubator or radiant warmer; avoiding drafts and cold environmental temperatures; keeping infant clothed in undershirt, diaper, and gown in order to increase resistance to nonevaporative heat loss; keeping head covered *because up to 60% of heat loss occurs this way.*

Provide warm oxygen 32° to 36° C.

Administer IV fluids at room temperature.

Monitor for and report the following signs and symptoms of hypothermia: poor feeding, increased or decreased spontaneous activity, weak cry, decreased muscle tone, difficult arousal, irritability, lethargy, cyanosis, pallor, respiratory distress, bradycardia.

Monitor the following laboratory values that may be affected by thermal instability: decreased serum pH level, which indicates presence of acidosis *because acidosis may result from increased oxygen demands to generate heat*; decreased blood glucose *because hyperglycemia may result from increased use of carbohydrate stores in an effort to generate heat.*

REFERENCES

Lawson L: Hypothermia and trauma injury: temperature monitoring and rewarming strategies, *Critical Care Nurse Quarterly*, 15(1):21, 1992.

Merenstein GB, Gardner SL: *Handbook of neonatal intensive care*, ed 3, St. Louis, 1993, Mosby.

Roncoli M, Medoff-Cooper B: Thermoregulation in low birth-weight infants, *NAACOG'S Clinical Issues*, 3(1):25, 1992.

Stevens T: Managing postoperative hypothermia, rewarming and its complications, *Critical Care Nurse Quarterly*, 16(1):60, 1993.

Thermoregulation, ineffective—cont'd

Thought processes, altered

CLINICAL CONDITION/ MEDICAL DIAGNOSIS	RELATED FACTORS
Borderline personality disorder Diabetes	Coping with feelings of distress Negative self-evaluation

---

Patient goals
Expected outcomes
    Associated nursing/collaborative interventions *and scientific rationale*

Achieve positive self-evaluation as evidenced by the following:

Maintains contact with mental health and medical systems

Reinforce appointment times for medical treatment. *Urging the patient to use the clinic contact as opportunity for helping self and taking responsibility for self is a way of promoting competencies of patient.*

Provide weekly contact to focus on events and teach tolerance of one's emotional state. *Becoming aware of one's own anger, disappointment, etc. enables patient to express emotions, and to then learn new ways to manage the range of emotions.*

Demonstrates cognitive ability to track the consequences of certain stressful events on emotions and thoughts about self.

Teach to monitor self in relation to causes of stress or problems and behaviors occurring as result of inaccurate thoughts, and to note the changes needed in modifying stressor, changing behavioral response to stressor, or changing automatic thoughts.

Assist to determine what is helpful, less helpful, and even harmful.

Use medications to manage or treat diabetes appropriately

Acknowledges inappropriate use of insulin to manage feelings of fear and desperation, and agrees to work on the issue

Set target or goal with patient of no insulin manipulation resulting in emergency room treatments for next 6 months.

Recognize that suicide attempts with insulin is a poor problem solving behavior and help patient develop more adaptive coping strategies.

Demonstrates the use of one or two coping strategies to handle feelings of distress

Teach coping strategies to focus on the behavior (e.g., recording of automatic thoughts, asking another about personal interpretations of situation, relaxation techniques, role playing) and to use cognitive processes (e.g., catching and stopping automatic thought, active problem solving).

Teach how to reward self in concrete ways (e.g., going to a special movie), as well as use of cognitive methods (e.g., "That was a good idea.").

REFERENCES

Beck AT: *Cognitive therapy of personality disorders*, New York, 1990, Guilford Press.

Chen A: Noncompliance in community psychiatry: a review of clinical intervention, *Hosp Community Psychiat* 42(3):282, 1991.

Lazarus RS: Why we should think of stress as a subset of emotion. In Goldberger L, Breznitz S, eds: *Handbook of stress: theoretical and aspects*, ed. 2, New York, 1993, Free Press.

Linehan MM, Heard HL: Dialectical behavior therapy for borderline personality disorder. In Clarkin JL, Marziali E, Munroe-Blum H, eds: *Borderline personality disorder: clinical and empirical perspectives* York, 1992, Guilford Press.

Robbins CJ, Hayes AM: An appraisal of cognitive therapy, *J Consult Clin Psychol* 61(2):205, 1993.

Taylor SE, Aspinwall LG: Coping with chronic illness. In Goldberger L, Breznitz S, eds: *Handbook of stress: theoretical and clinical aspects*, New York, 1993, Free Press.

Wasson EJ, Linehan MM: Personality disorders. In Bellack AS, Hersen MM, eds: *Handbook of behavioral therapy in psychiatric settings* New York, 1993, Plenum Press.

Thought processes, a tered—cont'd

Tissue integrity, impaired

CLINICAL CONDITION/ MEDICAL DIAGNOSIS	RELATED FACTORS
Venostasis ulcers	Venous pooling

Patient goals
Expected outcomes
> Associated nursing/collaborative interventions *and scientific rationale*

Attain tissue healing as evidenced by the following:

Reduced edema surrounding lesion
Skin color and temperature consistent with color and temperature of unaffected extremity
Intact skin of lower extremity
> Assess lesion for depth (partial or full thickness) and healing phase (e.g., granulation, epithelization).
> Remove constrictive clothing.
> Provide physiologic and aseptic environment for lesion.
> Consult physician concerning moisture-retentive dressings.
> Consult physician concerning medications (e.g., diuretic therapy).

Wound free of purulent and necrotic material
> Clean lesion with nonirritating solutions.
> Remove purulent drainage and necrotic tissue.
> Consult physician concerning debridement strategies.

Wound care performed by patient or significant other
> Teach patient or significant other to perform wound care and to detect symptoms and signs of infection or increased inflammation.
> Teach patient to avoid constrictive clothing (e.g., shoes, stockings, tight- waisted undergarments).

Circulatory exercises and postural maneuvers performed by patient

Demonstrate and assist patient in performing lower extremity exercises and deep breathing exercises sequentially, to activate skeletal muscle pump and respiratory pump in lying or standing position.

Elevate extremity when patient is in sitting position.

Teach patient to avoid crossing legs. *Gravity affects venous flow and lymph in the lower extremities. Crossing legs impedes venous return and promotes venostasis that leads to edema formation and impaired tissue perfusion.*

Develop an exercise schedule with patient that includes a comfortable combination of walking and rest periods and that avoids standing still for prolonged periods.

Consult physician about compressive stockings or pneumatic leggings. *If venous insufficiency is severe, long-term ambulatory elastic compression stocking therapy may be used to facilitate venous return and promote healing or prevent recurrence of ulceration.*

REFERENCES

Bishop JB, et al: A prospective randomized evaluator-blinded trial of two potential wound healing agents for the treatment of venous stasis ulcers, *J Vasc Surg*, 16(2):251-257, 1992.

Dickey JW: Stasis ulcers: the role of compliance in healing, *South Med J* 84(5):557-561, 1991.

Holloway GA, et al: Multicenter trial of cadexomer iodine to treat venous stasis ulcer, *West J Med*, 151(1):35-38, July 1989.

Kikta MJ, et al: A prospective, randomized trial of Unna's boots versus hydroactive dressing in the treatment of venous stasis ulcers, *J Vasc Surg*, 7(3):478-483, 1988.

Mayberry JC, et al: Fifteen year results of ambulatory compression therapy for chronic venous ulcers, *Surgery*, 109(5):575-581, 1991.

Motta GJ: How moisture retentive dressings promote healing, *Nursing 93*, 23(12):26-33, 1993.

Rubin JR, et al: Unna's vs. polyurethane foam dressings for the treatment of venous ulceration: a randomized prospective study, *Arch Surg*, 125(4):489-490, 1990.

US Department of Health and Human Services: Clinical practice guidelines Number 3—Pressure ulcers in adults: prediction and prevention, *AHCPR Publication No. 92-0047*, May, 1992.

Young JR, Terwoord BA: Stasis ulcer treatment with compression dressing, *Cleve Clin J Med* 57(6):529-531, September 1990.

Tissue integrity, impaired—cont'd

Tissue perfusion, altered (peripheral)

CLINICAL CONDITION/ MEDICAL DIAGNOSIS	RELATED FACTORS
Arterial occlusive disease	Interruption of arterial flow

> **Patient goals**
> **Expected outcomes**
>> Associated nursing/collaborative interventions *and scientific rationale*

Manifest decreasing signs and symptoms of tissue damage as evidenced by the following:

Decreased claudication, with warmth and good color of extremities, no ulcers

Encourage ambulation, if possible.

Instruct on exercise program of active or passive ROM to extremities every 2 hours as appropriate. *Exercise promotes adequate circulation and formation of collateral blood vessels.*

Keep legs level with or slightly lower than heart. *Gravity promotes arterial circulation and reduces pain.*

Avoid prolonged exposure to cold environmental temperature; room temperature should be 72° to 74° F. *Cold temperatures cause vasoconstriction.*

Avoid pressure on extremities by use of water mattress, foot cradle, keeping heels off bed.

Administer and teach patient about pain medication and agents that decrease blood viscosity.

Modify lifestyle to decrease signs and symptoms of peripheral vascular disorder as evidenced by the following:

Verbalizes knowledge of therapeutic measures

Assist patient in controlling risk factors. Instruct patient to:

- Stop smoking *because smoking constricts blood vessels, inhibits ability of blood to carry oxygen by*

increasing carbon monoxide levels, and results in
increased platelet adhesiveness and thrombus
formation

- Eat low fat–low cholesterol diet *because lipids
attach to the arterial wall, causing atherosclerotic
lesions*
- Exercise *because sedentary lifestyle decreases
arterial patency and prevents collateral circulation
from developing*
- Control blood pressure *because hypertension
causes a high-pressure arterial system, which
damages the intimal endothelium and makes it
more permeable to lipid penetration and plaque
formation*
- Use proper foot care, wear protective shoes,
and inspect feet daily

Instruct patient about signS and symptoms to
report to physician, such as cuts, rashes, ulcers,
reddened areas, increased pain.

Give patient list of community resources.

Discuss the patient's and significant others'
responses to the disease, such as anxiety,
powerlessness, depression and fears such as of
increased pain, inability to walk, and
amputation.

REFERENCES

Beaver B: Health education and the patient with peripheral vascular
disease, *Nurs Clin North Am*, 21(2):265, June 1986.
Burch KO: PVD: nurse-patient interventions, *J Vascular Nurs*, 9(4):13,
1991.
Crosby F, et al: Well-being and concerns of patients with peripheral
arterial occlusive disease, *J Vascular Nurs*, 11(1):5, 1993.
Herman JA: Nursing assessment and nursing diagnosis in patients
with peripheral vascular disease, *Nurs Clin North Am*, 21(2):219,
June 1986.
Hiatt W, Regensteiner J: Nonsurgical management of peripheral
arterial disease, *Hospital Practice*, 28(2):59, 1993.
Turner J: Nursing intervention in patients with peripheral vascular
disease, *Nurs Clin North Am*, 21(2):233, June 1986.
Warbinek E, Wyness MA: Designing nursing care for patients with
peripheral vascular occlusive disease—Part II: nursing assessment
and standard care plans, *Cardiovascular Nursing*, 22(2):6, 1986.

Tissue perfusion, altered (peripheral)—cont'd

Trauma, risk for (falling)

CLINICAL CONDITION/ MEDICAL DIAGNOSIS	RISK FACTORS
Degenerative joint disease	Sedentary lifestyle; household clutter; narrow, poorly lighted hallways

> **Patient goals**
> **Expected outcomes**
>> Associated nursing/collaborative interventions *and scientific rationale*

Increase activity level as evidenced by the following:

Obtains and uses a walker
Increases walking distance 10 feet per week
Walks outdoors when visitors or family members are willing to provide assistance

Refer patient for free loan of walker from community resource, e.g., church.

Develop with patient a plan to increase walking distance to tolerance level. *Increased activity will strengthen muscles and decrease risk of falling.*

Increase safety while maintaining an independent lifestyle as evidenced by the following:

Obtains information about "life-line" to summon help when needed
Negotiates with neighbors to check on him periodically.

Discuss with patient advantages of "life-line" over portable telephone to summon help. *Life-line enables the patient to summon help from any room and outdoors.*

Provide information about home health services to assist with ADLs as needed.

Adapt home environment to reduce risk of falling as evidenced by the following:

Obtains assistance from family members to sort and store items that are creating a hazard in hallways
Keeps an updated list of where items are stored

Hallways are clear and well-lighted
Collaborates with family to complete risk assessment profile

Assist patient with examination of hazards in environment.

Teach patient to keep flashlight at bedside in case of power failure during the night.

Educate patient and family members about risk factors that contribute to falls.

Use a "risk assessment for falls scale" to alert patient and family to internal and external risk factors.

REFERENCES

Hogue CC, Studenski S, Duncan P: Assessing mobility: the first step in preventing falls. In Gunk SG, Tornquist EM, Champagne MT, Copp LA, Wiese RA, eds: *Key aspects of recovery: improving nutrition, rest and mobility*, New York, 1990, Springer Publishing Co, pp 275-280.

Janken JI, Reynolds BA: Identifying patients with the potential for falling. In McLane AM, ed: *Classification of nursing diagnoses: proceeding of the seventh conference*, St. Louis, 1987, Mosby, pp 136-142.

Johnston JF: The elderly and fall prevention. *Applied Nurs Res*, 1(3):140, 1987.

McCloskey JC, Bulechek GM: Fall prevention. *Iowa intervention project: nursing interventions classification (NIC)*, St. Louis, 1992, Mosby, pp 253-254.

Morse JM: Nursing research on patient falls in health care institutions. *Annual Review of Nursing Research*, 11:299-316, 1993.

Ross JER, Watson CA, Glydenvand TA, Reinboth JAL: Potential for trauma: falls. In Mass M, Buckwalter KC, Hardy M: *Nursing diagnoses and interventions for the elderly*, Redwood City, CA, 1991, Addison-Wesley Nursing, pp 18-31.

Tinetti ME, Williams RF, Mayewski R: Fall risk index for elderly patients based on number of chronic disabilities. *Am J Med*, 1986, 80:430-434.

Whedon MB, Shedd P: Prediction and prevention of patient falls. *Image: J Nurs Scholarship*, 21:108-114, 1989.

Trauma, risk for (falling)—cont'd

Unilateral neglect

CLINICAL CONDITION/ MEDICAL DIAGNOSIS	RELATED FACTORS
Right-sided CVA with hemianopia	Disturbed perceptual ability

> **Patient goals**
> **Expected outcomes**
> > Associated nursing/collaborative interventions *and scientific rationale*

Have realistic awareness of perceptual deficit as evidenced by the following:

Verbalizes realistic estimation of degree of deficit, e.g., does not ignore or underestimate deficit
> Explain to patient that one side is being neglected. Encourage patient to share own perception and provide realistic feedback *to assist the patient to understand and acknowledge the condition.*

Be protected from injury as evidenced by the following:

Experiences no accidents
> Provide a safe environment by regularly orienting patient to environment; removing excess furniture and equipment; providing good lighting; placing call bell and frequently used objects on unaffected side within easy reach; keeping side rail up on affected side. *Structuring the environment to decrease hazards is essential to safety.*

Absence of injury resulting from deficit
> Supervise or assist in transferring and ambulating. Protect neglected side during activities and teach patient to assume this responsiblity; teach patient to check position of limbs on affected side *to prevent unfelt trauma.*
> Note perceptual deficit on patient record and in patient's room to inform caregivers. *Continuity of*

Unilateral neglect

safe care is enhanced when all caregivers are aware of the patient's perceptual deficits.

Acquire knowledge and skill to decrease or cope with deficit as evidenced by the following:

Responds to verbal, visual, and tactile cues to decrease neglect of affected side; scans and protects affected side

Teach patient to scan affected side; place clock or some frequently used item on side of deficit *to help establish a pattern of scanning.*

Use "cueing" to affected side (e.g., place red line in margin of books on affected side, small bells on limbs of affected side) and monocular patching of eye on unaffected side.

Spend time with patient, manipulating affected side and encouraging patient to use it. (1) Have patient handle ignored limbs on unaffected side. (2) Increase stimulation to affected side by touching or massage with scented lotion. *Verbal, visual, and tactile cues to decrease neglect of the affected side reinforce each other in enhancing perceptual functioning.*

Compensates for perceptual loss.

Assist compensation for perceptual deficit by arranging environment within patient's perceptual field.

Use visual and verbal communication regarding limb placement on affected side.

Demonstrates increased participation and independence in ADLs

Promote conscious attention, after initial stress, to neglected side by placing frequently used items on that side, position patient so that affected side is in view; talk to patient from that side. *Activities that direct attention to the neglected side can increase awareness and use of that side.*

Place food tray toward unaffected side; teach patient to rotate place periodically.

Encourage patient to perform ADLs such as toothbrushing in front of a mirror; supervise and give feedback.

Verbalizes feelings of progress in regard to perceptual deficit

Assess regularly for degree of deficit and adaptation to deficit; assess contributing factors.

Decrease confusing stimuli; avoid relocation; maintain consistency of caregivers and consistency of routine for self-care; explain procedures and treatment well in advance. *An established plan of care by consistent caregivers can decrease distortions in perception and subsequent disorientation.*

Include family in rehabilitation process *so that they understand it, support it, and can continue it in home environment.*

REFERENCES

Baggerly J: Sensory perceptual problems following stroke, *Nurs Clin North Am* 26(4):997, 1991.

Booth K: The neglect syndrome, *J Neurosurg Nurs* 14:38, 1982.

Butter CM, Kirsch N: Combined and separate effects of eye patching and visual stimulation on unilateral neglect following stroke, *Arch Phys Med Rehabil* 73:1133, 1992.

Hickey JV: The clinical practice of neurological and neurosurgical nursing, ed 3, Philadelphia, 1992, JB Lippincott.

Kalbach LR: Unilateral neglect: mechanisms and nursing care, *J Neuroscience Nurs* 23:125, 1991.

Warren M: A Hierarchical model for evaluation and treatment of visual perceptual dysfunction in adult acquired brain injury, Part 1 and 2, *Am Jour Occup Ther* 47(1):42, 1993.

Wyness MA: Perceptual dysfunction: nursing assessment and management, *J Neurosurg Nurs* 17:105, 1985.

Urinary elimination, altered

CLINICAL CONDITION/ MEDICAL DIAGNOSIS	RELATED FACTORS
Long-term use of a Foley catheter	Diminished urinary sphincter control; social isolation

Patient goals
Expected outcomes
> Associated nursing/collaborative interventions *and scientific rationale*

Establish a normal pattern of urinary elimination as evidenced by the following:

Adheres to established voiding schedule
Decrease in number of episodes of involuntary loss of urine

> Establish a regular voiding schedule with patient; start with every 2 hours.

> Teach and monitor use of voiding record *to identify changes in pattern of urination and decrease in involuntary loss of urine.*

> Teach and monitor use of pelvic floor exercises (PFEs).

> Provide written instructions:
> - Sit or stand without tensing muscles of legs, buttocks, or abdomen
> - Contract and relax circumvaginal muscles and urinary and anal sphincters for 3-4 seconds and repeat in a staccato fashion.
> - Do PFEs 25 to 30 times, three times a day. *PFEs strengthen the circumvaginal muscles, urinary sphincter, and external anal sphincter.*

Drinks 6 to 8 glasses of water per day

> Collaborate with patient to establish a pattern of fluid intake *to maintain hydration*, (e.g., 200 ml every 2 hours during day).

> Suggest patient drink 120 ml cranberry juice per day.

Skin in perineal area is clean and dry
No redness or discomfort in perineal area

Urinary elimination, altered

Teach patient protective skin care, (e.g., use Desitin ointment on skin in vulnerable areas).

Provide information about continence aids. *Use of continence aids helps to alleviate patient's anxiety and contributes to continence.*

Experience decrease in social isolation as evidenced by the following:

Makes short trips to family member's home
Reports increase in self-confidence
Contacts employer to plan for return to work

Encourage short trips to friends and relatives.

Suggest regular use of panty liners *to increase confidence.*

Assist patient with design of a plan for eventual return to work; help patient make initial contact with employer.

REFERENCES

Dowd TT: Discovering older women's experience of urinary incontinence, *Res Nurs Health*, 14(3):179-186, 1991

McCormick KA, Palmer MH: Urinary incontinence in older adults. *Annual Review of Nursing Research*, 10:25-53, 1992.

Palmer MH, Bone LR, Fahey M, Mamom J, Steinwachs D: Detecting urinary incontinence in older adults during hospitalization. *Applied Nursing Research*, 5(4):174-180, 1992.

Sampselle CM, DeLancey JO: The urine stream interruption test and pelvic muscle function. *Nursing Research*, 41(2):73-77, 1992.

Specht J, Tunink P, Maas M, Bulechek G: Urinary incontinence. In Maas M, Buckwalter KC, Hardy M: *Nursing diagnosis and interventions for the elderly*, Redwood City, CA, 1991, Addison-Wesley, pp 181-204.

Voith AM: Alterations in urinary elimination: concepts, research, and practice. *Rehabilitation Nursing*, 13(3):122, 1988.

Urinary retention

CLINICAL CONDITION/ MEDICAL DIAGNOSIS	RELATED FACTORS
Bowel resection; moderate prostatic hypertrophy	Disruption of usual voiding pattern; limited activity

Patient goals
Expected outcomes
    Associated nursing/collaborative interventions *and scientific rationale*

Reestablish usual voiding pattern as evidenced by the following:

Voids every 3 to 4 hours
Uses Credé maneuver to facilitate complete emptying of bladder (with physician's approval)
Verbalizes understanding of prostatic hypertrophy in development of urinary retention

Use 100% silicone catheter for indwelling catheter in immediate postoperative period.

Select appropriate catheter size. *Catheter that is too large obstructs seminal ducts and may lead to epididymitis or prostatitis; usual size is 16-18 French in male, French catheter scale: each gradation is $1/3$ mm. Catheter that is too narrow is difficult to insert and permits retrograde extension of bacteria.*

Teach patient methods to stimulate voiding: stroke lower abdomen or inner thighs; pour warm water over perineum; run water in sink; tap over symphysis pubis. *Stimulation of primitive reflexes facilitates voiding after removal of catheter.*

Teach patient and family the pathophysiology of prostatic hypertrophy in relation to urinary retention.

Adhere to health practices to prevent urinary infection as evidenced by the following:

Maintains adequate oral intake by taking 8 oz. of fluid with meals, between meals, and in early evening
Takes superphysiologic amounts of vitamin C, at least 1000 mg daily

Provide patient with oral and or IV intake of 2000-2500 ml unless contraindicated.

Teach patient and family to maintain acid urine with use of vitamin C or large quantities of cranberry juice. *Keeping urine acidic helps to prevent bladder infections.*

No signs or symptoms of infection after removal of catheter as evidenced by the following:

Reports absence of burning, frequency, and urgency
Urinalysis confirms the absence of bacteria in urine

Monitor patient for signs and symptoms of urinary tract infection.

Obtain daily urinalysis if catheter remains in for more than 48 hours.

Obtain midstream voided specimen 24 hours after removal of catheter and with any signs or symptoms of urinary tract infection, e.g., burning, frequency, urge incontinence.

Instruct patient and family to call physician if signs or symptoms of infection develop after discharge from hospital.

Increase level of activity as evidenced by the following:

Walks with assistance 4-5 times a day
Request pain medication 1/2 hour before walking in early postoperative period.
Stands to void or walks to bathroom after removal of catheter.

Collaborate with patient to establish increasing activity schedule.

Provide pain medication 1/2 hour before walking and initial voiding attempts after removal of catheter.

Have patient stand to void or walk to bathroom after removal of catheter.

REFERENCES

Kinney AB, Blount M: Effect of cranberry juice on urinary pH, *Nursing Research*, 28:287, 1979.

Kinney AB, Blount M, Dowell M: Urethral catheterization: pros and cons of an invasive but sometimes essential procedure *Geriatric Nurs*, 1:258, 1980.

McCloskey JC, Bulechek GM: Urinary retention care. In *Iowa Intervention Project: Nursing interventions classification (NIC)*, St. Louis, 1992, Mosby.

Voith AM, Smith DA: Validation of the nursing diagnosis of urinary retention. *Nurs Clin North Am*, 20:723, 1985.

Urinary retention—cont'd

Ventilation, inability to sustain spontaneous

CLINICAL CONDITION/ MEDICAL DIAGNOSIS	RELATED FACTORS
Chronic respiratory failure; respiratory muscle dysfunction/weakness	Imbalance between ventilatory capacity and ventilatory demand because of decreased capacity and/or increased demand

Patient goals
Expected outcomes
> Associated nursing/collaborative interventions *and scientific rationale*

Demonstrate decreased ventilatory demand as evidenced by the following:

Effective breathing pattern.
Respiratory rate within normal limits.
No accessory muscle use.
Ti/Ttot* and Vd/Vt* within normal limits
Normal lung compliance
Arterial CO_2 and O_2 concentrations within normal limits
Body temperature within normal limits
Work of breathing (measured) within normal limits
No air trapping at end of expiration (Auto-PEEP)*
Normal, clear breath sounds
> Set ventilator to maximize expiratory time (increase inspiratory flow rate or decrease delivered tidal volume). *This setting will decrease occurrence of air trapping or intrinsic PEEP, thus decreasing WOB.**
> Avoid excessive carbohydrate caloric intake.
> Monitor body temperature and treat fever.
> Maintain infection control procedures.
> *Decreased metabolic demands will decrease the ventilatory workload.*

* Abbreviations: *PEEP*, positive-end expiratory pressure; *WOB*, work of breathing; *ROM*, range of motion; *Ti*, inspiratory time; *Ttot*, total respiratory time; *Vd*, dead space; *Vt*, tidal volume.

Provide calm, quiet, and comfortable environment.
Teach relaxation and stress reduction techniques
Monitor acid/base status of body fluids and treat
alterations.

Anxiety, stress, hypoxemia, and acidosis increase
respiratory drive, thus increasing ventilatory demand
and WOB*. Avoiding these conditions decreases
demand and WOB.

Maintain airway patency and clearance by
checking size of endotracheal tube and
suctioning airway prn. *Decreased air flow*
resistance minimizes WOB.

Schedule physical activities and exercise routines,
as tolerated: up to chair, ambulate, assist with
hygiene, and active and passive ROM* and bed
exercise. *Prevent muscle deconditioning and provide*
patient with diversionary activities. Muscle decondi-
tioning will contribute to increased ventilatory
demand. Diversion helps decrease anxiety.

**Achieve optimal ventilatory capability as evidenced
by the following:**

**Maximal inspiratory and expiratory pressures within
normal limits**
Tidal volume and vital capacity within normal limits
Respiratory rate within normal limits

Assess nutritional status. Correct nutritional
deficits. *Optimal muscle performance depends on*
adequate supply of nutrients for energy production
and protein for muscle tissue repair. In addition,
malnutrition blunts respiratory drive.

Position to allow maximal thoracic excursion *to*
allow diaphragm to contract from optimum length
for maximum contractility.

Monitor acid/base status of body fluids and correct
alterations. *Alkalosis blunts respiratory drive.*

Monitor effects of sedative agents. *Sedatives can*
blunt respiratory drive.

*Abbreviations: *PEEP*, positive-end expiratory pressure; *WOB*, work of
breathing; *ROM*, range of motion; *Ti*, inspiratory time; *Ttot*, total
respiratory time; *Vd*, dead space; *Vt*, tidal volume.

Ventilation, inability to sustain spontaneous—cont'd

Promote normal rest/sleep patterns. Pace activities to allow rest periods. *Rest allows energy reserves to be replenished. Sleep deprivation blunts respiratory drive.*

Provide mechanical ventilatory support at a level that provides rest of respiratory muscles. Use appropriate settings. Apply appropriate mode of ventilation. *Rest is only specific treatment for muscle fatigue. Maximal rest allows complete recovery from fatigue. Improper ventilator settings, type, and cycling and high resistance valves and circuitry add to workload and prevent complete rest and recovery of muscle function.*

Provide inspiratory muscle training, if appropriate. *This increases strength and endurance, and prevents further deconditioning of respiratory muscles.*

REFERENCES

Benotti PN, Bistrian B: Metabolic and nutritional aspects of weaning from mechanical ventilation, *Critical Care Medicine*, 17:181-85, 1989.

Burns SM, Clochesy J, Goodnough-Hanneman S, Ingersoll G, Knebel AR, Shekleton ME: Weaning from long-term mechanical ventilation, *Am J Critical Care*, 4(1):4-22, 1995.

Geisman LK, Ahrens T: Auto-PEEP: An impediment to weaning in the chronically ventilated patient, *AACN Clinical Issues in Critical Care Nursing*, 2(3):391-7, 1991.

Gracey DR, Viggrano RW, Naessens JM, Hubmayr RD, Silverstein MD, Loenig GE: Outcomes of patients admitted to a chronic ventilator-dependent unit in an acute care hospital, *Mayo Clinic Proceedings*, 67:131-6, 1992.

Kastens VM: Nursing management of "Auto-PEEP", *Focus on Critical Care*, 18(5):419-421, 1991.

Marini JJ: The physiologic determinants of ventilator dependency, *Respiratory Care*, 31:271-282, 1986.

Marini JJ: Weaning from mechanical ventilation, *New Engl J Med*, 324(21):1496-1498, 1991.

Shekleton ME: Respiratory muscle conditioning and the work of breathing: a critical balance in the weaning patient, *AACN Clinical Issues in Critical Care Nursing*, 2(3):405-414, 1991.

Thompson KS, Caddick K, Mathie J, Newlon B, Abraham T: Building a critical path for ventilator dependency, *Am J Nurs Vol 91(7)*, July: 28-31, 1991.

Tobin MJ: Weaning from mechanical ventilation, In Simmons DH, ed: *Current Pulmonology*, vol 2, Chicago, 1990, Yearbook, pp 47-105.

Ventilatory weaning response, dysfunctional

CLINICAL CONDITION/ MEDICAL DIAGNOSIS	RELATED FACTORS
Acute respiratory failure	Physiologic and psychologic readiness to wean from mechanical ventilation

> **Patient goals**
> Expected outcomes
>> Associated nursing/collaborative interventions *and scientific rationale*

Achieve stable, optimal physiologic status as evidenced by the following:

Alert and rested appearance
Heart rate and rhythm, blood pressure, respiratory rate, tidal volume, electrolytes (especially K^+, Mg^{++}, PO_4), Hgb, Hct, arterial blood gases, weaning parameters, serum albumin, and albumin/globulin ratio within normal limits
Balanced intake and output
Weight stable and within target ideal body weight range
No complaints of dyspnea
Effective airway clearance; normal, clear breath sounds; minimal secretions
Effective breathing pattern: complete, equal, bilateral chest excursion and no paradoxical breathing
No complaints of pain

> Assess and monitor respiratory, hemodynamic, metabolic, hydration, and CNS parameters. *Ventilatory and hemodynamic stability and decreased metabolic demand help to minimize work of breathing.*
> Maintain proper ventilator settings. *Inappropriate settings can increase ventilatory workload and predispose respiratory muscles to fatigue. Appropriate settings promote rest of respiratory muscles.*
> Encourage adequate intake of food and fluids.

453

Provide nutritional supplementation as needed.
Obtain nutritional consultation.
*Normal muscle performance and adequate energy
supply depend on matching nutritional requirements
to metabolic needs.*

Promote normal rest/sleep patterns. Schedule
weaning trial in AM. Allow 1- to 2-hour rest
periods before weaning trial after other
activities. *Rest is necessary to replenish depleted
energy reserves and promote optimal muscle and
organ system function.*

Maintain airway patency and clearance:
- Check size of endotracheal tube
- Check placement of endotracheal tube
- Suction airway prn before weaning trial

*Decreased air flow resistance minimizes the work of
breathing.*

Position with head elevated, back straight from
waist (in chair, on side of bed, in high Fowler's).
*Maximal thoracic excursion allows increased lung
volumes, thus increasing ventilation to participate in
gas exchange.*

Promote comfort and relieve pain:
- Teach relaxation techniques
- Provide diversionary activities
- Administer analgesic medication.

*Discomfort and pain increase anxiety and cause
ineffective breathing patterns such as "splinted"
respiration or rapid, shallow breathing that increases
dead space.*

**Demonstrate feelings of control and independence
and minimal anxiety as evidenced by the following:**

Calm, relaxed appearance
Verbalizes understanding of weaning plans
States satisfaction with answers to questions
**Expresses minimal feelings of anxiety and
powerlessness**

Discuss weaning plan with patient and significant
others
Explain procedures to be followed.

Solicit and answer questions.

Reassure that continuous monitoring will occur during weaning trial.

Reassure that multiple weaning trials are normal and expected.

Explain alarm systems and all safety measures being implemented.

Increased understanding will promote cooperation with plan and increase belief in ability and motivation to succeed, as well as decrease anxiety about weaning trial.

During weaning trial: tolerate decreased ventilatory rate or level of pressure support or total discontinuation of mechanical ventilatory support as evidenced by the following:

Stable breathing pattern with minimal initial increase in respiratory rate and decrease in tidal volume

Stable blood pressure, heart rate, and rhythm

Stable arterial blood gas levels

Breath sounds clear

Quiet, comfortable breathing without complaints of dyspnea, fatigue, or excessive warmth or discomfort

Skin of face and peripheral extremities remains warm and dry and pink in color

Communicate confidence in patient's readiness and ability to wean.

Provide comfortable and calm lighting, temperature, and support persons.

These actions increase patient's level of confidence in self and decrease anxiety level.

Implement collaboratively developed individualized weaning plan that includes goals, methods, and time frames. *Use of a plan that incorporates weaning protocols agreed on by all health-care team members promotes consistency of approach and increases weaning success rate.*

Remain with patient and monitor status continuously during weaning trial. *Promote safety, because change can occur rapidly and may require immediate intervention.*

Suction airway prn during weaning trial *to maintain airway patency and decrease resistance to air flow, thus minimizing work of breathing.*

Provide fan at bedside. *Sensation of coolness and blowing air lessens feelings of shortness of breath.*

Communicate progress in achieving weaning goals to patient and significant others as weaning process continues. *Positive feedback increases motivation.*

REFERENCES

Birdsall C: Searching for the best weaning methods, *Critical Care Specialist*, 1:6-7, 1993.

Calhoun CJ, Specht NL: Standardizing the weaning process, *AACN Clinical Issues in Critical Care Nursing*, 2(3):398-404, 1991.

Goodnough-Hanneman S, Multidimensional predictors of success or failure with early weaning from mechanical ventilation after cardiac surgery, *Nurs Res*, 43(1);4-10, 1994.

Goodnough-Hanneman S, Ingersoll G, Knebel AR, Shekleton ME, Burns SM, Clochesy J: Weaning from short-term mechanical ventilation, *Am J Critical Care*, 3(6):421-441, 1994.

Henneman EA: The art and science of weaning from mechanical ventilation, *Focus on Critical Care*, 18(6): 490-501, 1991.

Jenny J, Logan J: Analyzing expert nursing practice to develop a new nursing diagnosis: dysfunctional ventilatory weaning response (pp 133-140). In Carroll-Johnson RM, ed: *Classification of nursing diagnoses; proceedings of the ninth conference*, Philadelphia, 1991, JB Lippincott Co.

Knebel AR: Weaning from mechanical ventilation: current controversies, *Heart and Lung*, 20(4):321-331, 1991.

Logan J, Jenny J: Interventions for the nursing diagnosis Dysfunctional ventilatory weaning response. In Carroll-Johnson RM: *Classification of nursing diagnoses: Proceedings of the ninth conference*, Philadelphia, PA, 1991, JB Lippincott Co, pp 141-147.

Sabau D, Sabo J, Kraus-Hargett J, Bearden E, Curnyn M, Solis RT: Therapist driven weaning protocol evaluation in the cardiovascular recovery room, *Critical Care Medicine*, 22(1):A226, 1994.

Violence, risk for: self-directed or directed at others

CLINICAL CONDITION/ MEDICAL DIAGNOSIS	RELATED FACTORS
Antisocial personality disorder	Antisocial character

Patient goals
Expected outcomes
    Associated nursing/collaborative interventions *and scientific rationale*

Experience a reduced probability for violence as evidenced by the following:

Verbalizes less aggression, decreases use of coercive or intimidating interaction style, verbalizes anger appropriately, refrains from harming self/others, and controls own behavior

Monitor patient for the following: verbal aggression (e.g., anger/shouting), coercive or intimidating interaction style, and physical aggression against self/others. *Early interventions in the preceding factors can prevent a serious violent episode.*

Observe for side effects of drugs/medications *because violence can be precipitated by them.*

Assess for evidence of past physical aggression against other/objects, life stressors, and family violence. *A past history or any of the preceding additional risk factors predisposes an individual to coping with life or obtaining a desired end through violence.*

Determine parental discipline patterns the client experienced. *The more abusive, the greater potential for violence.*

Avoid a tone of voice that suggests nagging, pessimism, indifference, or hostility. Also avoid direct confrontation and response to abusive language with abusive language. *Patients respond to these staff behaviors defensively (sometimes*

457

Violence, risk for: self-directed or directed at others

violently) *because they are perceived as a threat to the self.*

Avoid extensive eye-to-eye contact, especially when anger is intensifying. *Eye contact can be perceived as an assertion of dominance over the individual and can lead to defensive violence.*

Respond to questions asked by patient. *This increases the patient's feeling of worth and decreases the need for violence to obtain what is desired.*

Demonstrates positive regard for others, and demonstrates constructive coping skills in dealing with stress and frustration.

Monitor patient for the following: strong interest in and/or availability of weapons and ideas of persecution. *These are predisposing factors that can lead to violence.*

Monitor patient for a value system in which violence is viewed as an acceptable response, for perceptions of self and environment, and for variations in interpersonal perceptions. *If the perceptual variation is disturbing to the individual, violence may be used to force greater congruence of perceptions.*

Identifies therapeutic resources available to help change behavior and verbalizes need to decrease the use of violence

Provide one-to-one supportive counseling *to identify coping mechanisms and to recognize consequences of violent behavior.*

Provide nurse-group psychotherapy *to eliminate interpersonal dysfunctions, develop better communication skills, and foster socialization.*

Provide positive reinforcement of behaviors that help to decrease/control violent behavior *because this rewards the patient's attempts to use socially acceptable behaviors.*

Recommend or provide family therapy to *resolve family issues/conflicts and to empower the family in coping with and establishing sanctions for the violent family member.*

Provide health teaching in the following areas:

- Accepting accountability for own behavior (e.g., if patient injures self/others or breaks something, he/she must provide restitution within the limits of program)
- Recognizing impending violence and taking action for aborting the violent behavior
- Learning alternate coping mechanisms, such as negotiating skills, socially acceptable ways of expressing feelings of anger and hostility, and/or stress-reducing and relaxation skills. *Alternative coping mechanisms for stress or perceived threats decrease the need to use violence for coping.*

Responds to ward milieu nonviolently

Create a unit environment that is light, open, and uncrowded with a low noise level and adequate staffing *so that the patient can feel safe and know that the staff can control any violence that occurs. The low noise level decreases arousal/agitation as increases in these can lead to violence.*

Establish hospital unit norm against physical harm to self or others with set sanctions for infractions. *The expectation that violence will not be tolerated decreases violence.*

- Provide staff education on managing assaultive-aggressive behavior *to decrease probability of patient/staff injuries.*
- Provide staff training on what will be perceived as aggression/assaultiveness *to prevent the splitting of the staff by patient manipulation.*

Provide opportunities for aerobic exercises 3 to 7 times a week. *This uses a socially acceptable way of expressing angry feelings, decreasing agitation, and maintaining health.*

REFERENCES

AAN Working Paper: Violence as a nursing priority: policy implications, *Nurs Outlook,* 41(2):83, 1993.

Benson S, et al: Monitoring violence, *Nurs Times,* 88(11):16, 1992.

Larson L: High risk for violence: self-directed or directed at others. In McFarland GK, McFarland EA, eds: *Nursing diagnosis and intervention,* ed 2, St. Louis, 1993, Mosby.

Madula LN, Poggenpoel M: The experience of a community characterized by violence: implications for nursing, *J Adv Nurs,* 18(5):691, 1993.

Violence, risk for: self-directed or directed at others—cont'd

Morrison EF: A coercive interactional style as an antecedent to aggression in psychiatric patients, *Res Nurs Health*, 15(6):421, 1992.

Morrison EF: A comparison of perceptions of aggression and violence by psychiatric nurses, *J Nurs Stud*, 30(3):261, 1993.

Morrison EF: the measurement of aggression and violence in hospitalized psychiatric patients, *J Nurs Stud*, 30(1):51, 1993.

Roper M, Anderson N: the interactional dynamics of violence, part I: an acute psychiatric ward, *Arch Psychiatr Nurs*, 5:209, 1991.

Violence, risk for: self-directed or directed at others—cont'd

MEDICAL DIAGNOSES

with Associated Nursing Diagnoses

The following list of medical diagnoses is based on the Diagnostic and Related Groups* and the Diagnostic and Statistical Manual of Mental Disorders (DSM-IV).†

The specific diagnoses listed were chosen based on their prevalence in the patient population. The titles of some diagnoses were simplified to reflect commonly used terminology. Below each medical diagnosis is a list of associated nursing diagnoses.

*_Medicare DRG Handbook, 1992._ A joint publication by Health Care Investment Analysts, Inc. and Ernst and Young.

†American Psychiatric Association. _Diagnostic and Statistical Manual of Mental Disorders, DSM-IV, ed. 4_, Washington, DC, 1994, American Psychiatric Association.

Adjustment disorder with anxiety   DSM-IV 309.24

Anxiety
Coping, ineffective individual
Family processes, altered
Role performance, altered
Self-esteem, situational low
Sleep pattern disturbance
Social interaction, impaired

Alcohol abuse   DSM-IV 305.00

Anxiety
Coping, defensive
Coping, ineffective family: disabling
Coping, ineffective individual
Denial,ineffective
Family process, altered: alcoholism
Injury, risk for
Nutrition, altered: less than body requirements
Parenting, altered
Powerlessness
Role performance, altered
Self-esteem disturbance
Self-esteem, chronic low
Self-esteem, situational low
Social interaction, impaired
Thought processes, altered
Trauma, risk for
Violence, risk for: self-directed or directed at others

Amputation for circulatory system disorders, except upper limb and toe   DRG 113

Adjustment, impaired
Body image disturbance
Mobility, impaired
Skin integrity, impaired

Angina pectoris   DRG 140

Anxiety
Pain
Tissue perfusion, altered: cardiopulmonary

Anorexia nervosa   DSM-IV 307.1

Anxiety
Body image disturbance
Constipation
Coping, ineffective individual
Denial, ineffective
Fluid volume deficit, risk for
Nutrition, altered: less than body requirements
Self-esteem disturbance
Social interaction, impaired

Antisocial personality disorder   DSM-IV 301.7

Coping, ineffective individual
Decisional conflict (specify)
Parenting, altered, risk for
Role performance, altered
Social interaction, impaired
Violence, risk for: self-directed or directed at others

Attention-deficit/hyperactivity disorder, combined type   DSM-IV 314.01

Coping, ineffective individual
Growth and development, altered
Incontinence, functional
Mobility, impaired physical
Role performance, altered
Self-care deficit, dressing/grooming
Self-esteem disturbance
Self-esteem, chronic low
Sleep pattern disturbance
Social interaction, impaired
Thought processes, altered
Trauma, risk for

Autistic disorder   DSM-IV 299.00

Communication, impaired verbal
Injury, risk for
Nutrition, altered: less than body requirements
Personal identity disturbance
Role performance, altered
Self-care deficit, bathing/hygiene

Self-care deficit, dressing/grooming
Self-care deficit, feeding
Self-care deficit, toileting
Social interaction, Impaired
Thought processes, altered
Violence, risk for: self-directed or directed at others

Back problems   DRG 243

Mobility, impaired
Pain, chronic
Self-care deficit
Sleep pattern disturbance

Back (and neck) procedures   DRG 214

Adjustment, impaired
Body image disturbance
Mobility, impaired
Pain

Biliary tract disorders   DRG 207

Body image disturbance
Nutrition, altered: less than body requirements
Pain

Bipolar I disorder, most recent episode manic
DSM-IV 296.40

Anxiety
Coping, ineffective individual
Family processes, altered
Fluid volume deficit, risk for
Injury, risk for
Nutrition, altered: less than body requirements
Powerlessness
Role performance, altered
Self-esteem disturbance
Sensory perceptual alterations (specify)
Sleep pattern disturbance
Social interaction, impaired
Thought processes, altered
Violence, risk for: self-directed or directed at others

Bowel procedures, major   DRG 148

Airway clearance, ineffective
Infection, risk for
Nutrition, altered: less than body requirements
Pain

Bronchitis and asthma   DRG 96

Airway clearance, ineffective
Breathing pattern, ineffective
Gas exchange, impaired
Knowledge deficit

Bulimia Nervosa   DSM-IV 307.51

Anxiety
Body image disturbance
Coping, ineffective individual
Fluid volume deficit, risk for
Nutrition, altered: less than body requirements
Powerlessness
Self-esteem disturbance
Social interaction, impaired

Cardiac arrhythmia and conduction disorders
DRG 138

Activity intolerance
Anxiety
Cardiac output, decreased
Tissue perfusion, altered

Cellulitis   DRG 277

Pain
Peripheral neurovascular dysfunction, risk for
Skin integrity, impaired, risk for
Tissue perfusion, altered: peripheral

Cerebrovascular disorders, except transient ischemic attack   DRG 14

Adaptive capacity, decreased: intracranial confusion,
  acute
Injury, risk for
Self-care deficit

Thought processes, altered
Unilateral neglect

Chemotherapy, without acute leukemia DRG 410

Body image disturbance
Fatigue
Nutrition, altered: less than body requirements
Protection, altered

Chest pain   DRG 143

Activity intolerance
Anxiety
Breathing pattern, ineffective
Pain

Chest procedures, major   DRG 75

Airway clearance, ineffective
Pain
Skin integrity, impaired
Tissue perfusion, altered

Cholecystectomy, total   DRG 197

Infection, risk for
Nutrition, altered: less than body requirements
Pain

Circulatory disorders, except acute myocardial infarction, with cardiac catheterization
DRG 125

Injury, risk for
Pain
Peripheral neurovascular dysfunction, risk for
Injury, risk for
Tissue perfusion, altered

Circulatory disorders with acute myocardial infarction and cardiovascular compensation
DRG 121

Anxiety
Cardiac output, decreased

Pain
Tissue perfusion, altered

Circulatory system, operating room procedure
DRG 120

Cardiac output, decreased
Fluid volume deficit
Fluid volume excess
Tissue perfusion, altered

Cocaine dependency DSM-IV 304.20

Anxiety
Coping, defensive
Coping, ineffective family: disabling
Coping, ineffective individual
Denial, ineffective
Family processes, altered
Hopelessness
Knowledge deficit (specify)
Nutrition, altered: less than body requirements
Parenting, altered
Powerlessness
Role performance, altered
Self-esteem disturbance
Social interaction, impaired
Thought processes, altered
Violence, risk for: self-directed or directed at others

Connective tissue (and musculoskeletal) malignancy (and pathological fractures)
DRG 239

Injury, risk for
Mobility, impaired
Pain
Trauma, risk for

Coronary bypass with cardiac catheterization
DRG 106

Anxiety
Cardiac output, decreased
Fluid volume deficit, risk for

Infection, risk for
Knowledge deficit

Coronary bypass without cardiac catheterization
DRG 107

Anxiety
Cardiac output, decreased
Fluid volume deficit, risk for
Infection, risk for

Delusional disorder   DSM-IV 297.1

Communication, impaired verbal
Coping, ineffective individual
Role performance, altered
Sensory/perceptual alterations (specify)
Social interaction, impaired
Social isolation
Thought processes, altered
Violence, risk for: self-directed or directed at others

Dementia of the Alzheimer's type, with late onset, with delirium   DSM-IV 290.3

Anxiety
Caregiver role strain
Caregiver role strain, risk for
Communication, impaired verbal
Coping, ineffective individual
Denial, ineffective
Family processes, altered
Fear
Fluid volume deficit, risk for
Health maintenance, altered
Home maintenance management, impaired
Injury, risk for
Powerlessness
Role performance, altered
Self-care deficit, bathing/hygiene
Self-care deficit, dressing/grooming
Self-care deficit, feeding
Self-care deficit, toileting
Self-esteem disturbance

Sensory/perceptual alterations (specify)
Sleep pattern disturbance
Social interaction, impaired
Thought processes, altered
Trauma, risk for
Violence, risk for: self-directed or directed at others

Depersonalization disorder   DSM-IV 300.6

Anxiety
Coping, ineffective individual
Personal identity disturbance
Sensory/perceptual alterations (specify)
Social interaction, impaired
Thought processes, altered

Depressive disorder, major, single episode DSM-IV 296.20

Anxiety
Decisional conflict (specify)
Fatigue
Grieving, dysfunctional
Hopelessness
Nutrition, altered: less than body requirements
Nutrition, altered: more than body requirements
Powerlessness
Role performance, altered
Self-esteem, situational low
Self-mutilation, risk for
Sleep pattern disturbance
Social interaction, impaired
Social isolation
Thought processes, altered
Violence, risk for: self-directed or directed at others

Diabetes   DRG 294

Infection, risk for
Knowledge deficit
Nutrition, altered
Peripheral neurovascular dysfunction, risk for

Digestive disorders, miscellaneous (and esophagitis and gastroenteritis)   DRG 182

Fluid volume deficit, risk for
Nutrition, altered: less than body requirements
Pain
Swallowing, impaired

Digestive malignancy   DRG 172

Constipation
Diarrhea
Hopelessness
Nutrition, altered: less than body requirements

Digestive system diagnoses   DRG 188

Constipation, risk for
Diarrhea, risk for
Fluid volume deficit
Nutrition, altered: less than body requirements
Pain

Duodenal (and stomach and esophageal) procedures   DRG 154

Fluid volume deficit, risk for
Nutrition, altered: less than body requirements
Oral mucous membrane, altered
Pain

Dysequilibrium   DRG 65

Coping, ineffective individual
Energy field disturbance
Mobility, impaired
Self-care deficit
Sensory/perceptual alterations (kinesthetic)

Dyspareunia (not due to a general medical condition)   DSM-IV 302.76

Pain
Sexual dysfunction
Sexuality patterns, altered
Social interaction, impaired

Esophageal (and duodenal and stomach) procedures   DRG 154

Fluid volume deficit, risk for
Nutrition, altered: less than body requirements
Oral mucous membrane, altered
Pain

Esophagitis (and gastroenteritis and miscellaneous digestive disorders)   DRG 182

Fluid volume deficit, risk for
Nutrition, altered: less than body requirements
Pain
Swallowing, impaired

Femur (and hip) procedures, except major joint   DRG 210

Mobility, impaired
Pain
Peripheral neurovascular dysfunction, risk for
Skin integrity impaired, risk for

Gastroenteritis (and esophagitis and miscellaneous digestive disorders)   DRG 182

Fluid volume deficit, risk for
Nutrition, altered: less than body requirements
Pain
Swallowing, impaired

Gastrointestinal hemorrhage   DRG 174

Fluid volume deficit
Nutrition, altered: less than body requirements
Pain
Tissue perfusion, altered

Gastrointestinal obstruction   DRG 180

Infection, risk for
Nutrition, altered: less than body requirements
Pain

Gender identity disorder in adolescents or adults
DSM-IV 302.85

Body image disturbance
Personal identity disturbance
Role performance, altered
Sexual dysfunction
Sexuality patterns, altered
Social interaction, impaired
Social isolation

Headache and seizure   DRG 24

Injury, risk for
Pain
Sensory/perceptual alterations

Heart failure and shock   DRG 127

Activity intolerance
Anxiety
Cardiac output, decreased
Tissue perfusion, altered

Hip (and pelvis) fractures   DRG 236

Injury, risk for
Mobility, impaired
Pain
Self-care deficit

Hip (and femur) procedures, except major joint
DRG 210

Mobility, impaired
Pain
Peripheral neurovascular dysfunction, risk for
Skin integrity impaired, risk for

Hypochondriasis   DSM-IV 300.7

Anxiety
Body image disturbance
Coping, ineffective family: compromised
Coping, ineffective individual
Family processes, altered
Fear

Knowledge deficit (specify)
Pain, chronic
Role performance, altered
Social interaction, impaired

Insomnia, primary   DSM-IV 307.42

Anxiety
Fatigue
Role performance, altered
Sleep pattern disturbance
Social interaction, impaired
Thought processes, altered

Intermittent explosive disorder   DSM-IV 312.34

Coping, ineffective individual
Family processes, altered
Parenting, altered, risk for
Role performance, altered
Social interaction, impaired
Violence, risk for: self-directed or directed at others

Joint and limb reattachment procedures, major
DRG 209

Pain
Peripheral neurovascular dysfunction, risk for
Self-care deficit
Tissue perfusion, altered: peripheral

Kidney (and urinary tract) infections   DRG 320

Incontinence, urge
Pain
Urinary elimination, altered

Mental retardation, moderate   DSM-IV 318.0

Communication, impaired verbal
Coping, ineffective individual
Growth and development, altered
Home maintenance management, impaired
Injury, risk for
Role performance, altered
Self-care deficit, bathing/hygiene

Self-care deficit, dressing/grooming
Self-care deficit, feeding
Self-care deficit, toileting
Self-esteem disturbance
Social interaction, impaired

Metabolic, miscellaneous (and nutritional) disorders, without complications   DRG 297

Body image disturbance
Nutrition, altered: less than body requirements, risk for
Nutrition, altered, more than body requirements, risk for

Metabolic, miscellaneous (and nutritional) disorders, with complications   DRG 296

Body image disturbance
Knowledge deficit
Nutrition, altered
Skin integrity, impaired, risk for

Musculoskeletal (and connective tissue) malignancy (and pathological fractures) DRG 239

Injury, risk for
Mobility, impaired
Pain
Trauma, risk for

Neck (and back) procedures   DRG 214

Adjustment, impaired
Body image disturbance
Injury, perioperative positioning, risk for
Mobility, impaired
Pain

Nervous system disorders, degenerative   DRG 12

Confusion, chronic
Environmental interpretation syndrome: impaired
Memory, impaired
Mobility, impaired

Sensory/perceptual alterations
Thought processes, altered
Unilateral neglect

Nutritional (and miscellaneous metabolic disorders) without complications   DRG 297

Body image disturbance
Nutrition, altered: less than body requirements, risk for
Nutrition, altered: more than body requirements, risk for

Nutritional (and miscellaneous metabolic disorders) with complications   DRG 296

Body image disturbance
Knowledge deficit
Nutrition, altered
Skin integrity, impaired, risk for

Obsessive-compulsive disorder   DSM-IV 300.3

Anxiety
Coping, ineffective individual
Fear
Pain
Powerlessness
Self-care deficit, bathing/grooming
Self-care deficit, feeding
Skin integrity, impaired, risk for
Social interaction, impaired
Social isolation
Thought processes, altered

Pacemaker implant, permanent cardiac, without acute myocardial infarction, heart failure, or shock   DRG 116

Body image disturbance
Infection, risk for
Knowledge deficit
Self-care deficit, dressing/grooming

Pancreatic disorders, except malignancy
DRG 204

Knowledge deficit
Nutrition, altered: less than body requirements
Pain

Pathological fractures (and musculoskeletal and connective tissue malignancy)   DRG 239

Injury, risk for
Mobility, impaired
Pain
Trauma, risk for

Pelvis (and hip) fractures   DRG 236

Injury, risk for
Mobility, impaired
Pain
Self-care deficit

Pneumonia, simple and pleurisy   DRG 89

Activity intolerance
Airway clearance, ineffective
Gas exchange, impaired
Pain

Prematurity with major problems   DRG 387

Infant behavior, disorganized

Prematurity without major problems   DRG 388

Breast feeding, interrupted
Infant behavior, disorganized, risk for
Infant behavior, organized: potential for enhanced
Infant feeding pattern, ineffective
Parent/infant/child attachment, risk for

Prostatectomy, transurethral   DRG 336

Body image disturbance
Pain
Sexual dysfunction
Urinary elimination, altered

Pulmonary disease, chronic obstructive   DRG 88

Activity intolerance, risk for
Airway clearance, ineffective
Breathing pattern, ineffective
Gas exchange, impaired

Pulmonary edema and respiratory failure
DRG 87

Anxiety
Fluid volume excess
Gas exchange, impaired
Ventilation, inability to sustain spontaneous

Psychosis   DRG 430

Social interaction, impaired
Thought processes, altered
Violence, risk for

Red blood cell disorders   DRG 395

Activity intolerance
Fatigue
Gas exchange, impaired
Tissue perfusion, altered

Rehabilitation   DRG 462

Management of the therapeutic regimen, individual:
    effective
Mobility, impaired
Role performance, altered
Self-care deficit
Self-esteem, situational low
Skin integrity, impaired, risk for
Spiritual well-being, potential for enhanced

Reproductive system, female, reconstructive procedures   DRG 356

Body image disturbance
Pain
Sexual dysfunction
Sexuality patterns, altered

Respiratory infections and inflammations DRG 79

Activity intolerance
Airway clearance, ineffective
Breathing pattern, ineffective
Gas exchange, impaired

Respiratory neoplasms DRG 82

Anxiety
Gas exchange, impaired
Pain

Respiratory signs and symptoms DRG 99

Airway clearance
Breathing pattern, ineffective
Gas exchange, impaired

Respiratory system diagnoses with ventilator support DRG 475

Breathing pattern, ineffective
Gas exchange, impaired
Ventilation, inability to sustain spontaneous
Ventilatory weaning process, dysfunctional

Schizophrenia, catatonic type DSM-IV 295.20

Communication, impaired verbal
Family processes, altered
Injury, risk for
Nutrition, altered: less than body requirements
Role performance, altered
Self-care deficit, bathing/hygiene
Self-care deficit, dressing/grooming
Self-care deficit, feeding
Self-care deficit, toileting
Self mutilation, risk for
Sensory/perceptual alterations (specify)
Sleep pattern disturbance
Social interaction, impaired
Social isolation
Thought processes, altered
Trauma, risk for
Violence, risk for: self-directed or directed at others

Schizophrenia, paranoid type   DSM-IV 295.30

Communication, impaired verbal
Coping, defensive
Coping, ineffective individual
Family processes, altered
Loneliness, risk for
Personal identity disturbance
Role performance, altered
Sensory/perceptual alterations (specify)
Social interaction, impaired
Thought processes, altered
Violence, risk for: self-directed or directed at others

Seizure and headache   DRG 24

Injury, risk for
Pain
Sensory/perceptual alterations

Septicemia   DRG 416

Anxiety
Body temperature altered, risk for
Fluid volume deficit, risk for
Tissue perfusion, altered

Stomach (and esophageal and duodenal) procedures   DRG 154

Fluid volume deficit, risk for
Nutrition, altered: less than body requirements
Oral mucous membrane, altered
Pain

Syncope and collapse, with complications   DRG 141

Injury, risk for
Sensory/perceptual alterations
Tissue perfusion, altered: cerebral

Syncope and collapse, without complications   DRG 142

Injury, risk for
Sensory/perceptual alterations

Tissue perfusion, altered: cerebral
Trauma, risk for

Transient ischemic attack and precerebral occlusions   DRG 15

Anxiety
Injury, risk for
Thought processes, altered
Tissue perfusion, altered: cerebral

Urinary tract (and kidney) infections   DRG 320

Incontinence, urge
Pain
Urinary elimination, altered

Vascular disorders, peripheral   DRG 130

Injury, risk for
Pain
Peripheral neurovascular dysfunction, risk for
Tissue perfusion, altered

Vascular procedures, except major reconstruction without pump   DRG 112

Infection, risk for
Mobility, impaired physical
Pain
Tissue integrity, impaired

Vascular procedures, extracranial   DRG 5

Infection, risk for
Pain
Peripheral neurovascular dysfunction, risk for
Tissue perfusion, altered

Bibliography

NANDA proceedings

Gebbie KM, Lavin MA, eds: *Classification of nursing diagnoses: proceedings of the first national conference*, St Louis, 1975, Mosby-Year Book.

Gebbie KM, ed: *Classification of nursing diagnoses: summary of the second national conference*, St Louis, 1976, Clearinghouse, St. Louis Univ.

Kim MJ, Moritz DA, eds: *Classification of nursing diagnoses: proceedings of the third and fourth national conferences*, St Louis, 1982, McGraw-Hill Book Co.

Kim MJ, McFarland GK, McLane AM, eds: *Classification of nursing diagnoses: proceedings of the fifth national conference*, St Louis, 1984, Mosby-Year Book.

Hurley ME, ed: *Classification of nursing diagnoses: proceedings of the sixth conference*, St Louis, 1986, Mosby-Year Book.

McLane A, ed: *Classification of nursing diagnoses: proceedings of the seventh conference*, St Louis, 1987, Mosby-Year Book.

North American Nursing Diagnosis Association: *Classification of nursing diagnoses: proceedings of the eighth conference*, Philadelphia, 1989, JB Lippincott.

North American Nursing Diagnosis Association: *Classification of nursing diagnoses: proceedings of the ninth conference*, Philadelphia, 1991, JB Lippincott.

North American Diagnosis Association: *Classification of nursing diagnoses: proceedings of the tenth conference*, Philadelphia, 1994, JB Lippincott.

AHCPR Agency for Health Care Policy and Research; a federal agency within the U.S. Public Health Service, U.S. Department of Health and Human Services, responsible for the multidisciplinary development of clinical practice guidelines for selected conditions, e.g., incontinence, pain, depression.

critical thinking/diagnostic reasoning The cognitive process of collecting information, interpreting and clustering information, naming clusters, and formulating nursing diagnosis.*

defining characteristics Signs and symptoms indicating the presence of a nursing diagnosis.

diagnostic label Terminology used to name/label a nursing diagnosis.

DSM IV The fourth edition of the American Psychiatric Association's *Diagnostic and Statistical Manual of Mental Disorders*; the official manual of mental disorders clinically useful for making treatment and management decisions in varied clinical settings (p. xix).†

etiology Previous term for related factor.

expected outcomes Changes in patient behaviors resulting from nursing interventions.

functional health patterns Health patterns useful in assessing human functioning.

function level classification‡

    0 = Completely independent.

    1 = Requires use of equipment or device.

    2 = Requires help from another person for assistance, supervision, or teaching.

    3 = Requires help from another person and equipment device.

    4 = Dependent; does not participate in activity.

ICD-10-CM A clinical modification of the ICD-10 which serves as the official system in the United States for the classification of all diseases, injuries, impairments, symptoms, and causes of death.

life processes Events/processes occurring throughout the lifespan that are related to health status.

NANDA North American Nursing Diagnosis Association.

---

*Gordon M: From *Nursing diagnosis: process and application*, ed 3, St Louis, 1994, Mosby-Year Book.

†From American Psychiatric Association. *Diagnostic and statistical manual of mental disorders, DSM-IV-R*. ed 4, Washington, D.C., APA, 1994.

‡Code adapted from Jones E and others: *Patient classification for long-term care: users' manual*, HEW, Publication No. HRA-74-3107, November 1974.

nursing diagnosis   A clinical judgment about an individual, family, or community responses to actual and potential health problems/life processes. Nursing diagnoses provide the basis for selection of nursing interventions to achieve outcomes for which the nurse is accountable.*

patient goals/expected outcomes   Goals the patient will achieve fully or in part as a result of nursing interventions, along with changes in patient behavior, function, cognition, and affect, indicating goal achievement.

potential nursing diagnosis   Now referred to as at-risk nursing diagnosis.

qualifiers for diagnoses†

(Suggested/not limited to the following):

Acute: severe but of short duration

Altered: a change from baseline

Chronic: lasting a long time, recurring, habitual, constant

Decreased: lessened, lesser in size, amount or degree

Deficient: inadequate in amount, quality or degree, defective, not sufficient, incomplete

Depleted: emptied wholly or in part, exhausted of

Disturbed: agitated, interrupted, interfered with

Dysfunctional: abnormal, incomplete functioning

Excessive: characterized by an amount or quantity that is greater than necessary, desirable, or useful

Increased: greater in size, amount or degree

Impaired: made worse, weakened, damaged, reduced, deteriorated

Ineffective: not producing the desired effect

Intermittent: stopping or starting again at intervals, periodic, cyclic

Potential for enhanced: (for use with wellness diagnoses) made greater, to increase in quality or more desired

related factors   Factors contributing to an actual nursing diagnosis.

risk factors   Predisposing factors that increase vulnerability to the development of a nursing diagnosis (used with at-risk nursing diagnoses).

signs and symptoms   Objective manifestations and subjective sensation, including perception and feelings.

taxonomy   The science of classification (i.e., the study of the general principles of scientific classification).

*Approved at the Ninth Conference on Classification of Nursing Diagnoses.
†From NANDA: *Nursing Diagnoses: Definitions and Classification* 1994-1995, Philadelphia, NANDA.

Classification of nursing diagnoses by human response patterns*

Exchanging

Altered nutrition: more than body requirements.
Altered nutrition: less than body requirements.
Altered nutrition: potential for more than body requirements.
Risk for infection
Risk for altered body temperature
Hypothermia
Hyperthermia
Ineffective thermoregulation
Dysreflexia
Constipation
Perceived constipation
Colonic constipation
Diarrhea
Bowel incontinence
Altered urinary elimination
Stress incontinence
Reflex incontinence
Urge incontinence
Functional incontinence
Total incontinence
Urinary retention
Altered tissue perfusion (specify type), (renal, cerebral, cardiopulmonary, gastrointestinal, peripheral)
Fluid volume excess
Fluid volume deficit
Risk for fluid volume deficit
Decreased cardiac output
Impaired gas exchange
Ineffective airway clearance
Ineffective breathing pattern
Inability to sustain spontaneous ventilation
Dysfunctional ventilatory weaning response (DVWR)
Risk for injury
Risk for suffocation
Risk for poisoning
Risk for trauma

*From NANDA: *Nursing Diagnoses: Definitions and Classification 1994-1995*, Philadelphia, NANDA.

Risk for aspiration
Risk for disuse syndrome
Altered protection
Impaired tissue integrity
Altered oral mucous membrane
Impaired skin integrity
Risk for impaired skin integrity
Decreased adaptive capacity: intracranial
Energy field disturbance

Communicating

Impaired verbal communication

Relating

Impaired social interaction
Social isolation
Altered role performance
Altered parenting
Risk for altered parenting
Risk for altered parent/infant/child attachment
Sexual dysfunction
Altered family processes
Caregiver role strain
Risk for caregiver role strain
Altered family process: alcoholism
Parental role conflict
Altered sexuality patterns

Valuing

Spiritual distress (distress of the human spirit)
Potential for enhanced spiritual well-being

Choosing

Ineffective individual coping
Impaired adjustment
Defensive coping
Ineffective denial
Ineffective family coping: disabling
Ineffective family coping: compromised
Potential for enhanced community coping
Ineffective community coping
Family coping: potential for growth
Ineffective management of therapeutic regimen
    (individuals)

Noncompliance (specify)
Ineffective management of therapeutic regimen: families
Ineffective management of therapeutic regimen: community
Effective management of therapeutic regimen: individual
Decisional conflict (specify)
Health-seeking behaviors (specify)

Moving

Impaired physical mobility
Risk for peripheral neurovascular dysfunction
Risk for perioperative positioning injury
Activity intolerance
Fatigue
Risk for activity intolerance
Sleep pattern disturbance
Diversional activity deficit
Impaired home maintenance management
Altered health maintenance
Feeding self-care deficit
Impaired swallowing
Ineffective breastfeeding
Interrupted breastfeeding
Effective breastfeeding
Ineffective infant feeding pattern
Bathing/hygiene self-care deficit
Dressing/grooming self-care deficit
Toileting self-care deficit
Altered growth and development
Relocation stress syndrome
Risk for disorganized infant behavior
Disorganized infant behavior
Potential for enhanced organized infant behavior

Perceiving

Body image disturbance
Self-esteem disturbance
Chronic low self-esteem
Situational low self-esteem
Personal identity disturbance
Sensory/perceptual alterations (specify) (visual, auditory, kinesthetic, gustatory, tactile, olfactory)
Unilateral neglect
Hopelessness
Powerlessness

Knowing

Knowledge deficit (specify)
Impaired environmental interpretation syndrome
Acute confusion
Chronic confusion
Altered thought processes
Impaired memory

Feeling

Pain
Chronic pain
Dysfunctional grieving
Anticipatory grieving
Risk for violence: self-directed or directed at others
Risk for self-mutilation
Post-trauma response
Rape-trauma syndrome
Rape-trauma syndrome: compound reaction
Rape-trauma syndrome: silent reaction
Anxiety
Fear

Classification of nursing diagnoses by functional health patterns*

Health perception-health management

Health-seeking behaviors (specify)
Altered health maintenance (specify)
Ineffective management of therapeutic regimen (specify area)
Effective management of therapeutic regimen
Ineffective family management of therapeutic regimen
Ineffective community management of therapeutic regimen
Noncompliance (specify area)
Risk for infection (specify type/area)
Risk for injury
Risk for trauma
Risk for perioperative positioning injury
Risk for poisoning
Risk for suffocation
Altered protection (specify)
Energy field disturbance

Nutritional metabolic

Altered nutrition: more than body requirements or exogenous obesity
Altered nutrition: risk for more than body requirements or risk for obesity
Altered nutrition: less than body requirements or nutritional deficit (specify type)
Ineffective breastfeeding
Interrupted breastfeeding
Effective breastfeeding
Ineffective infant feeding pattern
Impaired swallowing (uncompensated)
Risk for aspiration
Altered oral mucous membrane (specify alteration)
Fluid volume deficit
Risk for fluid volume deficit
Fluid volume excess
Risk for impaired skin integrity or risk for skin breakdown
Impaired skin integrity

*Adapted from Gordon M: *Nursing diagnosis: 1995-1996*, St. Louis, 1995, Mosby-Year Book.

Impaired tissue integrity (specify type)
Risk for altered body temperature
Ineffective thermoregulation
Hyperthermia
Hypothermia

Elimination

Colonic constipation
Perceived constipation
Intermittent constipation pattern
Diarrhea
Bowel incontinence
Altered urinary elimination
Functional incontinence
Reflex incontinence
Stress incontinence
Urge incontinence
Total incontinence
Urinary retention

Activity-exercise

Activity intolerance (specify level)
Risk for activity intolerance
Fatigue
Impaired physical mobility (specify level)
Risk for disuse syndrome
Self-bathing—hygiene deficit (specify level)
Self-dressing—grooming deficit (specify level)
Self-feeding deficit (specify level)
Self-toileting deficit (specify level)
Diversional activity deficit
Impaired home maintenance management (mild, moderate, severe, potential, chronic)
Dysfunctional ventilatory weaning response (DVWR)
Inability to sustain spontaneous ventilation
Ineffective airway clearance
Ineffective breathing pattern
Impaired gas exchange
Decreased cardiac output
Altered tissue perfusion (specify)
Dysreflexia
Disorganized infant behavior
Risk for disorganized infant behavior
Potential for enhanced organized infant behavior
Risk for peripheral neurovascular dysfunction
Altered growth and development

Sleep-rest pattern

Sleep-pattern disturbance (specify type)

Cognitive-perceptual

Pain (specify type and location)
Chronic pain (specify type and location)
Sensory/perceptual alterations
Unilateral neglect
Knowledge deficit (specify area)
Altered thought processes (specify)
Acute confusion
Chronic confusion
Impaired environmental interpretation syndrome
Impaired memory
Decisional conflict (specify)
Decreased intracranial adaptive capacity

Self-perception—self-concept

Fear (specify focus)
Anxiety
Risk for loneliness
Hopelessness
Powerlessness (severe, moderate, low)
Self-esteem disturbance
Chronic low self-esteem
Situational low self-esteem
Body image disturbance
Risk for self-mutilation
Personal identity disturbance

Role-relationship

Anticipatory grieving
Dysfunctional grieving
Altered role performance (specify)
Social isolation or social rejection
Social isolation
Impaired social interaction
Relocation stress syndrome
Altered family processes (specify)
Altered family processes (alcoholism)
Altered parenting (specify alteration)
Risk for altered parenting (specify alteration)
Parental role conflict
Risk for altered parent-infant/child attachment
Caregiver role strain

Risk for caregiver role strain
Impaired verbal communication
Risk for violence

Sexuality-reproductive

Altered sexuality patterns
Sexual dysfunction
Rape trauma syndrome
Rape trauma syndrome: compound reaction
Rape trauma syndrome: silent reaction

Coping-stress-tolerance

Ineffective coping (individual)
Defensive coping
Ineffective denial
Impaired adjustment
Post-trauma response
Family coping: potential for growth
Compromised family coping
Disabling family coping
Ineffective community coping
Potential for enhanced community coping

Value-belief

Spiritual distress (distress of the human spirit)
Potential for enhanced spiritual well-being

AHCPR Clinical practice guidelines for selected conditions

Acute pain

The purpose of this guideline is to set "forth procedures to minimize the incidence and severity of acute pain after surgical and medical procedures and pain associated with trauma in adults and children." (p. iii)*

"The guideline emphasizes

- "A collaborative, interdisciplinary approach to pain control, including all members of the health care team and input from the patient and the patient's family, when appropriate
- "An individualized proactive pain control plan developed preoperatively by patients and practitioners (since pain is easier to prevent than to bring under control, once it has begun)
- "Assessment and frequent reassessment of the patient's pain
- "Use of both drug and nondrug therapies to control and/or prevent pain
- "A formal, institutional approach to management of acute pain, with clear lines of responsibility." (p. 2)*

Benign prostatic hyperplasia

"This Clinical Practice Guideline makes specific recommendations to identify both the most effective methods for diagnosing benign prostatic hyperplasia (BPH) and the most appropriate treatments for BPH based on patient preference and clinical needs." (p. v)†

The guideline has the following goals:

- "Identifying the most appropriate and effective diagnostic methods for detecting BPH and gauging its severity
- "Selecting the most appropriate treatment approach.

*From Acute Pain Management Guideline Panel. Acute Pain Management: Operative or Medical Procedures and Trauma. Clinical Practice Guidelines. AHCPR Pub. No. 92-0032. Rockville, MD: Agency for Health Care Policy and Research, Public Health Service, U.S. Department of Health and Human Services, Feb. 1992.

†From Benign Prostatic Hyperplasia Panel. Benign Prostatic Hyperplasia: Diagnosis and Treatment. Clinical Practice Guideline. AHCPR Pub. No. 94-0582. Rockville, MD Agency for Health Care Policy and Research, Public Health Service, U.S. Department of Health and Human Services, Feb. 1994.

"Motivation to seek active treatment will, for most patients, depend on the degree to which their symptoms bother them. The guideline details the relative benefits and harms associated with all diagnostic and treatment approaches, including watchful waiting." (p. v)*

Cataract

These guidelines focus "in general, on functional impairment of the patient with cataract and, in particular, on improvement in function as a result of treatment for the condition....Maintenance or restoration of autonomy through appropriate treatment to remove the disability, therefore, becomes the goal of the guideline." (p. 1)†

"To facilitate a broad approach to the care of persons with functional impairment due to cataract, this guideline covers the following subjects:

- "The process of caring for a patient with functional impairment due to cataract should start when a visual disability is recognized. This should lead finally to consultation with an appropriate surgeon to make or confirm a diagnosis and provide appropriate treatment.
- "The setting for surgery should be where a patient can receive quality care in a safe environment, ideally close to his or her home or support system.
- "The decision to perform cataract surgery is generally made by judging the effect of the cataract on the patient's visual and overall function and assessing the patient's visual needs, after a thorough consideration of the potential risks associated with surgery.
- "Modern cataract surgery is safe and effective in restoring vision in patients with cataracts.
- "The components of postoperative care include patient education, evaluation of the condition at discharge, and postoperative visits and examinations."

*From Benign Prostatic Hyperplasia Panel. Benign Prostatic Hyperplasia: Diagnosis and Treatment. Clinical Practice Guideline. AHCPR Pub. No. 94-0582. Rockville, MD Agency for Health Care Policy and Research, Public Health Service, U.S. Department of Health and Human Services, Feb. 1994.

†From Cataract Management Guideline Panel. Cataract in Adults: Management of Functional Impairment. Clinical Practice Guideline, Number 4. Rockville, MD. U.S. Department of Health and Human Services, Public Health Service, Agency for Health Care Policy and Research. AHCPR Pub. No. 93-0542. Feb. 1993.

The purpose of this guideline is "to assist primary care providers (e.g., general practitioners, family practitioners, internists, nurse practitioners, registered nurses, mental health nurse specialists, physician assistants, and others) in the detection and diagnosis of depressive conditions." (p. iii)*

The guidelines include the following:

- "Despite the high prevalence of depressive symptoms and full major depressive episodes in patients of all ages, depression is underdiagnosed and undertreated by primary care and other nonpsychiatric practitioners, who are paradoxically, the providers most likely to see these patients initially.

- "Primary mood disorders include both depressive (unipolar) and manic-depressive (bipolar) conditions.

- "Major depressive disorder (sometimes called unipolar depression) is characterized by one or more episodes of mild, moderate, or severe clinical depression without episodes of mania or hypomania (i.e., low-level mania).

- "Depression may co-occur with nonpsychiatric medical disorders or with other psychiatric disorders; it may also be brought on by the use of certain medications.

- "Major risk factors for depression include a personal or family history of depressive disorder, prior suicide attempts, female gender, lack of social supports, stressful life events, and current substance abuse.

- "The social stigma surrounding depression is substantial and often prevents the optimal use of current knowledge and treatments.

- "The cost of the illness in pain, suffering, disability, and death is high.

- "Given the strong evidence that treatments are effective, third-party coverage for the diagnosis and treatment of depression should be equal to that available for other medical disorders." (p. v)*

*From Depression Guideline Panel. Depression in Primary Care: Volume 1. Detection and Diagnosis. Clinical Practice Guideline, Number 5. Rockville, MD. U.S. Department of Health and Human Services, Public Health Service, Agency for Health Care Policy and Research. AHCPR Publication No. 93-0550, April 1993.

Appendix C

Depression: treatment

The purpose of this guideline is "to assist primary care providers (e.g., general practitioners, family practitioners, internists, nurse practitioners, registered nurses, mental health nurse specialists, physician assistants, and others) in the...treatment of major depressive disorder." (p. iii)*

The guideline includes the following:

- "Once major depressive disorder is diagnosed, interventions that predictably decrease symptoms and morbidity earlier than would occur naturally in the course of the illness are logically tried first.

- "The key initial objectives of treatment, in order of priority, are (1) to reduce and ultimately to remove all signs and symptoms of the depressive syndrome, (2) to restore occupational and psychosocial function to that of the asymptomatic state, and (3) to reduce the likelihood of relapse and recurrence.

- "Given the strong evidence that treatments are effective, third-party coverage for the diagnosis and treatment of depression should be equal to that available for other medical disorders." (p. v)*

Pressure ulcers

"The purpose of this guideline is to help identify adults at risk of pressure ulcers, to define early interventions for prevention, and to manage Stage I and pressure ulcers." (p. 1)[†]

The guideline includes the following goals:

- "Identify at-risk individuals needing prevention and the specific factors placing them at risk.

- "Maintain and improve tissue tolerance to pressure in order to prevent injury.

- "Protect against adverse effects of external mechanical forces: pressure, friction, and shear.

- "Reduce the incidence of pressure ulcers through educational programs." (pp. 3-5)[†]

* From Depression Guideline Panel. Depression in Primary Care: Volume 2. Treatment of Major Depression. Clinical Practice Guideline, Number 5. Rockville, MD. U.S. Department of Health and Human Services, Public Health Service, Agency for Health Care Policy and Research. AHCPR Publication No. 93-0551. April 1993.

[†] From Panel for the Prediction and Prevention of Pressure Ulcers in Adults. Pressure Ulcers in Adults: Prediction and Prevention, Clinical Practice Guideline, Number 3. AHCPR Publication No. 92-0047. Rockville, MD: Agency for Health Care Policy and Research, Public Health Service, U.S. Department of Health and Human Services. May 1992.

Appendix C

Sickle cell disease

The purpose of this guideline is to set forth "a comprehensive program for identifying, diagnosing, and treating newborns and infants with sickle cell disease and recommends education and counseling strategies for their parents." (p. v)*

These guidelines include the following:

- "The panel recommends screening all newborns regardless of racial or ethnic background for sickle cell disease.

- "When feasible, laboratory testing should be linked to other neonatal screening programs to facilitate specimen collection, identification, and handling.

- "Pneumococcal infections in infants with sickle cell anemia and sickle B-thalassemia account for significant morbidity and mortality. It has been documented unequivocally that these infections are reduced significantly by the administration of twice-daily oral penicillin.

- "Education services should be offered to all parents of infants who are identified with a hemoglobin abnormality. These services should be nondirective and conducted in an environment conducive to the free exchange of information." (pp. 2-4)*

Urinary incontinence

"The purpose of this guideline is to improve reporting, diagnosis, and treatment of UI, reduce variations in clinical practice; educate health professionals and consumers about this condition; and, finally, encourage further biomedical, clinical, and cost research on UI." (p. xi)†

"The guideline provides practice recommendations in three areas:

- "Identification and evaluation

*From Sickle Cell Disease Guideline Panel. Sickle Cell Disease: Screening, Diagnosis, Management, and Counseling in Newborns and Infants. Clinical Practice Guideline No. 6. AHCPR Pub. No. 93-0562. Rockville, MD: Agency for Health Care Policy and Research, Public Health Service, U.S. Department of Health and Human Services, April 1993.

†From Urinary Incontinence Guideline Panel. Urinary Incontinence in Adults. Clinical Practice Guideline. AHCPR Pub. No. 92-0038 Rockville, MD: Agency for Health Care Policy and Research, Public Health Service, U.S. Department of Health and Human Services. March 1992.

Appendix C

The identification and documentation of UI can be improved with more thorough medical history taking, physical examination, and recordkeeping.

- "Selection of appropriate therapy

    ...techniques such as bladder retraining and pelvic muscle exercises are effective, low risk interventions that can reduce incontinence significantly in varied populations...[indicates] what drugs can be used effectively for certain types of incontinence, including doses and possible side effects.

- "Education of health professionals and the public

    ...the public [is] advised to report incontinence problems once they occur and be informed that incontinence is not inevitable or shameful but is a treatable or at least manageable condition." (pp. xi-xii)*

*From Urinary Incontinence Guideline Panel. Urinary Incontinence in Adults. Clinical Practice Guideline. AHCPR Pub. No. 92-0038. Rockville, MD: Agency for Health Care Policy and Research, Public Health Service, U.S. Department of Health and Human Services. March 1992.

Appendix C

Index

Italic entries indicate corresponding nursing care plans.